Psychedelics a Psychotherapy

"A remarkable collection of sophisticated psychedelic therapists and integration specialists sharing new methods, new models, and theoretical underpinnings for both. What makes this volume invaluable is the wide range of solutions that the writers have come up with for helping and healing. There is a richness of ideas and case histories here, and no matter what your orientation is, you're going to learn many other ways your own work might go."

JAMES FADIMAN, PH.D., MICRODOSE RESEARCHER,
AUTHOR OF *THE PSYCHEDELIC EXPLORER'S GUIDE,*
AND COAUTHOR OF *YOUR SYMPHONY OF SELVES*

"This authoritatively written and beautifully illustrated book explores perfectly the complexities and benefits of interweaving these disparate subjects into a platform of hope for our patients with unremitting mental disorders. A highly recommended read for practitioners, patients, and anyone with a keen eye on the contemporary development of psychedelic culture and medicine."

BEN SESSA, MBBS, MRCPSYCH, CHIEF MEDICAL OFFICER
AT AWAKN LIFE SCIENCES, INC., AND PSYCHEDELIC THERAPIST

"This new book provides a rich education for those seeking wisdom about the deepest varieties of psychotherapy."

ROBIN CARHART-HARRIS, PH.D., HEAD OF CENTRE FOR
PSYCHEDELIC RESEARCH AT IMPERIAL COLLEGE LONDON

"As psychedelic drugs reintegrate themselves back into our lives how are we, in turn, to reintegrate them? This timely book will serve as a roadmap to those who walk this path, bringing together indigenous cultural knowledge and modern psychotherapeutic thinking to illustrate an ancient process of deepening inner awareness that so many feel has such contemporary potential to heal."

JAMES RUCKER, PH.D.,
HONORARY CONSULTANT PSYCHIATRIST AT THE
SOUTH LONDON AND MAUDSLEY NHS FOUNDATION TRUST
AND NIHR CLINICIAN SCIENTIST FELLOW AT
KING'S COLLEGE LONDON

"This edited collection of articles by seasoned experts in psychedelic-assisted therapy fills a critical gap. This book covers what every therapist needs to know in order to be competent in helping clients integrate their psychedelic experiences."

DAVID LUKOFF, PH.D.,
PROFESSOR OF PSYCHOLOGY AT SOFIA UNIVERSITY

"A valuable collection of experiential discoveries and research findings. A guide for those who would fathom how the competent use of psychedelics may facilitate healing and illumine the dynamics and mysteries of human consciousness."

WILLIAM A. RICHARDS, PH.D.,
PSYCHOTHERAPIST AT THE JOHNS HOPKINS CENTER
FOR PSYCHEDELIC & CONSCIOUSNESS RESEARCH
AND AUTHOR OF SACRED KNOWLEDGE

"This groundbreaking volume is essential reading for all practitioners in the healing professions, especially those whose primary focus remains the biological facets of mental health. A paradigm shift—toward a deeper model of the human being recovering the soul, the feminine, and our need for a profound sense of social belonging and embeddedness in nature—is absolutely essential. Our multifaceted crisis can only be resolved through the kind of integrative approaches advanced here: those that start from the inner dimension and its corresponding outer expressions."

DAVID LORIMER, MA, PGCE,
PROGRAM DIRECTOR AT THE SCIENTIFIC AND MEDICAL NETWORK
AND EDITOR OF PARADIGM EXPLORER

"I could not be more appreciative for the publication of *Psychedelics and Psychotherapy*. It should be essential reading for anyone interested in maximizing the healing potential of expanded states of consciousness and is a MUST for anyone considering the path of becoming a psychedelic therapist, sitter, or guide. These are the wise voices of dedicated and well-seasoned practitioners."

DIANE HAUG, MA, LPCC, SENIOR STAFF MEMBER WITH
GROF TRANSPERSONAL TRAINING AND
CODIRECTOR OF GROF LEGACY PROJECT USA

"An important book that unites the current vogue for medical application of psychedelics with the deeper spiritual understanding of humanity as interconnected, which is denied by the illness model of mental well-being. Psychedelics are identified as a means to face and heal the inner pain behind mental breakdown, and the theme is illustrated from a variety of therapeutic perspectives—using multiple ways of exploring expanded consciousness—the whole enlivened by the inclusion of artwork arising from the process."

ISABEL CLARKE, CONSULTANT CLINICAL PSYCHOLOGIST,
EDITOR OF *PSYCHOSIS AND SPIRITUALITY,* AND AUTHOR OF
MADNESS, MYSTERY AND THE SURVIVAL OF GOD

"This rich, brilliant anthology is a must-read resource for anyone interested in psychedelic-assisted psychotherapy, covering areas such as preparation and integration, the use of evocative music, mandala drawing, bodywork, and archetypal astrology."

RENN BUTLER, AUTHOR OF *PATHWAYS TO WHOLENESS*
AND *THE ARCHETYPAL UNIVERSE*

"Read and Papaspyrou have years of experience in the field of healing with expanded states of consciousness and, with keen observation of what is needed as psychedelics enter the mainstream, have chosen wise authors and essential topics to include in this book. *Psychedelics and Psychotherapy* reflects the multi-dimensional experience of both client and therapist in psychedelic therapy and the subtle issues that arise. This book is essential reading for those just joining this important healing work. Veterans in the field will appreciate the skillful articulation of the differences between psychedelic therapy and ordinary therapy, especially regarding training, ethical awareness, presence, and supervision in supporting the inner healing intelligence of clients in the therapeutic alliance."

KYLEA TAYLOR, LMFT,
AUTHOR OF *THE ETHICS OF CARING*

"A wonderful mind-expanding book that has renewed my compassion, enthusiasm, and curiosity for the therapeutic experience. Authors with deep experience write beautifully about the transformative nature and process of psychedelic therapy."

RACHEL GIBBONS, PSYCHOANALYST, GROUP ANALYST,
CONSULTANT PSYCHIATRIST, AND
ORGANIZATIONAL CONSULTANT

"An important, timely, and rich collection that should interest anyone with a serious interest in psychedelics."

JEREMY NARBY, ANTHROPOLOGIST AND
AUTHOR OF *THE COSMIC SERPENT*

"Research and reports of users in this field are gaining increasing awareness, yet the voice of those therapists who offered therapy is seldom heard. A rich, thorough resource of practitioners awaits the reader; collectively, they represent hundreds of years of experience in this growing field."

MANUEL AICHER, PSYCHOTHERAPIST

Psychedelics and Psychotherapy

The Healing Potential of Expanded States

Edited by

TIM READ and

MARIA PAPASPYROU

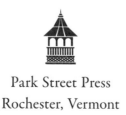

Park Street Press

Rochester, Vermont

Park Street Press
One Park Street
Rochester, Vermont 05767
www.ParkStPress.com

Text stock is SFI certified

Park Street Press is a division of Inner Traditions International

Cataloging-in-Publication Data for this title is available from the Library of Congress

ISBN 978-1-64411-332-5 (print)
ISBN 978-1-64411-333-2 (ebook)

Printed and bound in the United States by Lake Book Manufacturing, Inc. The text stock is SFI certified. The Sustainable Forestry Initiative® program promotes sustainable forest management.

10 9 8 7 6 5 4 3 2

Text design by Debbie Glogover and layout by Virginia Scott Bowman
This book was typeset in Garamond Premier Pro with Caslon used as the display typeface

To send correspondence to the author of this book, mail a first-class letter to the author c/o Inner Traditions • Bear & Company, One Park Street, Rochester, VT 05767, and we will forward the communication, or contact the author directly: Tim Read at **walkingshadows.tr@gmail.com** and Maria Papaspyrou at **https://towardswholeness.co.uk**.

Contents

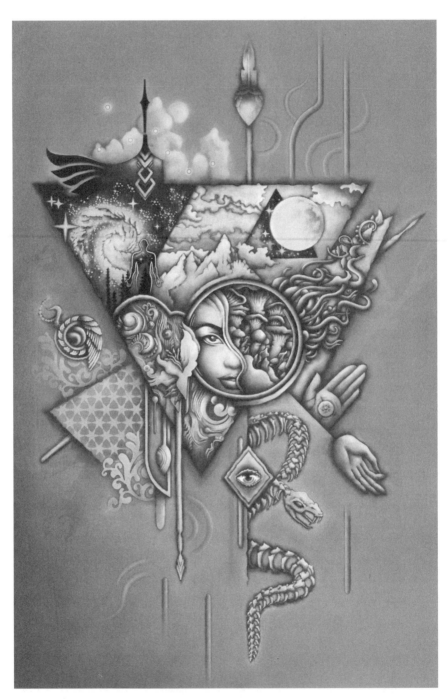

Manifold by Stuart Griggs.

Psychedelics as a Pathway to the Self

Gabor Maté

P lant medicine work is becoming increasingly popular with Westerners seeking to heal physical illness or mental anguish or to gain a sense of meaning amid the growing alienation in our culture. The main reasons why people are turning to plant medicines and other psychedelic modalities are twofold. First, mental health illnesses are burgeoning in our societies. Anxiety is the fastest growing diagnosis on both sides of the Atlantic while more and more people become depressed. The loss of community and the pain of dislocation and alienation are social contributors to the rise in mental discomfort. Second, there is a nearly complete failure of the Western medical system in dealing with the crisis of mental health; we not only fail to understand mental illness but are fundamentally in denial about the unity of the human soul, mind, and body, as well as in denial about the social nature of human beings. Because Western medicine tends to look upon mental illness as a largely biological problem, prevention of and responses to it are often inadequate, which has driven people to look for solutions outside the mainstream. We can add a third reason: the search for spiritual realization.

As a Western-trained doctor, I have long been aware of modern medicine's limitations in handling chronic conditions of mind and body. For all our astonishing achievements, there are a host of ailments whose ravages we physicians can at best alleviate. In our narrow pursuit of a cure, we fail to comprehend the essence of healing. We tend to see people's illnesses as isolated, accidental, and unfortunate events rather than as the outcomes of lives lived in a psychological and social context; illness is the body's expressions of experiences, beliefs, and lifelong patterns of relating to self and to the world. Mainstream medical practice largely ignores the role of emotions in the physiological functioning of the human organism. Yet the scientific evidence abundantly shows that people's lifetime emotional experiences profoundly influence health and illness. And since emotional patterns are a response to the psychological and social environment, disease in an individual always tells us about the multigenerational dynamics that the person was born into, as well as the broader culture in which that person's life unfolds.

Such a holistic understanding informs many aboriginal wisdom teachings. The ceremonial use of ayahuasca, for example—like all plant-based indigenous practices around the world—arises from a tradition of seeing the mind and body as inseparable in sickness and in health. I have witnessed people overcome addictions to substances, sexual compulsion, and other self-harming behaviors. Some have found liberation from chronic shame or the mental fog of depression or anxiety. I know others who have healed from autoimmune diseases like rheumatoid arthritis and multiple sclerosis. Where is the healing coming from?

Plant medicines and other psychedelic substances are not drugs in the Western sense of a compound that attacks pathogens such as bacteria or obliterates malignant pathological tissue. Nor are they a chemical, like antidepressants, that alters the biology of a diseased nervous system. And they are far from being a recreational substance ingested for escapist purposes. In their proper ceremonial setting, under compassionate and experienced guidance, the plant—or, as tradition has it, the spirit of the plant—puts people in touch with their repressed pain and trauma, the very factors that drive all dysfunctional behaviors. Consciously experiencing our primal pain loosens its hold on us and may set us on the path toward healing. The very word *healing* means wholeness, and we become whole when we reconnect with ourselves. This book showcases how mind, body, and spirit come together to tell the stories of our wounds and to cosupport our path toward healing.

The addictive power of substances is a myth. Contrary to popular belief, the addictive power does not reside in the drug itself; it resides in something that creates a susceptibility, invariably some trauma. The effect of the substances—how they are used and what purposes they serve in human life—depend very much on the context: the set and the setting. Addiction to drugs is about lowering consciousness, but healing substances within the right set and setting, as exemplified by aboriginal ceremonial practices, elevate consciousness. Often, the setting for recreational drug use is some dingy bar or back alley or a living room with a bunch of buddies wanting to get high. The setting for using plant medicines is a ceremony with shamans who have been through training that is not for the fainthearted or with psychologically adept guides who have faced their own wounds and darkness. In addiction, substances are used regularly or daily as a form of escape. Plant medicines and other psychedelic substances are not meant for daily use. They are used consciously in a ceremonial setting as a way of opening the doors of perception. Like plant medicines, psychedelics also need the appropriate context if they are to be an appropriate medicine. Each chapter in this book explores a particular setting and offers insights into the care and consideration that goes into holding the space. It exemplifies that the settings and formats are varied, but the knowledge, experience, and wisdom that is needed to support and hold the space is the common ground that supports the healing potential of expanded states.

It takes a lot of work to wake up as a human being; it's a lot easier to stay asleep. Trauma wires us to escape emotional pain and rely on short-term solutions, like addictions or other adaptations, or even therapies that address the symptoms rather than the causes. But self-awareness is the bottom line, the only way to truly address trauma. When we wake up, we are able to address childhood issues that have traumatized us and made us vulnerable to addictions or any other compensations. We usually arrive at this place after a lot of pain, when something happens that forces us to face up to the fact that our lives aren't working as they should. It is through our discomfort that we start seeking solutions.

Plant medicines can create deep insights and openings to the psyche and may also allow people to reexperience inner qualities they have lost connection to, such as wholeness, trust, love, and a sense of possibility. People quite literally remember themselves. The documented unity of mind and body means that such experiential transformation, if genuine, can powerfully affect the hormonal, nervous, and immune systems and organs such as the brain, bowels, and heart. Hence the healing potential of the plant seen through the lens of Western science.

Plant medicines and other psychedelic treatments can reveal the psychological baggage that you have carried all your life, and when you acknowledge this baggage, you realize it is not an inevitable and inextricable part of yourself. You can finally put it down. All the pain and all the meanings that you have created from that pain, all the ways you see yourself, and all the interpretations you have made of the world because of early experience can drop away, and you can just be in the present. That's very powerful. Psychedelic experiences may also reveal, or at least allow you to glimpse, your full potential as a loving and connected human being. Having a deep experience of your true self can be tremendously healing, so it's not surprising that some people working with these medicines come to realizations through these experiences that go deeper than their usual consciousness permits. When we find a way to reach shut down parts of ourselves, when we recognize our deep sources of suffering and what we are running away from, or when we realize ourselves as a meaningful and genuine part of a larger unity that is unshakeable no matter what, we have connected to a core self. In the right context this is a very deep experience.

Because psychedelics can connect us to our experiences of suffering in such visceral and deep ways, sometimes people have had what they call a bad experience. A bad experience usually means two things are happening. First, the personality and mind of the person who has taken the psychedelic are judging the experience. His personality was developed in the first place to help him escape the pain; his personality is his compensation, and it is wired to avoid the suffering. I would say that perhaps he didn't have a bad experience but rather had an experience where he felt pain or was in touch with a lot of fear, maybe even terror—pain and terror he had been carrying inside himself and running away from all his life. To experience it is not a bad thing; it is only bad if the person has no means to understand, digest, and contextualize the experience. The pain, fear, or terror coming up only surfaces because it is already there. It is better to be aware of it and revisit it with the awareness, strength, and mind of an adult rather than remain in denial about it.

Second, when someone has had a "bad experience," he usually didn't have the right guidance in the appropriate context. These journeys run so deeply that it is essential we navigate them while being held and guided by people who are experienced and wise in guiding us. Really, there are no bad experiences; there are only difficult experiences whose meaning we haven't divined and haven't had the guidance to understand and integrate into our life.

The intention for these experiences has to be seeking the truth. If the truth at that moment is painful, that is great. Once we realize the degree of pain and fear we each carry, it takes us back to our experience as an infant. Underneath that fear, there's the connected self who knows no fear. What is there to be afraid of when you are connected to everything?

Then the challenge becomes how to incorporate and integrate that experience into your life. This book stresses the importance of integration. The insights of an experience will not be enough. They will need to be integrated into daily life, and that takes daily work. The post-ceremony integration is at least as important as the experience itself. Otherwise, we will be impelled to just keep going back looking for the same experience over and over again, and nothing will have necessarily shifted. The openings, insights, and realizations that we might encounter in a ceremony is when the work begins. The medicine ceremony is an inquiry. What arises in that space will have to be understood somehow in order for us to be able to make use of it. Integration is a practice. These experiences can give us deep but possibly evanescent glimpses of our true self. The ongoing work is to keep returning to the true self and clearing out all the accumulated debris that we have taken on since early infancy. Those that seek to use these medicines will ultimately need to address their traumas. Like every other kind of spiritual work, the medicines will open the doors for us, but it is then up to us to walk through those doors, and then we have to continue to walk through those doors as part of our everyday lives. The work of integration might be different for everybody, but it does involve some disengagement from the daily grind, some time that is devoted to your core essence or to exploring it.

In addictions we use the word *recovery,* which means finding something that you have lost. Whatever you find couldn't have been destroyed, and it must have been there all along otherwise you couldn't have found it. What people recover when they recover from addictions is themselves. How do we lose ourselves, why is it so difficult to reconnect, and how do these plant experiences facilitate this reconnection? That question leads to the very essence of trauma because it is trauma that makes us disconnect in the first place. Peter Levine says, "In short, trauma is about loss of connection—to ourselves, to our bodies, to our families, to others, and to the world around us. This loss of connection is often hard to recognize, because it doesn't happen all at once. It can happen slowly, over time, and we adapt to these subtle changes sometimes without even noticing them" (Levine 2008, 9).

Therefore, trauma is not the external event that happens; it is the impact of the event, which is the lost connection to yourself. Had your experiences not resulted in a disconnection from the self, then you would not have been traumatized. The loss of connection itself is an adaptation: *If it is so painful to be myself, I better disconnect. If it is so painful for me to be aware of my gut feelings and to be able to assert, manifest, and declare them, I better disconnect.* And then we spend the rest of our lives trying to compensate for this disconnection through addiction or by developing certain personality patterns that will somehow get us indirectly what we didn't get in the first place: the love that would have allowed us to connect to ourselves.

Because we couldn't be ourselves in the face of so much pain and vulnerability, we cover up our wounds, we close our hearts, we don't know how to love ourselves or others, and we no longer have pleasure or joy. The same adaptations that helped us initially survive then become our burden, our separation and alienation from the world. This doesn't only happen on an individual level; it happens on a societal level. We live in a society that is profoundly alienated and validates our invalidity—our false self—and rewards us for our compensatory mechanisms. The capitalist economy depends on your false sense of self. That's why even those people who do the work of reconnecting with themselves while in ceremony with a substance or practice discover that the real difficulty is not in having these experiences but in manifesting their insights in daily living when the world is so intent on robbing them of the very truth of things.

The problem is that before our minds create the world, the world creates our minds. And so we have to go back to who we were before the world created our mind. This is where the plant medicines are so important and useful for they take us on a journey of great depth and help us reconnect. This book captures that depth and offers a range of voices that address and explore the journey into remembering who we have been all along, beneath the pain and alienation. Thomas Merton talked about surrendering, conquering ourselves, or allowing the spirit to conquer us. The self-conquest is not a willful act of self-abnegation but an actual surrendering to something greater than we are. He says: "In order to gain possession of ourselves, we have to have some confidence of victory. To keep that hope alive we must usually have some taste of victory. We must know what victory is, and like it better than defeat" (1958, 19). At the very least, this work with the plant spirits can give us a taste of that victory, a glimpse of ourselves, a glimpse of a deeper reality, and that can be the beginning of the path to healing.

Into the Deep

Integrating Psychedelics and Psychotherapy

Tim Read and Maria Papaspyrou

Freud famously described dreams as the royal road to the unconscious, and this seems to be even more true in describing the psychedelic experience. Our central assumption as editors is that while psychedelic states offer unequalled access to the deep psyche, this is usually not in itself enough; to make full use of their power, there needs to be traction, an engagement with process, a working through. The psychedelic experience is not so much a magic bullet as an evolving relationship with our inner world, a journey that ripens over time.

In this book, we use the terms *psychedelic state* or *expanded state* as umbrella terms to describe experiences with psychedelic substances and Holotropic Breathwork. We do not discuss in detail other expanded states accessed through spiritual practice or psychological crisis, although we believe that they can open similar territories of the psyche (Evans and Read 2020). We pay attention to Holotropic Breathwork as developed by Stanislav and Christina Grof, after his clinical research with LSD was made illegal, as a natural method for the induction of psychedelic states. Holotropic Breathwork, using hyperventilation with evocative music in a highly supportive setting, has been the only legal way in which people can access psychedelic experiences in most countries around the world and has been an indispensable resource for training people in supporting psychedelic states.

THERAPEUTIC USE OF PSYCHEDELICS

Stanislav Grof, the psychiatrist and pioneer of LSD psychotherapy, often says that when working with expanded states, the first thing is to leave behind whatever we think we have learned about treatment—our task is simply to fully support the process. We may bring our expertise to the preparation, the setting, and the integration, but in the session itself, the participant is the expert of his or her own experience.

The setting of the healing space and the trajectory of the process can vary greatly. Most people today have their initiatory experiences in recreational settings that often set the scene for further intentional explorations. The chapters that follow describe the variety of settings within which this work is currently unfolding. From shamanic settings, to clinical research settings, to underground psychedelic work, to Holotropic Breathwork, to harm-reduction settings, to psychotherapy settings, there is a flourishing of creativity and enthusiasm for the healing potential of expanded states. In some settings the work is done entirely within the ceremonial space without any formal integration input. Some clinical research is based on the magic bullet approach with minimal postsession integration while other settings favor an approach that has the long-term trajectory of explorative psychotherapy. There may be times when a diagnostic label is useful so that a psychedelic treatment is tailored to that condition, as in MDMA-assisted psychotherapy for post-traumatic stress disorder.

For people who seek resolution for deep-seated issues, there is a real question as to whether short-term work with expanded states can lead to lasting change. Grof's (1975) clinical LSD study with psychiatric inpatients with neurotic conditions suggests that it does not. After one supported LSD session, he found little evidence of lasting positive change, and some patients deteriorated. In a follow-up study (1975) where his patients' LSD sessions were supported by psychotherapy (dose was increased incrementally from 100 mcg and the number of sessions ranged from fifteen to one hundred over the course of up to a year), he discerned an emerging pattern. Various trauma-laden *complexes*— psychic structures that gather together similar feeling-toned elements— were successively processed. But there was a deeper layer to their healing process. Grof made the crucial discovery that much of his patients' experience in the LSD sessions originated from a primitive layer of the psyche that lies outside conscious memory and carries a powerful emotional quality of annihilatory anxiety, death, and rebirth, forming the nucleus of our key complexes.

Such early primitive experience can only be accessed reliably in expanded states, and the purification process where these early traumas are reexperienced and processed is challenging and often takes repeated exposure and subsequent processing. This is where the power of this work lies, and we feel this points to a possible evolution of psychotherapy and psychiatry. Healing work inevitably involves an encounter with our deep wounds; expanded states allow us access to those parts of psyche that we really need to work with and are so difficult to access in ordinary consciousness. The difficult and overwhelming experiential material described as a *bad trip* in an uncontrolled setting is a precious opportunity that facilitates healing in a controlled setting. Contrary to mainstream psychological methods, in work with expanded states the wounds and symptoms are not to be suppressed, fragmented, and avoided; they are to be invited, amplified, felt through, and processed.

Going even deeper in the psyche, expanded states often open us to *transpersonal* experiences, with a range and variety that feature prominently in this volume. This transpersonal layer of the psyche, which often has a numinous tone, tends to reveal the limitations of our conventional paradigms of mind; indeed, consciousness is revealed to be more complex than we had previously imagined. The first generation of psychedelic explorers were drawn to the Sanskrit and yogic traditions of India in their attempts to chart this territory, while the current generation has been looking primarily west, to the shamanic traditions of the Americas. Inevitably, the emergent second generation of psychedelic thinkers borrow from the first generation but are also developing distinctive voices and perspectives of their own. One of the aims of this book is to showcase the variety and complexity of these voices, alongside current best practices and some of the theories underpinning this work. We think that theoretical models of psyche can help us navigate the psychedelic experience, but we should not confuse the map for the territory. This danger cannot be overstated: overreliance on our favored models may constrict our perspective and limit our capacity to observe and respond to that which lies beyond our conceptual framework.

COVID-19: MICROBE AND ARCHETYPE

This book has been long in gestation but came to fruition in the time of the coronavirus pandemic of 2020. For us as editors, and for many of the contributors, we did much of the labor of creation during this extraordinary period of lockdown and pestilence. We suggest that the pandemic has held an archetypal intensity that bears close comparison with a challenging psychedelic experience. By *archetype* we refer to the primary colors of meaning, the universal principles, the unchanging and inherited Platonic forms of our collective human experience (Read 2014). An amplified intensity of meaning has developed during the pandemic that has a quality of constriction and suffocation, an encounter with death and the emergence of *shadow*.

The concept of shadow has an important role in this book. Shadow represents those parts of ourselves that we repress from our conscious awareness, the aspects of ourselves to which we are deaf and blind. The transformative process involves us learning to hear and see ourselves in new ways—metaphorically speaking. Psychedelics help us see more deeply into the psyche, and this process inevitably brings an encounter with shadow, which may bring friction between the part of us that wants to surrender and the part of us that resists. Surviving the tension and moving through this process inevitably brings vitality and purpose to those exiled and forgotten parts of ourselves that in turn infuse and rekindle our life force.

The coronavirus has initiated a collective journey into our shadow. The time of lockdown and isolation has been an opportunity for many of us to look within and reflect deeply on our lives—on what truly matters and on what needs to change. The turbulence offered by the pandemic has challenged the status quo, offering the opportunity for transformative change through the death of redundant collective ego structures and the birthing of new ways of being in the world together. This death-rebirth dynamic is an archetypal theme that plays a central role in our collective psyche as evidenced by our mythic history—the crucifixion, Odin, Osiris, Innana, Persephone, Dionysus, Adonis, Baldr, Quetzlcoatl, Izanami, to name a few. So we consider the coronavirus pandemic to be an invitation to a collective death-rebirth process by activating some of our archaic psychic structures, thus opening a deeper layer of transformation to the more obvious socioeconomic and health challenges.

Synchronicities are meaningful coincidences where an internal experience and an external event meet in a way that has a profound effect on the person that experiences them. A synchronicity is a numinous experience that originates in the archetypal realm and initiates an awakening to a deeper order. There is a synchronicity between the coronavirus pandemic and the most crucial issue of our times—the environmental crisis and the urgent battle to save our planet. From this planetary perspective, it seems clear that we cannot continue preying on Mother Earth. We need a fundamental restructuring of our relationship with her and a remembering of our interdependence and interconnection with the forces of life that she is the very source of. We imagine coronavirus emanating from Earth as a manifestation of the archetypal feminine, in her darker regenerative form. She appears like a goddess, she has the world in her thrall, people fall before her, the engines of commerce are quietened, the oceans and skies are stilled, and the air becomes clear and fresh. Our planet can take a breath. Nature reclaims her rightful space. From the archetypal cosmology perspective developed by Richard Tarnas (2006) and articulated by Becca Tarnas in this volume, there is another compelling synchronicity between the rare alignment of Saturn, Pluto, and Jupiter in the sky and the coming together of the archetypal principles held by these planets: constriction, turbulence, and confrontation with shadow on a global scale.

As with any psychedelic experience, in our collective emergency we should honor the possibility of growth and learning, holding an enquiring mind-set, attending to the set while maintaining a safe setting and working on the integration. When psychedelics are used with an intentional mind-set and we process material from the deeper parts of the psyche, the challenge is how *not* to return to how we were before. We embrace the possibility of growth through change. Although insights may arise with clarity in an expanded state, they can so easily slip away, and the work lies in harvesting the fruits of the journey. This is what is meant by the term *integration*.

If we apply the same consideration to the pandemic, then we have a collective opportunity to develop new paradigms, new perspectives, and new ways of relating to one another and our planet. Our future may depend on our ability to navigate our collective darkness and emerge renewed. Coronavirus will not lead to the sudden transformation of the human race but has offered us an opportunity to fundamentally reorient. The rebirth will require deep collective inner work and courage. At the same time, the renaissance of interest in psychedelic substances as potent agents of change is gathering momentum. The walls of prohibition and the public conditioning that resulted from the War on Drugs are beginning to crumble. We suggest a further synchronicity between this psychedelic renaissance and the urgent need to transform our paradigms, much like for our predecessors in the 1960s. The deep psychic change that can follow intentional and integrated psychedelic use, we believe, can be part of the solution.

A COMING TOGETHER

We live in times when collective divisions and polarizations have become painfully obvious. Inequalities of class, race, privilege, wealth, and opportunity seem to be widening. We seem to be collectively *acting out* rather than thinking through. Instead of processing our existential anxieties, we vote for populists who offer us easy solutions to complex issues. But the great currents of meaning that disturb us do not simply go away, and even if we avert our gaze, the collective currents and undertow of unprocessed shadow will still find a way of making themselves known to us. The coronavirus pandemic offered a fertile ground for our collective shadow to emerge; one example is the way in which the Black Lives Matter movement has mobilized and directed our attention to matters of race, our unconscious assumptions, and how much work we need to do to truly partner with one another as human beings. This has immediate relevance for the field of psychedelic work and for the work that still lies ahead of us if we are to make this field inclusive and equitable. What would it be like for a descendant of slaves to surrender to an expanded state with white therapists? How can we avoid retraumatization even if we feel we hold the best intentions? Is it even possible to really face the pain together? How can this work be truly inclusive, rather than simply another manifestation of privilege?

We offer the *archetypal feminine* as one model of transformative change. Although the term *toxic masculinity* is frequently used, we feel that this term causes condemnation and shame, which may divert us from working with what really requires attention. We prefer the term *wounded masculine* and recognize that the challenge is to work with the inner woundedness in order to weaken its outer manifestations. Our current period of history seems to highlight aspects of the wounded masculine: the patriarchal leaders whose narcissistic lack of compassion is revealed by the pandemic; the predominance of socioeconomic models based on competitiveness, power, and domination; the deeply ingrained sexist structures; the persecution and retraumatization of refugees; and a phallic rapacious approach to the planet. This contrasts with the archetypal feminine qualities of nourishment, partnership, and connection, with emphasis on relationship and harmony. This is a complex area; the archetypal qualities of masculine and feminine do not map directly onto gender. These are psychic structures and qualities we all hold within ourselves, whether we are men or women. Nor should we identify the masculine archetype as holding predominantly negative qualities and the feminine devoid of wounded and toxic manifestations. The masculine archetype of the father is just as needed in our times. The need is to restore the feminine and the masculine archetypes to their true vital essence and hold them in complementary balance with each other. This need is urgent.

Psychedelics seem to facilitate this rebalancing by restoring key qualities of the archetypal feminine, a potential that has been termed *femtheogenic* (Papaspyrou 2015, 2019) and can support a movement toward vibrant, cocreative, ecologically minded people and, by extension, societies. The history of the psychedelic movement shows how evangelical enthusiasm, naive idealism, and irresponsible use can undermine the grounded sober appraisal of potential benefits. But we can see, perhaps, how a gradual exposure of greater numbers of people to psychedelics with appropriate set, setting, and integration will add to the conversation in a way that may have some positive sociopolitical consequences as an outcome of our healing process.

Psychedelics have been termed sacred medicines because of their transcendent qualities. While the term *spiritual* carries baggage, the transpersonal aspect of the psychedelic experience cannot be dismissed, no matter how much we emphasize the science. Psychedelics tend to awaken people to a bigger picture, one that gives fresh perspectives to the concerns of their everyday lives. The spiritual emergence that often flows from such awakenings is beautiful to experience and to witness. It is one of the greatest gifts of working with expanded states of consciousness. Many of us believe that numinous encounters are essential for supporting humanity's shift from egocentricity and ethnocentricity to the true global, ecosystemic consciousness required to save our planet.

The Opening Circle

Tim Read and Maria Papaspyrou

Humans have come together since our time began to seek both healing and answers for those existential questions that have always preoccupied us about life, death, and our place in the greater scheme of things. Such seeking often takes place in our sacred spaces where we meet together in a spirit of peace, compassion, and connection. These days, in ceremonies and retreats, we usually begin with an opening circle, a place of introductions but also an invitation to this sacred space, the place of receptive opening, of gentleness, of love, of holding, of softly being together while we travel alongside one another in search of growth and wholeness. We believe that this mindset is the fundamental requirement for any work in psychedelic states, and we invite you to join us in this spirit.

The chapters in this anthology are a conversation about how to best provide a container for the dual process of opening and healing. As with most conversations, there are different voices and perspectives, a creative coming together that is greater than the sum of its parts. No conversation is ever complete; there may be some important voices that are absent, but any good conversation gathers momentum and goes on to inform other conversations. We have deep gratitude for those who have contributed to this volume and honor their presence and the gifts that they offer. Our authors were chosen not only for their wisdom and expertise but also, especially, for their human qualities, their heart, their essential decency, and the quality of their presence. These are humans who are in dedicated service to fellow humans, to this work, and to this field. This is indeed a labor of love.

Andrew Feldmar opens with a powerful statement about the fundamental importance of the collaborative therapeutic relationship in the psychedelic encounter: human to human, soul to soul, but absolutely not expert to patient. His vignettes offer a valuable perspective on selection criteria for psychedelic psychotherapy. Rachel Harris follows, discussing the importance of integration from a psychotherapeutic lens and the power of expanded states for reparative attachment work. She offers reflections on plant medicines as cotherapists in the psychotherapy space.

Jerome Braun, a Jungian analyst in private practice, discusses how his psychedelic experiences and training alongside Amazonian healers have enriched his own inner work, deepening his development and growth as a psychotherapist. Maria Papaspyrou addresses psychedelic integration in private practice with a Jungian focus, discussing both the challenges and the ethics involved, illustrating with clinical vignettes. Scott Hill continues the Jungian theme offering Donald Kalsched's perspective on trauma as a way of understanding challenging psychedelic experiences. He explores his own psychedelic experiences and the difficulties that arise when such inner encounters remain unintegrated. Tim Read develops the theme of challenging psychedelic states with a model that brings together psychodynamic and Grofian theoretical frameworks with a focus on processing early trauma, the importance of mourning, and complications of transpersonal experience.

The two chapters that follow, chapters 7 and 8, discuss work with expanded states in underground settings. Friederike Meckel Fischer provided underground psychedelic psychotherapy for selected clients in weekend workshops. She describes the use of substances, the power of the group process, and the importance of direct interventions by the therapist during the medicine session. Lisa Marie Jones discusses her training as an underground psychedelic therapist, the range and dosage of substances, constellation and ancestral work, and the issue of therapist intake.

We then move to a discussion of Holotropic Breathwork with a focus on integration, somatic aspects, facilitator presence, and work with trauma. Marianne Murray begins, in chapter 9, with a description of Holotropic Breathwork retreats, focusing on how the structure and flow of the setting supports the integration process. Holly Harman discusses the essential qualities of facilitator presence, the art of *not doing,* and the bodywork aspect of the healing work. Ingrid Pacey brings her unique experience of both Holotropic Breathwork and MDMA-assisted therapy in her long experience of working with survivors of sexual abuse. This segues into Shannon Carlin's chapter describing the MAPS (Multidisciplinary Association for Psychedelic Science) protocol for MDMA-assisted psychotherapy for post-traumatic stress disorder (PTSD), the cultivation of trust, and the concept of inner healing intelligence. Jo O'Reilly and Tim Read follow with a chapter that explores MDMA-assisted psychotherapy for PTSD from a psychoanalytic perspective. They discuss transference issues, the significance of disrupted attachment patterns, and how this treatment may address early developmental trauma as well as PTSD.

The chapters that follow explore the work with specific substances. In chapter 14, Daniel McQueen, a passionate advocate of cannabis as a psychedelic tool, discusses how modern blends of cannabis when used skillfully can mimic the classical psychedelics while holding some important advantages—not least legality in many states. Natasja Pelgrom who has walked the medicine path for many years, brings a shamanic perspective to her work with 5-MeO-DMT and discusses what is required of shamanic practitioners to become clear channels for their healing work. Svea Nielsen brings us her experience with iboga in various settings. She describes both micro-dosing and flood sessions, special precautions, dietary matters, and the impact of the iboga plant on withdrawal symptoms and addictions. A chapter by Deanne Adamson also discusses addiction and outlines the preparation and integration methods offered by her coaching team to people that are trying to work through their addictions with the support of psychedelic experiences.

The creative dimension of the psychedelic state is an indispensable part of the healing process, and the following two chapters attest to its significance for the integration process. In chapter 18, Bruce Tobin explores the idea of meaningful versus aesthetic art and offers specific art therapy exercises for use in the integration phase; his chapter has an extensive vignette with illustrations. John Ablett has been cultivating a Holotropic Breathwork practice for many years using mandalas for his integration. He explores how these have deepened his process and discusses aspects of his own personal journey.

A chapter on psychedelic crisis work follows by Nir Tadmor who has founded Safe Shore, a harm reduction initiative that operates in festivals in Israel. He brings a flavor of the front line in such spaces with the rewards and challenges of holding space for people outside the usual pathways of referral and consent. Leor Roseman, who is part of a team that carried out a research study on ceremonial groups comprised of Israeli and Palestinian participants, discusses the potential of such experiences for supporting reconciliation. He focuses on the relational aspects of these medicines as a complement to the focus on inner work.

The next two chapters come from a transpersonal perspective. Becca Tarnas describes the seminal work of Stanislav Grof and Richard Tarnas in archetypal astrology and recounts a personal vignette to explore how this deeper layer of meaning can provide a unique lens for the integration of psychedelic experiences. Chris Bache writes about the challenges of integration involved in his twenty-year visionary journey using high doses of LSD. This extraordinary piece of spiritual exploration delves deeply into the mind of the universe.

The book concludes with three chapters that discuss professional development for those working in this field. Renee Harvey explores the considerations involved in training the next generation of psychedelic therapists and what the future holds for psychedelic professionals. The chapter cowritten by Tim Read, Michelle Baker-Jones, Sven

Kimani, Jonny Martell, Roberta Murphy, Ashleigh Murphy-Beiner, and Rosalind Watts discusses the use of reflective space and supervision for shared learning. This is a collective piece with case vignettes by therapists who participated in the study on psilocybin and depression at Imperial College London and therapists at Synthesis retreats in the Netherlands with Tim as their supervisor. We conclude with a chapter by Maria Papaspyrou discussing the ethical matters surrounding work with expanded states alongside the wider ethics of the field at this precise moment of moving toward mainstreaming.

Our hope is for this book to inspire and generate ideas and further projects, propelling this ongoing dialogue forward as this field develops and unfolds.

1

On the Therapeutic Stance during Psychedelic Psychotherapy

Andrew Feldmar

The meaning of the word *parrhesia,* which first appeared in Greek literature by Euripides, implied *telling the truth to power and at the same time apologizing for the telling.* The apology was to protect the speaker from the wrath of power—from being burned at the stake or beheaded. It can be translated as *free speech,* and I think the word can also refer to the psychoanalytic notion of *free association,* as used by Freud. According to Michel Foucault (1983), "etymologically, 'parrhesiazesthai' means 'to say everything'—from 'pan' (everything) and 'rhema' (that which is said). The one who uses parrhesia, the parrhesiastes, is someone who says everything he has in mind: he does not hide anything but opens his heart and mind completely to other people through his discourse."

In this chapter I attempt to tell my truth to the powers that are forming during these heady days of psychedelic renaissance. More and more training programs are springing up, but I think that the skill of the psychedelic therapist can be transmitted only through apprenticeship. It's a very complex task to actually be there with someone who is in an altered state of consciousness. The possibility of alienation, the possibility of making things worse, is enormous. So, the gains are high, but the dangers are also great. I think the only way to make sure that in the future, when these substances will be legal, that they will not cause harm is to focus not on the drugs themselves but on the relationship between the therapist and the patient.

In 2001, my paper "Entheogens and Psychotherapy," in which I explored the potential therapeutic uses of psychedelics and described my own experiences with LSD, was published, and I was punished for it in the summer of 2006 when I was googled at the border between Canada and the US and denied entry (read about it in Solomon 2007). Because of the politics of fighting for the acceptance and legalization of psychedelics, plant medicines, entheogens, and empathogens, I am afraid that an ethos has developed that will consider these exceptional substances just like common pharmaceuticals. The emphasis is on the power of the substance, not on the relationship between the patient and the therapist. Protocols are being manufactured, as if the interactions could be standardized and controlled. Experts are created, selection criteria are invented, optimal musical backgrounds are offered, as if these were scientific matters. Psychotherapy has nothing to do with psychology nor with psychiatry or medicine. Aristotle already knew that what he called the *practical sciences,* such as ethics and politics, had nothing to do with the *productive* (medicine or architecture) or *theoretical* (mathematics or physics) *sciences.* We are making a terrible category mistake when we pretend that psychotherapy is productive or theoretical in any way. There are no blueprints for who I should be at the end of therapy, and the encounters are fully in the here and now, which have to be negotiated situation by situation, moment by living moment. Psychotherapy is ethics (how we treat each other) and politics (the art of accruing and maintaining sufficient personal power so I can do what I want and not what I don't want, power *to* not power *over*).

R. D. Laing defined psychotherapy as "an obstinate attempt of two people to recover the wholeness of being human through the relationship between them" (1965, 63). Treatment is how we treat each other. The introduction of a psychedelic, entheogen, or empathogen into the therapeutic relationship will heighten awareness of the other, awareness of how much we flow into and through each other. The therapist cannot hide; any attempt to do so will be noticed, as well as any one-upmanship, power game, falseness, tone of certainty, fear, desire, distancing, objectification, persuasion, coercion, or criticism. The therapist needs to cultivate and practice desirelessness, *just* listening, love, spontaneity, and candor. There cannot be a protocol to follow, programmed music played, orders given. The therapist should feel at home within the altered state of consciousness of the patient during the session. The therapist, if moved and guided by previous experience, needs to feel free to partake of the sacrament offered to the patient and still honor the responsibility of containing the patient in a safe, secure, and trustworthy manner.

Love takes delight in the other as the other is, in his or her *is-ness*. Love desires nothing. Love is a relating behavior that allows the other to be a *legitimate* other, with whom one can coexist. You know you are loved when you feel freer in the company of the other than when you are alone. Love is opening to the possibility of enhancing the life of another. It is not just a feeling, an attitude or thought, a sentiment. Love confers survival benefits on the other, makes the other's life easier and richer, as judged by the other. The proof of love is in the recipient. Love lets the other be, with some care and concern.

The patient wants to know if the therapist is benevolent or malicious. Friend or foe. The healing moment can be the one when I am defenseless, at your mercy, and you could kill me, hurt me, shame me, humiliate me—but you don't. Trust cannot be created by fiat. It's the result of shared experience. Trust can never be earned. It has to be advanced. It can be broken by promises not kept, by betrayal, by lies. The worst traumas are caused by betrayal. The disaster of feeling captured and tortured (enduring unwanted, unchosen experiences), all trust broken, feeling forsaken, any hope of justice, love, and care annihilated, this cataclysm leaves alarms ringing in the background of the rest of the innocent victim's life. They are locked into constant high arousal. They are not really *living*; they are in *survival mode*.

Judith Lewis Herman (1992) thinks, and I agree completely, that all so-called mental illnesses are varieties of terror left behind by having been betrayed, unprotected, hurt, tortured, and silenced. She talks about the first phase of therapy, which she calls "establishing some measure of safety, security and trust between the therapist and the patient," and she emphasizes that this takes as long as it takes, sometimes minutes, at times years. MDMA, with its propensity to bring one into the present, to exit shame, and to open the heart, is useful in shortening this phase of therapy if, and only if, the therapist happens to be genuinely loving and trustworthy. In altered states I find it's best to be guileless, no tricks, no deception, for any falseness, manipulation will be perceived and, if denied, could retraumatize the patient. The aim of the therapist cannot be *to help*. If the patient finds the encounter helpful, that's a bonus, but it's best if the therapist isn't helping intentionally. Keeping company, containing, ensuring safety and connection when sought for, paying careful attention, and surrendering to what the situation calls for—these are worthy goals for the therapist.

Moments of communion—blessed moments when, for example, two dancers surrender to the music and move like one, neither leading nor following, experiencing themselves as parts of something greater than either of them—are hoped-for moments of fusion. Destructive shortcuts to oneness—for example, "let the two of us be one and let that one be me!"—are to be avoided. It's best if both the therapist and the patient heed Marion Milner's (1950) dictum: the only proper function of the will is to will not to will. Visualize the will as a snake, and make it bite its own tail (as in the symbol of the ouroboros).

All of the above applies to psychotherapy in general; it's just that in psychedelic psychotherapy, any deviation from this *radical* or back-to-the roots approach (as in *radic,* meaning "root") could cause deep hurt and panic, especially if deviations are not immediately acknowledged and remedied. The choices of the patient must be honored without judgment by the therapist: whether the patient becomes silent or converses with the therapist, wants music or silence, or physical contact or distance. The therapist follows, accompanies, supports; the therapist never leads. The model is that of the midwife rather than the obstetrician. Receptive, maternal support rather than active, expert heroics.

Sophisticated biochemical, genetic, and surgical treatments induce patients to yield decisions about their suffering to experts. We have to be careful not to add to this list psychedelic treatments. To appear all-knowing, the expert, the therapist promotes transference rather than resolving and helping to end it. Transference is the mistaken belief that the other knows. Children think their parents know. The end of transference is when we realize that nobody knows. A sad and painful and frightening moment, but it helps in the emancipation of the patient (Rancière 1991).

An Argentinian psychotherapist, Juan, proposed to climb Cerro Aconcagua, over twenty thousand feet high, with his patient Miguel (Lingis 2018). Dangerous. Juan had attempted the climb twice before and had been unsuccessful, the climb incomplete. Hippocratic oath: *first do no harm.*

Juan and Miguel took four weeks off work. It took four months of preparation. Their progress was difficult; Juan wondered if Miguel would survive. The summit was visible. It began to snow, and they came to a halt. They decided to turn back. It took them four days to descend to base camp. The therapist said nothing of what happened to them. No talking cure. No interpretation. No explication. The mountain drove them off. "Impassioned states, that totally fill and throb in mind and body, disconnected from, disconnecting the experience and knowledge and enterprises of the past" (Lingis 2018, 65). Such states can be transformative. Psychedelic psychotherapy is comparable to Juan's and Miguel's adventure. Nothing is certain. There are dangers.

Perhaps it's best if the therapist partakes of the sacrament of the psychedelic as well as the patient. A psychedelic-assisted session is a trip, not unlike the one Juan and Miguel went on. A joint undertaking of two into the unknown, uncontrollable, unpredictable, dangerous, and exciting. Two equals an "us." At most, the therapist is the more experienced Sherpa, perhaps the lead climber. How could the patient move toward emancipation if the therapist exempts himself from sharing the altered state of consciousness? If the therapist is cold sober, the patient might feel observed, objectified, manipulated. If both the therapist and the patient ingest LSD, it's OK if the therapist has half the amount of the patient or less. After all, the therapist has the role of containing the patient. The patient has no responsibility for containing the therapist. Inevitably, there occur these very human moments when the patient looks into the therapist's eyes and says, "Are you for real?" or "Do you care?" or "Will you hurt me?" What is the therapist going to say? Whatever the therapist answers, it won't matter. Words are not going to persuade anybody of anything. There are issues of shame, there are issues of trust, there are issues of betrayal that I think only come to surface, can only be resolved, when the therapist risks everything by being unabashedly himself.

Sándor Ferenczi, one of the, to me, most palatable, sympathetic psychoanalysts, said you need only two qualifications to be a good therapist: you have to have zero ambition and a lot of time. Well, I say that that's precisely what the psychedelic therapist needs: zero ambition and a lot of time. Because the moment the patient feels that it's the therapist who is driving the session, the whole session is derailed. It's absolutely essential that the therapist follows the patient rather than the other way around. Any guide with therapeutic zeal can do untold harm. One of the pseudoscientific questions that arises in psychedelic therapy is: How do you select your patients? What are the selection criteria? Well, as far as I have been able to ascertain, there aren't any. Self-selection, I would say, is probably the best criterion. I have never suggested to anybody to do an LSD session. I only respond to people who say, "I'm going to do one." So self-selection. Because anything else, any other criterion or restriction, basically shows the therapist's fear, his need to cover his own ass, to avoid being held responsible by the authorities. Actually, what's going to happen is totally unknown and unpredictable. Coming into psychology from the sciences, I was astonished by the misuse of statistics (Bakan 1967) and the misguided scientism that was the order of the day. It was stated that the aim of psychology was to *control and predict human behavior* (Johnson 1971). Good luck! I will tell two little stories that illustrate the dangers of pretending to know selection criteria. Under current prejudices, neither of the two patients in my stories would have been allowed LSD psychotherapy.

Mary was a roughly fifty-year-old woman, very depressed. She was in a mental hospital when there were still mental hospitals in Vancouver. And she was in a locked ward. She received several courses of electroconvulsive therapy, and she was on major antipsychotics. She had attempted suicide four times. Her psychologist at the hospital, who was a patient of mine, for some odd reason thought that she could benefit from seeing me. So, it was the psychologist who transported this woman to see me twice a week for fifty-minute sessions. For three long months, this woman came in, sat down, didn't move a muscle, never looked at me, and just sat there. Three months, twice a week. Who am I to say anything to her? I thought at first. I welcomed her and there we sat. After a while, I began to notice that I'm thinking things that I probably wouldn't be thinking if I were alone, if I wasn't in her presence. Now, those thoughts, which I thought arose because I was with her, I started to verbalize. I even joked that she was my analyst because she was quiet and I was speaking. She didn't crack a smile. To cut a long story short, her first words to me were spoken after three months and totally surprised me because by then I expected that she would never speak. She said, "I'm afraid of you." I said, "What could I possibly do that would be harmful to you?" She said, "You might take my freedom away from me." I said, "How?" She said, "I'm afraid I won't feel free to commit suicide if I continue this." I didn't think that was such a bad thing. So that's how it began.

We engaged in regular, unassisted psychotherapy for about three years, during which time she weaned herself off all medication. What we came to was that she lived in a 24/7 soap opera. From the time she was born, she wanted to be the good child of her parents, be the good student at school, and then the good wife to her husband. Then she said she didn't want any children, but her husband insisted, so she had to be the good mother to her children. She was very keenly aware that no one was interested in her. Everybody was interested in the mother, in the daughter, in the wife. I had to make very sure that I didn't expect her to be a good patient. It would have been one more load on her shoulders. Clearly, her attempts at suicide were to escape the 24/7 soap opera. I mean, imagine yourself having to perform 24/7, and there is no way out, no way to get offstage, except, she thought, by offing yourself. I could understand. The only alternative I could offer her was that maybe there is a way to be authentic and not have to play anything or anybody without having to kill yourself. I wasn't sure, but at least it seemed to me worth trying before she really annihilated herself.

And then she had the bright idea that she was going to take LSD. I thought she was either brave or foolhardy, but I was willing to accompany her into the unknown. First session, absolutely nothing happened. She got even gloomier than before. A month later, she said, "I'm doing it again." I say OK. It works, she cried. She had a horrendous experience of abandonment. She saw me walking away from her. She said, "All I see is your back, and you're leaving." Now, that opened something up. That opened up a trauma that she hadn't talked about before. She was three years old, in Germany, where her family was stationed, when they got the order to go back to Canada, and her parents suddenly thought, "We haven't even seen Europe." So, she was three years old and they put her with a German nanny. In her words, they "parked me like luggage." The older children and the parents went off for a six-week tour of Europe. Of course, the German woman who looked after her didn't want any crying, didn't want any tears, so, from that moment on, she felt she was a piece of shit because gold you take with you, shit you leave behind. She got the message. She thought I, too, would leave her sooner or later. It was a very dark, sad, traumatic LSD session.

A month later, I thought she was going to kill herself for sure. It was clear between us that suicide prevention wasn't my job, and it was clear even between her husband and me that if he wanted to protect her he would have to keep a twenty-four-hour vigil. I couldn't do that. She informed me that she was doing a third and last LSD trip before ending her life and—guess what?—she came out of that episode smiling and laughing. In terms of Stanislav Grof's four stages of birth— bliss inside, no exit, bloody battle, bliss outside—she came out in bliss outside, and she conceived a way of being where she didn't have to play any roles, and she wasn't too frightened that her husband wouldn't have anything to do with her, her children wouldn't have anything to do with her. Because that was her fear, that unless she performed the roles, no one would tolerate her. Now, this was over ten years ago, and she is still perfectly well. She is living a very creative and happy life. She performs occasional grandmother functions, which she used to dread but now embraces because she is in control of it. She doesn't play the grandmother; she is the grandmother. Once a year, she sends me a little note: "Love you, and hate you!"

• • •

The second story illustrating the uselessness of selection criteria is about Lana, a woman I worked with for at least four years. She was diagnosed with multiple personality disorder. She was a fifty-five-year-old woman who would suddenly, in front of my eyes and ears, turn into a seven- year-old boy.

I thought she was pulling my leg. Around that time, I was going around saying and teaching that multiple personality disorder was iatrogenic. Patients just performed that to entertain their therapist. But it wasn't so. So, I wanted to look up the literature on what to do with somebody who is so split. And then I resisted the urge, and I thought she's going to teach me. Her multiple personality disorder is not like anyone else's.

So that's how we proceeded. The little boy taught me everything. The little boy knew everything. He was the repository of all the memories of torture and sexual abuse that she went through in her childhood. She knew nothing about the boy. She remembered nothing of the abuse. Occasionally, she would come in as the woman. She would say hello, the boy would come out, and at the end of the session, she would come out and write the check and sign it and ask, "What did we do?" But, of course, when I offered to tape-record the session, she would have none of it. It took a while, but magically, the two personas integrated.

Physiologically she manifested some very interesting phenomena. She wore glasses with a very strong prescription. When the boy came out, the boy took the glasses off, and he had perfect vision. She was allergic to peanut butter. The boy could polish off half a bottle of peanut butter and show no symptoms. If she had a cold and took aspirin, he would call me up and say she was overmedicating him. After he disappeared, blended into her, because she was slowly able to receive all the information that he was the repository of, she had to change her glasses; her new prescription was half as strong as the original.

After that, for about five years, she was fine and lived her life and worked. And then she phoned me up and said she was going to do some LSD. I thought, What if the boy comes out again? But that was my worry, not hers. I mentioned it to her, but she said, "Well, then we'll deal with him." Her reason was that she thought that her life was a little bit gray, not enough color in it. She felt that some creativity in her could be loosened up, that there was still some stultifying fear. Again, to cut a long story short, she had a very deep LSD session. At one point she was crying, and there was snot and tears all over her face, and I, without thinking, wiped her nose with my handkerchief. She later identified that moment as life changing. She said nobody had ever done that for her. This allowed her to feel the grief of never having been cared for, of never having been loved. It's the smallest things that can make the biggest difference, and these actions cannot be programmed. They somehow have to happen. One has to allow for them.

Often, when either a patient or therapist plan for programmed music during a session, they never get to it; they find they don't want it. Silence seems to be much more important during an LSD session than music. The music is, I think, for the sake of the therapist. It keeps you the expert. I once proposed to a gathering of psychedelic therapists that, if they felt they needed music during a session, they ask the patient to bring his or her music instead of programming it themselves or, if the session is being done in the patient's home, they let patients select what they want to listen to. The answer was something like, "But most people we work with have such poor musical education. They wouldn't know what to select." How supercilious, how stultifying.

R. D. Laing wrote:

> We are afraid of our souls, of our souls becoming alive. We are *psycho phobic*. I submit that until we experience our selves, and our world, as one, we are terrified to do so. What we call our consciousness, what we call our mental states, are nothing else than our experience of the world, or the world of experience, or, just simply, our experience. Schizoid minds create a schizocosmos. As long as we remain in this state of apartness from ourselves, from one another, from the cosmos, we can only yearn for the healing of the mind/body, subject/object, self/other, self/cosmos splits and cut-offs which characterize our schizoid experience. Real health is characterized by the realization of the fact that all is one, that all is in each, as each is in all. (1987, 78–79)

Psychedelic psychotherapy, at its best, can heal both therapist and patient. We are all in the same boat; there is no *us* and *them*, the painful illusion of being skin-encapsulated egos.

2

Ayahuasca and Psychotherapy

Rachel Harris

Years ago, in a land far away, I was talking with a Jungian analyst about his female client whose mother had died when she was a child. It seemed clear to me, a young therapist at the time, that this woman should have a female therapist. I blithely made my point with the kind of confidence only an inexperienced therapist is naive enough to express. The older therapist, steeped in the wisdom that Jungians attain after listening to thousands of dreams, patiently responded, "Yes, it will be the woman in me who heals her."

After decades in private practice, I often reflect back upon this snippet of conversation that turned out to be formative. The analyst exemplified how it's the relationship that heals as opposed to the specific therapeutic technique (Wampold 2015), and it's what we bring from our personal depths to that relationship that makes all the difference.

At some level, this is the essence of psychedelic psychotherapy. As therapists, we have to be able to meet our clients in those mysterious realms that both open from within and also blast into outer space. We have to know how to access these mystical territories within ourselves in order to connect with our psychedelic clients who are exploring these otherworldly worlds. We have to know in our bones what they're talking about. It's the mystical traveler in ourselves that we must bring to the therapeutic relationship.

Does this mean the therapist has to have personally attended an ayahuasca ceremony? Does the therapist have to be in her own healing process with this psychedelic medicine, attending regular ceremonies? Yes and no. Is this absolutely a requirement? No. A therapist can gain access to these states of consciousness in a variety of ways. Does it make a difference if the therapist has her own personal relationship with the spirit of ayahuasca? Yes.

We have now officially left the realm of evidenced-based treatments.

The spirit of ayahuasca may be referred to in different ways depending upon context—as a generic *unseen other*, as *Grandmother Ayahuasca*, or as a *cosmic serpent*. When I asked in a study of ayahuasca use in North America, "Do you have an ongoing relationship with the spirit of ayahuasca?" 74 percent of people reported yes (Harris and Gurel 2012). If both the therapist and the client have such a relationship with this mysterious plant spirit, the whole nature of the therapeutic alliance is qualitatively transformed.

Ayahuasca differs from many of the other psychedelics in that the plant spirit remains in the body long after the psychedelic effect fades or even the biochemical markers disappear. The sensation is that an *intentional other* has entered your body to scan your energy field, to balance, align, and repair your vibrational patterns. This is the shamanic healing process, and it continues, albeit with less intensity, for weeks or even months following a ceremony. Gorman (2010) captured this sensation with the title of his book *Ayahuasca in My Blood*. The medicine is not literally in the blood, but this phrase describes the lived experience of the presence of ayahuasca at a cellular level, at the level of DNA (Tafur 2017), which becomes a permanent aspect of the felt somatic sense.

The presence of ayahuasca in the therapist's body and energy field changes the process of therapy. The therapist's inner world is expanded into shamanic realms, imaginal landscapes, and the further reaches of the unconscious. The therapist is a knowledgeable traveler through these realms, experienced in maintaining equilibrium in the face of extraordinary emotions and psychedelic experiences. This enhanced inner capacity, with its access to the numinous, allows for a deeper and broader connection between the unconscious of the therapist and that of the client. Jung (1969, para. 544) described this elusive dynamic in the therapeutic relationship as "soul must work on soul."

Recent work on intersubjectivity in neuropsychoanalysis describes this implicit connection (Schore 2011) as the therapist attunes nonverbally to the client on a moment-to-moment basis (Spezanno 2005). The therapeutic healing process is alive and present in both their bodies and energy fields. The process of therapy unfolds via implicit communication, nonverbal resonance, and somatic responsiveness between two human beings, beyond their roles as therapist and client. This implicit, embodied, and unconscious realm is ayahuasca's prime territory, and the presence of the medicine creates a deeper connection between therapist and client, replete with mystery and meaning. The two share an appreciation for other realities and sources of insight and wisdom. At this level, cognitive behavioral techniques or analytical interpretations are irrelevant at best and harmful at worst. With ayahuasca present in both therapist and client, our understanding of the therapeutic alliance must be transformed.

PERSONAL EXPERIENCE

I must admit I've been hesitant to state unequivocally that it's better to see a therapist who has her own relationship with the spirit of ayahuasca. This is hardly a requirement in graduate school or for professional licensing. But I have experienced both sides of this equation and think it's a critical aspect of the therapeutic relationship.

During research interviews for my ayahuasca study (Harris 2017), which admittedly bordered on brief psychotherapy, I could feel in the person-to-person connection when the spirit of Grandmother Ayahuasca arose in each of us and connected us at another level. I often asked the other person if they could sense her arrival, and they usually could. This otherworldly bond deepened our conversation and trust in each other as we talked about experiences that are difficult to capture in words or are outright ineffable.

I emailed a request to interview one of my research subjects five years after he had completed the questionnaire from that same study (Harris 2017, 289–98). He agreed, and we talked on the phone. I wanted to follow up with him because he had had a complex relationship with Grandmother Ayahuasca, feeling guilty that he hadn't lived up to her recommendations. He had not attended an ayahuasca ceremony during that five-year period, and he continued to feel guilty. Fairly soon into our exploration of his relationship with this plant spirit, I asked him if he felt her presence in the moment, as we were speaking. He said yes, almost immediately. I agreed and could feel our connection deepen into our shared mystery.

It's as though there's a third-party present, a cotherapist for me and a supportive presence for the interviewee. Acknowledging my sense of the presence of ayahuasca between us is healing for the person I'm interviewing because it affirms their relationship with this plant spirit. Such recognition is important in our Western culture since the experience of the presence of a plant spirit is outside our consensus reality. Yet, it's a significant aspect of the ayahuasca healing process that continues well after the ceremony ends.

On the other side of this equation, I've been seeing a Jungian therapist who has studied Hawaiian shamanism and even has an intimate connection with Hawaiian goddesses. I can sense that she's connected to those particular spirit realms; however, as I'm not, I don't join her in that other world. She understands these unseen realms, but that's not the same as a shared energetic connection. We still have a good working relationship in therapy, and I have clearly benefited; at the same time, I know she cannot enter into my experiences with Grandmother Ayahuasca.

From an indigenous point of view, this concept of shared spirit realms is an accepted reality. Shamans can see into participants' visions during ceremonies and guide them through these other worlds. Also, shamans have been known to impart teachings to their protégés by appearing in their nighttime dreams. The medicine seems to open a link that allows for this level of communication.

ATTACHMENT RELATIONSHIP

The 74 percent of people in my research study who reported an ongoing relationship with the spirit of ayahuasca described "a consistent presence in my life," an ever-present guide and source of wisdom, both supportive and loving. A few people wrote that this was the first time they felt truly loved in their lives even though at times it was a tough love. They felt the spirit of ayahuasca always had their best interests at heart, "showing me how to forgive myself, how and why I should live healthier." One person answered that the "relationship felt like a parental bond" and he "felt loved." Another wrote, "She is my mother" (Harris 2017).

These quotes describe an attachment bond, the kind of affective relationship between baby and primary caretaker. The key elements of an attachment bond are that the child seeks to be close to the attachment figure, experiences distress at separation, turns to the attachment figure in times of stress, and feels that the attachment figure is a secure base from which the child can explore the world (Bowlby 1969). The descriptions of a personal relationship with the spirit of ayahuasca meet these criteria in the same way that Kirkpatrick has said that people with a personal relationship with God are also in an attachment relationship (2005).

Moreover, these attachment relationships with an unseen other have the capacity to repair old attachment wounds from childhood (Granqvist, Mikulincer, and Shaver 2010). People who grew up with parents who were not consistent, attuned, or responsive fall into avoidant, anxious, or disorganized attachment categories. They struggle with emotional dysregulation and have difficulty managing relationship distress. The narrative of their life story lacks coherence, purpose, and meaning, and they seem to have a diminished capacity for self-reflection and insight. About 50 percent of the population falls into these categories of insecure attachment.

In a relationship with an unseen other, these people heal enough to shift attachment categories and achieve an earned security attachment category with a better prognosis for long-term relationships and a coherent life story (Siegel 2010). Without equating the spirit of ayahuasca with God, both kinds of relationships are with an unseen other and are filled with a love that is always available.

When the experience of being loved peaks during an ayahuasca ceremony, it's as if the universe embraces us with love. This is such a healing revelation, filling us with radiant light, that we emerge the next morning with great gratitude for Grandmother Ayahuasca. Receiving cosmic love in ceremony changes the person in a profound and permanent way. A mortal therapist, even with a strong therapeutic alliance, cannot cajole the heavens to open up and shower the golden light of love onto a client sitting in her office.

Veronica was in her early thirties but had not quite gained traction in her life. It wasn't that she was lost; she just didn't have the healthy self-confidence to find a way to move forward. Veronica didn't have a college degree or independent career, so she got by on minimum hourly wages. She had been in an abusive relationship that took years to escape and was currently working on her recovery.

"Grandmother Ayahuasca is there for me in a way that no one else ever was. I can call on her day or night and she'll respond. She's always there and loving. So, for the first time in my life, I feel lovable," Veronica said, as she explained her relationship with the spirit of ayahuasca.

As a therapist, I couldn't help but ask myself if this was a textbook case of spiritual by-passing. Is Veronica relying on her relationship with an unseen spirit instead of working on healthy and realistic relationships with potential mates? Certainly, some people escape the developmental challenges of so-called real life by retreating into the spirit world and imagining personal fulfillment.

I didn't think this was the case with Veronica. Instead, I saw her gathering her shattered sense of self into a new identity that deserved to be loved. Her relationship with Grandmother Ayahuasca was giving her a more positive foundation, allowing her to shift to a secure attachment category that would surely enable her to make better relationship choices in life. People who feel lovable create different life trajectories than people who don't feel lovable, and Veronica was, in a sense, starting over.

For Veronica, ayahuasca ceremonies were taking the place of psychotherapy. Ideally, she could benefit from both, with therapy supporting and expanding her sense of being lovable and the ceremonies deepening her relationship with Grandmother Ayahuasca. But she couldn't afford psychotherapy. Like a good-enough mother, ayahuasca can continue to heal Veronica so she can move forward with her life.

RUPTURE IN THE THERAPEUTIC PROCESS

Even with the presence of ayahuasca and a strong therapeutic alliance, it's inevitable that a glitch will occur in the therapist-client relationship. One or the other will feel misunderstood, diminished in some way, and possibly frustrated, disappointed, or upset with the other. This disconnection is called a rupture in the moment-to-moment relationship between therapist and client, and it usually means that one or the other's unconscious has been tweaked (Ginot 2012). It can be as small an interaction as:

Client after an ayahuasca ceremony, with awe: "The lights were incredible, like fireworks!"

Therapist, slightly impatient: "Yes, but what did you learn?"

A better response from the therapist would have simply been "uh-huh," a neutral acknowledgment to allow the client to continue to share. But this particular therapist happens to value insight and achievement, and she wanted to get into the depth work immediately. Her timing was off. A very simple rupture.

Client, startled by the abrupt shift, stutters: "I'm not sure, I just wanted to enjoy the beauty."

Therapist, realizing she's out of step: "I'm sorry, I rushed you. Please go on."

Client, accepting the repair: "Yes, the lights were different this time. I could feel them streaming into my body."

The rupture was not only about timing; it was in the wrong modality. "What did you learn?" requires a cognitive answer with linear thinking. Lights streaming into a body comes from the shamanic realm where miracles happen beyond explanation. Note the seamless shift from seeing the lights to the somatically based experience of feeling the lights enter the body. A therapist without ayahuasca experience might at best consider "light streaming into a body" to be a metaphor. A therapist with experience recognizes that this is a direct description of the process of healing.

The challenge is how quickly therapists can catch themselves when they're out of attunement. And then how quickly they can repair the disconnection and reconnect with the client.

From an intersubjective perspective, a rupture reflects both the client's and the therapist's psychic structure, what Bowlby (1969) called an internal working model. We have all constructed our egos to protect us and ensure our survival. Whatever our attachment experiences, we learned very early how to predict and understand our environment, how to survive and pursue a felt sense of safety (Pietromonaco and Barrett 2000). The egoic architecture we develop is typically rigid, unconscious, and reactively stubborn.

A rupture in the therapeutic relationship can entangle both the therapist's and the patient's ego. How the therapist responds in that moment can determine the course of treatment. Therapeutic skill is essential along with personal humility. In this moment, it is who the therapist is that is of utmost importance. How much awareness does the therapist have of her own psychic architecture and recurring patterns? How much flexibility does she have within her own ego structure to sidestep her most reactive patterns and find an elegant pathway to reconnection with the client?

It's tempting to think that if the therapist is experienced with ayahuasca, then surely she is aware and flexible enough to respond artfully to the client. There's plenty of research showing an increase in cognitive flexibility with psychedelics (Carhart-Harris et al. 2014). On the other hand, we all know people who have been sitting in ceremonies for years and are still stuck in their familiar, repetitive patterns. It's our responsibility as therapists to catch ourselves in the moment when a rupture occurs and titrate a response specific for that client.

Ayahuasca gives us the objectivity and space to dis-identify with our feelings and thoughts so that we have a split second not to react but to consciously choose how to respond. This is what integration looks like, whether in our roles as psychotherapists or in our everyday lives. This is how we change our habitual patterns of perceiving and behaving.

INTEGRATION

My favorite bumper sticker reads "Don't believe everything you think," a practical summary of dis-identification, especially if we extend the message to: "Don't believe everything you think or feel."

Our default mode network (DMN), the neural network that occupies 60 percent of waking time with our personal narratives, anxieties about the future, ruminations over the past, and other everyday worries, constitutes our habitual patterns of thinking and feeling (Carhart-Harris and Friston 2010). Implicit learning during the first few years of life established these neural pathways in order to survive and hopefully thrive in our family of origin. These habitual thoughts and feelings constitute our core issues, or *early maladaptive schemas,* defined as "broad pervasive themes regarding oneself and one's relationship with others, developed during childhood and elaborated throughout one's lifetime" (Young and Klosko 1993). These themes are the architectural building blocks of our self-construction and the self-reinforcing content of the DMN.

One person described his core issues this way: "I mean as a kid, you come to all these conclusions that aren't necessarily right, but they help you survive in the moment. And then you spend, as far as I can tell, the rest of your life unpacking those poor coping mechanisms to see where they do and/or where they don't serve you."

The good news is that this engine fueling our psychic status quo, the DMN, is disrupted during an ayahuasca ceremony, as well as with other psychedelic experiences. In other words, the DMN is quieted, so the morning after the ceremony we feel freer from our chronic internal monologue and self-critic, experience greater inner spaciousness, and, hence, have the chance to reset our internal programming or recalibrate our psyche.

The Navajo recognize this moment in the way they greet a person returning from a vision quest. "For four days after the conclusion of the ceremony, the patient is considered, by family and friends, as if he or she is a Holy Person and given an opportunity to focus, evaluate, interpret, and experience a new self" (Kaptchuk 2011). Our psychic architecture is deconstructed in ceremony, and we have the opportunity to reimagine ourselves with spiritual maturity and conscious discernment.

Integration following an ayahuasca ceremony consists of the practice of catching ourselves when we fall into old patterns of thinking and feeling and choosing to respond differently.

Here are different ways people describe the reprogramming opportunity that ayahuasca ceremonies offer: "I don't take my moods so seriously anymore." "I've always struggled with anxiety and depression, but I'm more accepting of them now." "While I still get frustrated at times, I now have more space between action and reaction to respond in a more level-headed, caring way . . . usually."

In the psychological literature, this particular internal shift is described by a multitude of terms, such as decentering, meta-awareness, cognitive distancing, and self-distance perspective (Bernstein et al. 2015). Interestingly, neurological studies are finding that this same enhanced self-awareness occurs with both psychedelics and meditation (Dahl, Lutz, and Davidson 2015). From a clinical point of view, it's the integrative discipline of daily self-awareness practice that maximizes a psychedelic experience.

INDIGENOUS
AND WESTERN HEALING

There has been some resistance to psychotherapy in the ayahuasca communities in Western countries. It's not uncommon for people to assume that ceremonies, alone, will heal all their psychological issues. "Ayahuasca is my therapist." "I don't believe in psychotherapy; I believe in ayahuasca." And the ubiquitous, "One night of ceremony is worth ten years of psychotherapy."

One ayahuasca user described his attempts at psychotherapy: "The couple of times I tried psychotherapy, I never felt a real connection with the therapists I found. The traditional psychotherapy approaches seem too simplistic to capture how I think and feel. They're also devoid of physical and loving connections that feel healing in real life."

Admittedly, a healing ayahuasca ceremony is a hard act to follow for any psychotherapist, but those trained in cognitive-behavioral approaches consistently strike out. For ayahuasca-experienced people who have plumbed the depth of their souls in the darkness of night, such concrete approaches to therapy might almost feel insulting.

Yet, some people are beginning to realize that sitting in ceremonies doesn't solve all their issues. One forty-something man who had attended over one hundred thirty ceremonies wrote, "I still had unusual challenges in other areas of life, particularly around my personal relationships." This man decided to try psychotherapy, found a sympatico therapist, and realized that psychotherapy can offer additional healing, different and complementary to ayahuasca ceremonies.

It's important to note that working therapeutically with ayahuasca does not follow the same pattern as other psychedelics where research protocols focus on a mystical or ego dissolution experience with minimal therapeutic support. People attend ceremonies repeatedly over months or years. It's possible to have both weekly therapy sessions and multiple ceremonies occurring over the same period of time. The two containers safely hold the person, allowing for in-depth exploration of unconscious patterns as well as the mysteries of the universe. In this way, psychotherapy can inform ceremonial experiences, and ayahuasca can inform the therapeutic process.

I received one message from Grandmother Ayahuasca in a ceremony that I immediately took into my therapist's office: "Your childhood history is worse than I thought. That's why you can't do what I said." I was both disturbed by this psychological evaluation from a plant spirit and relieved that she understood my inability to follow her advice. In my therapy session, her message evoked greater compassion and forgiveness for myself.

In ayahuasca ceremonies and psychotherapy, the challenge is to weave together insights, downloads, visions, and mystical experiences in order to translate them into greater wisdom and loving-kindness in daily life. In both processes, we move from inner experiences to our lives in the outer world and back again. The ease with which we move between states of consciousness, the material and imaginal worlds, and indigenous and modern cultures can lead to the healing of the soul we all seek.

3

Impact of Personal Psychedelic Experiences in Clinical Practice

Jerome Braun

Psychedelic medicines make me a better Jungian psychoanalyst. What an unconventional comment to say as a Jungian analyst; yet, in truth, I now admit it after having an ongoing and intricate relationship with indigenous healers who reside in the depths of the Peruvian Amazon. Beginning in 2017, three sacred plant medicine healers (two men, called *curanderos,* and one woman, a *curandera*) of the Shipibo people have been sharing with me their parents', grandparents', and unseen ancestors' lineage of healing rites, natural pharmacological remedies, psychedelic medicines, and invaluable wisdom. At times, their wisdom and therapeutic capacities seem to surpass Western psychological methods of healing, yet their knowledge of the plant medicines' effects on human psychology also parallel Jungian concepts of the psyche.

In addition to the psychedelic medicine of the ayahuasca vine (*Banisteriopsis caapi*) cooked with chacruna leaves (*Psychotria viridis*), the curanderos teach me to work with other sacred plants of their Shipibo traditions that are not psychedelic. These "helper" plants to ayahuasca-chacruna have extraordinary psychological and transcendental capacities, for example: piñón colorado or bellyache bush (*Jatropha gossypiifolia*), a bush related to the poinsettia and used for enhancing receptivity to plant spirit guides and clairvoyance for healing; renaquilla (*Clusia rosea*), a vine that transforms into a master tree and is used for both physical and psychological strengthening; and zapote renaco (*Ficus americana* subsp. *guianensis*), a gigantic tree that tops the jungle canopy and is healing medicine to fortify the heart and soul. The Shipibo healers' sacred songs, ayahuasca-chacruna ceremonies, and sacred helper plants have infused into my Jungian psychoanalytic practice an exponential increase in intuitive functioning, deeper understanding of healing trauma in my clients and myself, an immeasurable increase of synchronistic and parapsychological moments with clients, provided astute clinical consults about clients' conditions and treatment procedures, developed in me a deeper trust in the reality of an inner healer in each of us, and introduced me to superior intelligences exceedingly wise beyond this human realm. What follows is one of the numerous experiences I had while working with the Shipibo healers.

I had just returned from one of my trips to the Amazonian healing center, where I had spent time working with renaquilla tree medicine. I was sitting in a therapy session with one of my clients, listening intently to her. Suddenly a vision of three snakes hanging on a branch of a tree appeared over her right shoulder. The vision was merely a flash, and then a detailed scene appeared in my mind's eye of a little girl in a basement being abused by a nondescript adult. It took me by surprise, and the scene had nothing to do with what my client was sharing at the time. In the right moment, I shared with her the scene of the little girl, and she gasped. She said she had never told anyone about what had happened to her, which was related to that basement scene. She asked how I knew that because we had never talked about it in therapy. She had held that shameful secret within herself for decades. I simply asked her to share more about what it meant to her. The results deepened her healing process and our therapeutic relationship.

The healing medicines work through images, visions, intuition, and living symbols, such as the vision of the three snakes, including downloads of transpersonal and transrational information that surpass conventional ways of thinking. Prior to working with the Shipibo healers, psychedelics, and healing plant medicines, I had never experienced this type of mysteriously intuitive transmission of client information.

EARLY WORK WITH CLIENTS ON PSYCHEDELIC DRUGS

For over two decades I have offered psychotherapy in private practice in San Francisco, California, during which time I trained at the C. G. Jung Institute in Kusnacht, Zurich, Switzerland, and became certified as a Jungian analyst. In the past, my interests in psychedelic drugs were solely focused on what a conventional psychotherapist may diagnose and treat: trauma, dependency, and addiction. I had no interest in trying psychedelics off the streets or through underground neoshamanic gatherings. My paradigm was heavily impacted in my youth by the War on Drugs campaigns of the 1970s and 1980s, initiated by Richard Nixon to shut down the first psychedelic wave, followed by Nancy Reagan's antidrug campaign of Just Say No. To this day, I can picture in my mind's eye the 1980s TV commercial by the Partnership for a Drug-free America of a man holding a sizzling hot iron skillet, dropping a cracked egg into it, instantly frying the egg, and then stating, "This is your brain on drugs." As any Jungian may attest to, images possess immense power to impact behaviors.

I was living in one of the hubs of the underground psychedelic renaissance, Northern California, when increasing numbers of people began seeking out my Jungian psychoanalytic practice in 2016. Many had undergone psychedelic journeys and sought Jungian psychotherapy to understand their life-changing experiences. A few clients initiated therapy after being traumatized during their psychedelic experiences. I became increasingly curious about how to understand my clients' experiences, which included raw archetypal material, core mythological themes, terrorizing shadow elements, contact with their dead relatives, and numinous experiences. These kinds of experiences did not easily fit into their predominantly rational and empirical paradigm.

In between psychotherapy sessions, some of my clients participated in underground psychedelic ceremonies or sacred medicine work in other countries. I witnessed rapid, radical, and therapeutic changes in these clients—far exceeding the rate of growth and improvement of my other clients. Their level of anxiety, depressed mood, and psychological suffering improved significantly, and the positive changes seemed sustained over time. These changes were astounding and truly radical, in other words, reaching to the root of their complexes. Their remarkable recovery directly challenged the cultural images inculcated in my psyche from the '70s and '80s, and I had to confront my assumptions about psychedelics.

I searched for ways to frame within a Jungian context my clients' reports of remarkable and undeniable recoveries and sometimes paranormal and mystical experiences. To date, I have found only one specific reference to psychedelics written by C. G. Jung. In Jung's correspondence with Victor White, an English Dominican priest, Jung warned against taking LSD and mescaline, writing that these drugs would provide unfettered access to unconscious material, more than needed and exceeding that from dreams and intuition (1976, 172–73). It's noteworthy that Jung did disclose to White that he knew little about psychedelics.

Jung's lifework was rooted in dialectical communication with the manifestations of the unconscious through dreams, intuition, visions, synchronicity, and psychic entities. Jung had his own relationship with Philemon, his spirit guide. Interestingly, Jungian concepts paralleled my clients' psychedelic experiences. Clients recounted their encounters with their deceased loved ones, experiencing archetypal material previously unknown to them, and communication with beyond-human intelligent benevolent beings. Surprisingly, what began to emerge in my research was that psychedelics and Jungian psychology parallel and crisscross one another. Searching for answers within a Jungian framework about my clients' psychedelic experiences—in conjunction with my personal dreams, intuition, and synchronistic events—led me to working with indigenous healers in the Amazon. One year before beginning with the Shipibo traditional medicine work, I had what Jungians call a "big dream."

> My dream began with a healer sitting comfortably cross-legged on the ground, eyes closed, and mouth slightly open, with innumerable small black spiders busily crawling in and out of his mouth, down his neck, and across his bare chest. In the dream, I felt captivated without any repulsion. I watched curiously and in awe. Then a wooden fence appeared between the healer and me. Many people gathered round to look at the healer, too. People picked up apples on the ground near the fence and tossed them toward the fence. My dream-ego instinctively picked up one of the red apples and threw it, hitting the central slat of the wooden fence. The apple passed magically through the slat, landing on the other side of the fence, causing the spiders to scurry rapidly and in unison toward the apple, biting off bits of the apple and carrying the apple pieces back to the healer's mouth. "Oh!" I said to myself in the dream, "That's how he eats without harming any spiders!" I woke up.
>
> I felt elated upon waking. Spending many months, contemplating and amplifying the dream images, I never fully understood it. It was not until I found myself in the Amazon years later, beginning an ongoing close relationship with indigenous healers and their families, that I understood that the dream was a foretelling of my relationship with the curanderos and psychedelic medicine work.

NEW PARADISE

Situated on the banks of the Ucayali River in the eastern Peruvian Amazon is a small indigenous community called La Comunidad Nativa Nuevo Paraíso or, briefly in English, New Paradise. Throughout the day, the Shipibo healing center is serenaded by an endless symphony of birdsong reverberating overhead and punctuated by monkey vocalizations in the distance. The bird songs are constant while the sun shines but pause during the roars of torrential rainstorms. The nights give way to the croaking, squawking, and ribbiting of the loudly communicative frogs. Rarely is there ambient silence.

Two curanderos and one curandera (Maestros Nelson and Javier and Maestra Anita) facilitate medicine ceremonies for up to six people per visit at their healing center. In addition to the healers, apprentices assist during ceremonies, and sometimes locals attend the healing ceremonies.

A restricted diet, called *la dieta,* is required, beginning two weeks before the ceremonies commence and continuing for two weeks after the last ceremony. Dieta, a diet based on Shipibo tradition, consists mainly of beans, rice, plantain, fish, and poultry and prohibits salt, sugar, caffeine, pork or other bloody meats, alcohol, and sexual activities of any kind. This diet of simple nourishment cleanses the internal physical body so the spirits of the plants will feel welcome to inhabit the person's body during ayahuasca-chacruna ceremonies.

Beyond the inconveniences of a restricted diet, increased awareness of my psychological attachments to and habits with food became glaringly evident. Dieta is an invaluable teaching in itself. Additionally, the dieta preparatory period for ceremony exponentially enhanced my dream life. Dieta is an important component of the development of surrender and, paradoxically, the strengthening of one's will to be centered and intentional, in preparation for challenges and discomforts during psychedelic medicine journeys.

On the night of the ayahuasca-chacruna ceremony, the curanderos blow *mapacho,* sacred tobacco, to clear the space of malevolent forces. One at a time, the participants approach the curanderos; the ayahuasca-chacruna brew is poured into a shot glass and handed to each participant. The participant expresses gratitude to the curanderos and to the sacred medicine, blows intentions into the ayahuasca-chacruna brew, and then consciously accepts and drinks the psychedelic medicine. At some point, one of the curanderos or the curandera is moved to begin singing a series of sacred songs, *icaros,* which mysteriously initiates psychedelic processes and healing energies. The icaros are initially sung to the whole group, creating a sacred circle and protective energetic field around the group. Next, each healer sits in front of a participant, singing a series of healing icaros individually tailored to that person's issues. Six to eight hours after the start of the ceremony, calm and rest ensue: the dominant sounds of nature—warm breezes rustling the leaves, frog ribbits, and nearby monkey calls—return to the ceremonial hall.

The icaros are fundamental to the healing process and tailored specifically to each participant's illness, traumas, psychological constitution, and ancestral lineage. In the Shipibo tradition, the ayahuasca-chacruna medicine is *not* the sole focus for healing. The brew is viewed as a powerful agent that opens the portals for the curandero or curandera to access the healing energies beyond this conventional empirical realm. Upon accessing these other realms, the Shipibo healers channel through their icaros energetic healing into the participant to realign the person's imbalances.

Traditionally, the healers drink ayahuasca-chacruna in ceremony while the patients do not. The ceremony has been tailored to Westerners visiting their healing center, with the participants drinking the brew, but the curanderos introduce a small amount initially and increase the amount incrementally, if needed, to avoid "blasting" the participants into the hinterlands of the cosmos. The goal is about healing not psychedelic obliteration. The curanderos' healing sequence is first to cleanse the physical body. In subsequent ceremonies they may increase the dosage and work on psychological traumas and the participant's lineage. Then, they may change the dosage for soul clearing; however, over the course of several ceremonies the healers' focus is to reduce risks of traumatization from the psychedelic medicine. Interestingly, the healers may decrease the dosage in subsequent ceremonies due to the efficacious healing powers transmitted through the curanderos and their icaros. In essence, Shipibo traditional healing is an inextricable composite of the ayahuasca-chacruna medicine, dieta, icaros, and the curandero's or curandera's channeling of healing energies guided by various plant spirits.

In addition to ayahuasca-chacruna, the Shipibo have thirty-seven sacred plants, which are not psychedelic but have properties of clairvoyance, parapsychology, and direct psychological downloads of wisdom. During one of my stays at the center, the maestros provided me with the opportunity to drink the medicine of piñón colorado, which enhances intuition and opens the capacity to receive teachings from the other plant spirits. Fasting from food for a minimum of three days is required when working with the other sacred plants, and the tradition consists of sitting alone day and night in solitary ceremony with the sacred "helper" plant medicine.

> In my first nighttime ceremony with piñón colorado, sitting on the floor in meditation inside my thatched roof hut, after an hour of inner silence, I felt a presence enter the hut. I looked up, and a distortion appeared in part of the wall and ceiling as if a convex lens about the size of a three-foot-long by two-foot-wide oval lens was hovering from the ceiling. Suddenly, there was a download of nonverbal information conveyed to me. "Jerome, your heart is broken, and you need to work on these things." The presence proceeded by relaying eight points that I needed to work on. In hindsight, I already knew six of these personal shadow issues—after twenty years of Jungian analysis, thanks to my analysts and a lot of my inner work—but I was unaware of the last two points! The download ended by conveying: "Now, lead with your heart." The vision disappeared, restoring the visual shape of the wall and ceiling to their customary shape.

Perhaps it is an unbelievable story, and prior to working with the Shipibo healers and psychedelics, if a client would have told me such a story, I may not have fully believed it either, thinking that these are merely projections of the imagination from the personal unconscious. Since piñón colorado's directive to lead with my heart, however, my predominant reliance on intellectual analysis has stepped down from its oversized pedestal, clearing ample space and increased trust of feelings, intuitive downloads, visions, and communications from intelligences beyond consensus reality.

PSYCHOTHERAPY
AND POSTPSYCHEDELIC INTEGRATION

For over two decades of offering psychotherapy, I have searched for effective interventions to help my clients heal their debilitating core negative complexes rooted in seemingly intractable, pervasive, relationship-ruining patterns. These destructive and life-inhibiting patterns stem from seemingly impenetrable identity complexes, such as never measuring up, feeling like a failure or fraud, identifying themselves as despicable, and, even worse, believing that the universe would be a better place without them. Talk therapy sometimes falls short of transforming core self-identity wounds. No matter the intervention or my sincere intention to help, some clients' wounds and negative core complexes seem immutable to shifting to an integrated knowing that they're not that underlying core identity of not-being-enough or that it *does* matter that they're here in this incarnation on this planet. Psychedelic medicine and postceremony integration with psychotherapy can transform these types of core identity wounds.

Integration is a commonly used nomenclature for postpsychedelic therapeutic sessions in circles of the psychedelic renaissance. The term *integration*—bringing back psychedelic material to ego-consciousness—can sometimes be misleading. Although integration connotes retrieving other elements to fold back into oneself, postpsychedelic therapy in Jungian analysis provides an additional orientation that focuses on expansion of one's ego-complex. For example, from a Jungian perspective a symbol revealed in a psychedelic journey is not merely "integrated" into ego-consciousness after ceremony but is related to as a living entity. In Jung's words, "A symbol always presupposes that the chosen expression is the best possible description or formulation of a relatively unknown fact, which is none the less known to exist or is postulated as existing" (1971, para. 814). A symbol is a living entity that cannot be reduced to explanations but invites a mutual relationship with it. The snake archetype has been an ongoing living symbol for me since initiation into working with ayahuasca-chacruna. The snake appears in its animal form; however, it simultaneously provides me with ongoing beyond-explanation psychic guidance.

> *To share an example, I was sitting in session with a male client who relies on hyperintellectual functioning and is highly defended against feelings. Suddenly, I had a vision of a snake flying in the air, and the snake flew through the window into the room aiming for my head. It was so real that I reflexively ducked my head as it passed. I quickly looked at my client, who was talking about work, wanting to see if he noticed the involuntary ducking of my head. He did not seem to notice; however, he shifted topics at that moment and revealed for the first time in over a year of analysis his deep-seated, primary fear in life. Prior to this moment, my client avoided talking about emotionally vulnerable parts of his psyche. He proceeded to express other emotional material he had never expressed in previous therapy sessions, and subsequent sessions have continued to deepen in a less intellectually defended, more personal, and more emotionally congruent manner.*

The snake in this vision could be mistakenly reduced to simply the animal that slithers on the ground or ascribed to mere imagination; however, its appearance had a deep psychological impact on both the client and myself that was beyond explanation. To quote Jung: "A symbol really lives only when it is the best and highest expression for something divined but not yet known to the observer. It then compels his unconscious participation and has a life-giving and life-enhancing effect" (1971, para. 819).

Some experiences from psychedelic sessions would be better explored not as integration into ego-consciousness as much as being in a dialectical relationship with the archetypal Self. In Edward Edinger's invaluable book *Ego and Archetype,* he described a fundamental process of ego development in relation to Self. Edinger, a Los Angeles Jungian analyst, expounded on Erich Neumann's concepts of the ego-Self axis.

To summarize Edinger's concept, he posited that the ego-Self axis consists of four developmental phases (1992, 6):

1. Uroboric state in which the ego-complex is fully subsumed in the Self
2. Emerging ego in which the ego-complex begins to become aware of itself and form itself while being subsumed within the Self
3. Advanced stage of development in which ego-consciousness differentiates itself from Self and is partially conscious of both ego and Self
4. Total separation of ego and Self yet connected by an ego-Self axis, hence a conscious dialectical relationship between a healthy, independent ego and Self

Edinger emphasized that this is a nonlinear process. "As this cycle repeats itself again and again throughout psychic development it brings about a progressive differentiation of the ego and the Self" (1992, 7). Edinger's concepts describe par excellence the dysregulation and reintegration processes of psychedelic medicine sessions and healing.

In my clinical and personal experiences, I find various types of postpsychedelic therapy for both integration and expansion processes. Postpsychedelic healing processes are cyclical, periodic, not linear, and consist of the following:

1. Debriefing and sharing with others the journeyer's experiences, creating meaning and new narratives
2. Participating in psychotherapy to deepen the psychedelic experiences, creating authentic personal understanding, meaning, and relationship with living symbols
3. Bringing new information into everyday life by amplification, psychological association, and repetition of the material creating new neuronal patterns, for example, through journaling, ritual, art, song, prayer, and the Jungian technique of active imagination

4. Occasionally receiving psychiatric medications due to severely adverse reactions or trauma caused during a psychedelic session
5. Metabolization, in other words, taking no further action because what was once a distressing issue or complex is completely resolved during a psychedelic session, leaving merely a memory of the event without any attached negative affect previously associated to the past event or memory
6. Experiencing transcendental and numinous events, resulting in an expansion of ego-consciousness

In my opinion, psychotherapy with a psychedelic-aware psychotherapist seems to be a requisite for postpsychedelic integration. Psychedelics as an adjunct to psychotherapy can be deeply healing, especially for depression, anxiety, and trauma. That holds equally true for prepsychedelic sessions to prepare for and enhance harm reduction.

Characterizing psychedelics as either good or bad hardly encompasses the complexity of the real therapeutic and medicinal attributes of psychedelics. Although psychedelics have great therapeutic value, it is important to acknowledge occasional adverse reactions to a psychedelic session; this topic warrants further research and attention from our psychotherapeutic communities working with clients who undergo damaging or traumatizing psychedelic experiences. In my experience, clients' traumatic experiences result less from the psychedelic medicine itself and more from an inappropriate set and setting, especially related to insufficient client or facilitator preparation or, worse, malfeasance on the part of a facilitator. On the other hand, psychedelic medicines more often offer extraordinary relief and healing unavailable through other means, including talk therapy in some cases.

A final note, regarding numinous experiences: when clients recount their numinous experiences, their sharing of these transcendental experiences is deeply powerful, beyond ego reality, potentially transformative for both the client and therapist, and warrants *not* being interpreted, in my clinical opinion. The numinous experience is beyond conceptualization. Reverent attention without intellectualization of the clients' precious gift of being visited by what's-beyond-ego allows the continuation of the presence of the beyond, the higher self, or *superior intelligences,* as I call them. It then enters into the sacred healing space of therapy, a temenos. In psychotherapy, this is a protected psychic field that surrounds the therapist and client, allowing the presence of the divine to be revealed to both psychotherapist and client. Intention to create a temenos, be it in psychotherapy or a psychedelic session, allows yet deeper experiences of the presence of superior intelligences to touch our human realms beyond what we can imagine. Interpretation pins down the client's experiences of a sacred visitation, like pinning a blue morpho butterfly onto a classification board. To the contrary, in a manner of reverence, postpsychedelic psychotherapy can support the client's conscious and direct communication with the inner healer, personal mystical guides, and archetypal Self.

For the most part, I have witnessed in my psychoanalytic practice that my clients' psychedelic medicine sessions in the *right* setting and with the *right* facilitator directly address their core wounds, with efficacy, immediacy, and sustained lasting healing results. Moreover, in my experience, the psychedelics of ayahuasca-chacruna in conjunction with my wise Shipibo guides have opened a portal to intelligences beyond my ego-complex. An ego-dominant orientation is shedding away, sometimes with excitement and curiosity, at other times with startling unfamiliar experiences, but all with confidence in the superior intelligences who are guiding me in psychotherapy sessions with clients, as well as in my day and nighttime realms beyond imagination.

4

Psychedelics in Private Practice

The Highs and Lows of Integration

Maria Papaspyrou

Psychology is ultimately mythology, the study of the stories of the soul.

JAMES HILLMAN

The shifting discourse around psychedelic substances from drugs to medicines and from getting high to getting healed has revived psychotherapy's interest in the healing potency of transpersonal experiences, made integration central to psychedelic practices, and encouraged people to seek support for their experiences in expanded states. Some arrive in therapy pushed by circumstance, after a traumatic or retraumatizing experience that requires processing. Others enter by choice, curious to explore and integrate their expanded experiences, in support of their healing and growth. As therapists, we offer a safe container that can hold the unfolding of a deep psychic reorganization.

In psychedelic states people often report dazzling and intricate visuals, but beyond the psychedelic aesthetics, people experience an opening to an incredibly powerful and wise healing field. The ceremonial context is a serious introspective space, at times easy to navigate and nourishing and at times treacherous and devouring. Some of the material that surfaces through such experiences can be encounters with an archetypal world, telepathic experiences, or bizarre dreamlike sequences that are difficult to decipher and can overwhelm consciousness. People report finding themselves in inner landscapes that might be flooded with memories from early life, or from what may seem like past lives, or even from lives that other people have lived. Some of their experiences might fill them with mystical awe, while others might bring them to the very edges of darkness and madness. Some people experience leaving their human consciousness and embodying an animal or plant consciousness, dissolving boundaries of all kinds and expanding in multiple directions. The profound emotional, physical, and energetic release during such a journey can range from ecstatic joy to primal terror, and yet most, upon their return, seem to retain a deep trust, if not reverence, for the wisdom of this space. There are those, however, who return terrified, fragmented, and broken. For many, this is indeed a heroic journey within and beyond. Most people will encounter these experiences without any working knowledge of the psyche, and this is where the spaces we offer as therapists can be of relevance and use.

Psychotherapy's foundational and core premise has been the strengthening of the conscious mind through the assimilation of the unconscious. It is a healing system that is fluid in translating the symbolic and archaic language of the unconscious into meaningful narratives. The clinical models of dream interpretation, free association, active imagination, and creative explorations are very relevant in the work of psychedelic integration, as is knowledge and understanding of transpersonal experiences, shadow work, trauma work, and attachment. Psychedelic integration therapists also need to understand the importance of set and setting as well as the effect of different substances on a physiological, psychological, and spiritual level.

Psychedelic experiences mediate between our conscious and unconscious worlds. By bringing unconscious material from the deep abode of one's Self into the surface of consciousness, they open up channels of communication between the two that can support our psychological journey toward greater integration and wholeness.

THE PSYCHEDELIC DREAM FUNCTION

A psychedelic experience carries messages rich in symbolic language and quality. In psychedelic integration, we have to work with the language of the psyche—the symbolic, mythopoetic, and archetypal layers of our being. As with dreams, the visions, myths, and symbols that spontaneously emerge in expanded states from one's depths are imbued with meaning and express vital psychological information. They carry into consciousness thoughts, intuitions, and feelings that were deeply buried within. "The underlying, primary psychic reality is so inconceivably complex that it can be grasped only at the farthest reach of intuition, and then but very dimly. That is why it needs symbols" (Jung 1966a, para. 345).

Symbols hold meaning that is indefinite and can only be understood by approximation. In integration work, we circle around these messengers creatively in order to awaken their inherent potential. We invite the person's own responses and associations to the material at hand and resourcefully work alongside the client to develop the images, symbols, and archetypes to their full effect. There is not one valid interpretation; numerous potentialities exist to help us get closer to aspects of the Self that have been shrouded from awareness. The image making and symbolic and linking functions are about bringing forms and metaphors to life and helping us cultivate deeper connections to our inner worlds.

The process of meaning extraction that lies at the heart of psychedelic integration is aligned with the principles of dreamwork. While the psychedelic experience is often more embodied, the terrain of both is our deep unconscious. Interestingly, however, psychedelic experiences don't usually take the form of many common dreams, such as falling, taking an exam, or being naked in a public space;

the emotional tone of such common dreams arise through different sequences in expanded states, for example through the death-rebirth cycles or through encounters with shadow that might give rise to feelings of shame or inadequacy. Clarissa Pinkola Estés (2003) discusses eight kinds of unusual dreams (described below), which in psychedelic states are quite common motifs.

- **Precognitive dreams** are dreams that seem to have arrived from a future point in time that might inform the dreamer about something that is yet ahead of him.
- **Apparition dreams** are palpable visitation dreams where the dreamer might meet, engage with, or receive a message from people who have died who she may or may not know. They come as psychic allies to offer the dreamer information, guidance, or reassurance.
- **Lucid dreams** are dreams where the dreamer feels awake within a dream, able to consciously engage with the dream images and spaces he is immersed in and ask for guidance.
- **Disembodied voice dreams** are where the dreamer is advised by a voice that exists separately from a body, or a voice that might carry no sound at all but the dreamer feels enfolded in its message.
- **Sexual dreams** are fully embodied sensual experiences that might culminate in orgasm.
- **Dreams of deep silence** are dreams that land the dreamer in a space of a deep silent void. The silence might be meditative, healing, and restorative, or deadening and frightening, as a voiceless cry for help.
- **Speaking in tongues** are dreams where the dreamer speaks words in a language she has never heard before (a phenomenon that in waking life is known as glossolalia); in certain cases, these words may turn out to exist.
- **Waking dreams** are visions in a hypnagogic or somnambulant state during which the dreamer watches moving images, like in a cinema.

I would add to this list *psychedelic dreams* of being held and cradled by an archetypal and transpersonal entity, giving psychedelic dreamers a tangible, visceral, and embodied experience of being safely contained.

While I have come across all of these types of *dreaming* in psychedelic integration, I have encountered few of them while working with common dreams. Perhaps we could assume that these dreams are nearer to transpersonal experiences, emanating from the collective unconscious as opposed to commonly occurring dream themes that might be arising from the personal unconscious. This would follow the distinction of *big dreams* versus *little dreams;* concepts that Jung borrowed from the Elgoni tribe in Kenya. Psychedelic dreams are, perhaps, nearer to big dreams in that they often arise from the collective unconscious, feel significant, purposive, visionary, archetypal, and mystical, and act as a portal or a wake-up call for the dreamer. While at times these motifs when encountered in expanded states will be clear in their scope and purpose—such as a message delivered by an apparition—at other times they will be open and available for amplification, exploration, and interpretation. The messages they carry from the deep unconscious, or from what might feel like a much greater source, can revive aspects of our lives that require attention, sometimes by bringing resolutions or clarifications of the past and sometimes by bringing resources for, or even from, the emergent future. They are communicating an unconscious reality, and if they seem irrational, it is only because we lack the means to understand them. Psychedelic experiences, like dreams, take form through our lives and need to be understood within the ancestral, biographical, and present-day context of a person's life. When such material is worked through within a therapeutic framework, it can help us develop further stability, resilience, and ego-strength through assimilating a little more of our unconscious into consciousness.

PSYCHEDELIC PRACTICE
AND PSYCHOTHERAPY

I call psychedelic practice a conscious and intentional engagement with psychedelic states at irregular intervals, leaving enough spaces for integrating the material that emerges, with a focus on supporting one's process of healing and growth, while retaining a critical inquiry over one's use of psychedelic agents and states. Psychotherapy and psychedelic states hold many principles and elements in common and complement each other, in some cases better than others. Their synergy works best when people are willing to truly engage with their expanded states in order to do the deeper inner work required and bring the material that emerges from their experiences into the therapeutic space for exploration, interpretation, and embedding. When this happens, the work is truly inspiring and moving and attains a greater depth.

Elli was in therapy for almost a year along with working with plant medicines. She held a close connection between our work and her own psychospiritual psychedelic practice, keeping the two as an integrated whole.

Elli was attending to broken attachment bonds in her family line, determined to change the intergenerational script that had infiltrated her own current family. At one point during our work, her mother developed a life-threatening condition, bringing Elli up against unresolved feelings that she had learned to suppress and avoid.

At the age of five, Elli was separated from her mother, who had become unable to look after her. Elli felt a rising anger and great difficulty in being with her mother; the potential ending of her relationship with her mother resurrected the earlier separation her younger self had experienced. As a way of attending to the early separation, I had suggested to Elli that she write a good-bye letter to her mother as her five-year-old self. But however much she tried, she was unable to move through her defenses and make contact with her early pain, confusion, rage, and fear.

A month later, Elli participated in an ayahuasca ceremony, taking that incomplete good-bye as her intention. In her medicine journey, Elli made some space on her mattress for an apparition of me to sit by her, as she bravely faced that day at the airport as her five-year–old self, where she was standing on the precipice of an enormous loss. She clearly saw her mother as unable and unavailable to emotionally attend to her and to their separation. She ran the scene through her mind's eye again and again, with her courageous young self intent on honoring that ending. Elli came to a deep realization that her creative way of coping with the separation as a child was to symbolically and emotionally fit her mother inside herself and carry her along wherever she went. The medicine was telling her that though this helped soften her feelings of fear, aloneness, and abandonment, it also created an entanglement between her and her mother that misdirected her from her own unique path in life. A vision appeared of a beautiful white alabaster statue, which she instinctively knew was not her. She started chipping and breaking it bit by bit until it revealed its contents inside: a bright golden girl, rescued and recovered from the false self that had developed around her. She "heard" the message: "Everything loves her."

Elli's experience was emotional, visceral, embodied, visual, symbolic, creative, concrete, and spiritual; it supported her sense of inner connectedness and moved her toward rediscovering a more authentic and undefended sense of Self. By instinctively summoning my presence for support during her journey, she brought continuity between her work in psychotherapy and her work in expanded states. That night, Elli mourned her early maternal loss and the consequent loss of parts of herself. This opened a softening compassion toward her mother alongside a deeper acceptance of her mother's illness and physical decline and a deep sadness for the loss ahead. Elli was starting to claim love in her life in new ways from the people that mattered to her. This was a very significant juncture in her work and one that was beyond reach in ordinary consciousness. In altered states she was able to lay aside the layers of deeply ingrained patterns and defenses, becoming available to meet herself more fully.

PSYCHEDELIC TELEOLOGY

When working with a confusing and disorienting experience, we need to grapple with its underlying purpose. As Jung (1966a) theorized, the conscious and the unconscious have a compensatory relationship; what is excluded from consciousness is delegated to our unconscious, forming a counterweight and a tension between the two, which every now and then requires a bit more of our unconscious to be received and assimilated by consciousness for balance to be restored. The more excluded and repressed the unconscious, the more dangerous and unpredictable it becomes; this danger diminishes with integration. And while therapy is not always necessary for integration, it becomes necessary when the immensity of these experiences is so difficult to deal with that the ego becomes overwhelmed and loses its sense of ground and direction. In clinical practice, we often find that what has made a psychedelic experience particularly challenging is an inadequately held space and/or earlier unresolved trauma that has resurfaced into consciousness in ways that are indigestible. It is a return to a time when the psyche experienced a fragmentation, and the resurfaced material attempts a resolution that was aborted a long time ago.

Sarah, a woman in her forties, arrived to therapy after a distressing ayahuasca ceremony. During the ceremony her internal experience was initially blissful. She experienced opening up to a sacred healing space that made her feel powerful and omnipotent. However, at some point she started noticing outside reflections that didn't match her internal experience. She saw people from the ceremonial circle looking at her with judgment and fear, and gradually the space on the outside started to feel menacing. Sarah panicked and began to separate herself from the group. She became aggressive toward the others, projecting her terror onto them. They responded by trying to calm and restrain her into safety. The tension between Sarah and the group took frightening proportions, until eventually Sarah ran out of energy, just before the ceremony ended.

When Sarah arrived in my office for therapy, she reported feeling deeply shaken, mostly by her experience with the group. She felt strongly that her own inner journey was beautiful but perhaps too powerful for those around her. For Sarah, the good was held on the inside, while the group was left holding the difficult, the unsafe, and the disturbed.

Sarah's key association with the emotional tone and character of the experience was from childhood. When Sarah was eight years old, she was playing with her younger sister outside their house when her sister had a fatal accident. While they were having fun in their inner world, tragedy struck from the outer world. The inside, her young psyche, was too tender to negotiate what had happened, and it managed this experience by splitting: a psychological defense that protects the individual from unbearable feelings by dividing the world in absolute terms (good versus bad), thus losing the capacity to hold ambiguity, complexity, and nuance. This defense had followed Sarah throughout life and into that ceremony itself, where it played out with her projecting her split-off difficult and unresolved feelings onto the group.

Sarah was shaken and in deep grief, embarking on her journey of trying to piece herself together, trying to bring what she saw on the outside and what she felt on the inside into greater cohesion. Processing what had emerged in the ceremony had moved her toward mourning all that was lost within a split second and all that followed: the loss of her sister and the upending of the family order; her grieving unavailable parents and her unconscious attempts to fill the void her sister left both within the family and within herself through addictions and an eating disorder; and the trail of dramatic relationships that had followed her since. While none of this became clear for Sarah during the ceremony itself, what she experienced became a catalyst for opening the emotional dam of suppressed feelings and misdirected emotional energy. Had Sarah not accessed support after the ceremony, this experience would have just been another episode in a series of wounded encounters, without resolution or breakthrough. To bring all these parts into consciousness is a truly courageous act; it required Sarah to reassess her life on a fundamental level. As we often see in deep work, once we realize we no longer need to defend ourselves, the emotional and psychic energy we used to maintain our defenses becomes available to us and we can use it in new ways.

The process of integration needs to be supported by a resilient ego that can do the assimilating. If the ego is overwhelmed, then our first task is to revive its capacity to integrate. Sometimes people return from these journeys experiencing intense states of boundary dissolution, physical energy releases, auditory and visual hallucinations, and derealization and dissociation, often accompanied by terrifying existential, archetypal openings that threaten to tear them apart. In the clinical space, this is not the time for emotional digging. This is the time for slowing down, holding, containing, grounding. Our primary task in such instances is to support the person to return to a sense of self that can sustain him in everyday life. Maintaining a predictable and repetitive schedule with regular meals and adequate sleep in a supportive environment provides an essential container for supporting this process. Avoiding substances and spiritual practices for a time as well as engaging in bodywork may further help the client ground.

Our conscious attitude toward the unconscious will be a significant factor in this process. If we view the unconscious as a devouring darkness that is meaningless and purposeless, then we amplify its potential to be so. If we recognize and relate to the unconscious for its potential to release darkness in service of growth, then we can center and realign it to its true force and potential. A difficult psychedelic experience carries dormant wisdom in its process. If we fail to receive its message and support its process, we are likely to re-encounter the process again, until a deeper balance is restored.

SHADOW WORK

Through psychedelic use, sometimes the fragments of Self that emerge to be processed and integrated constitute what Jungians call the personal shadow, a space in our unconscious psyche that holds all the unacknowledged, denied, neglected, and rejected parts of who we are. Here we relegate the parts of us that threaten to unstitch our domesticated ego structures. Our sense of Self remains limited, while we identify with qualities we wish to embody, at the expense of others we learn to repress. For some the shadow will be the darkness that completes their light, while for others it might be the light that completes their darkness. Never fully aware of all that we are, a lot of us exists unclaimed in the depths of Self.

An encounter with our shadow is a painful gift from our depths that can facilitate the release of suppressed emotion. In shadow work, the persona falls away, and we make contact with a truer but perhaps messier sense of Self. To integrate one's shadow is to embrace one's fuller Self, and here the task is not to process and eliminate the shadow—for the spirit, like the body, will always cast a shadow—but to become aware of it and consciously relate to it. When we are freed to embrace and operate from a deeper and broader sense of Self, more of our energies and resources become available, bringing us to greater presence and therefore intimacy with ourselves and the world around us.

Helen, a woman in her late thirties, had an experience with ayahuasca where she revisited her abortion from a decade earlier, a loss that in real life she had never mourned or processed. In her journey she had a vision where she was met by the soul of her unborn child, held in an amniotic sac made of pure universe. In that instant she felt the enormity of her choice and made contact for the first time with her profound grief that belonged to that long-ago event. Helen spent the rest of that journey loving her unborn child and trying to forgive herself for not being the person she thought she was, an evening during which she slowly and painfully accommodated a fuller sense of Self.

Helen, in her integration work, was processing her encounter with her personal shadow and unmourned loss. While grieving, she also felt a sense of completion, as if reunited with a part of herself that had also been aborted. It took time for the new parts of Self she had discovered to fit comfortably, and her process moved in waves, alongside her grief.

As she mourned her unborn baby and her old sense of self, a renewed passion and direction was being born, bringing her fertile energies in service of her creative visions.

It is usually the disturbing and dark that is repressed. Sometimes the darkness that returns belongs to others and has been inflicted on us. People sometimes seek psychotherapy after having encountered visions that contain scenes of early childhood abuse. They return from these experiences disoriented and confused about whether or not these visions are real memory traces, and their process can remain stuck on this question for a long time. As therapists, we cannot determine whether they have encountered an objective truth and do not need to: we are there to work with the significance of such images emerging and being held in the psyche, which indicate an important truth of some kind, whether objective or subjective. We often find that people feel relief when we acknowledge and validate their visions on their own merit, giving them permission to honor their experiences and to begin engaging with the material in meaningful ways.

THE SPACE IN BETWEEN SPACES

A psychedelic journey can offer valuable and significant insights that support the unlocking of deeply ingrained patterns. But often insight by itself is not a sufficient force of change, and psychedelic experiences can't replace the necessity for our inner work. If we outsource our healing and growth to psychedelics without making the effort to support and integrate these experiences, abdicate responsibility, and adopt a passive stance toward our unconscious, we are taking an enormous risk in allowing unprocessed experiences to dictate our choices and our life trajectory. To genuinely transcend our wounds, defenses, and early conditioning, it is essential to maintain our responsibility of bringing back the gifts of the imaginal world into a relationship with everyday life.

In our clinical practice, we need to be aware of how these states have the potential both to facilitate psychospiritual growth and to undermine that very process through psychedelic bypassing. A psychedelic experience can leave people in a state of ego inflation with a defensive attachment to these states. It can leave people possessed by archetypal energies in a way that separates them from their true nature and can create a dependence on expanded states for filling the void of an unsatisfactory life, which then stalls any movement of change in the real world. While psychedelic experiences are certainly not short of creative and healing potential, in the therapeutic space we need the maturity and clarity of occupying a space that bridges the split between the proponents and the opponents of these substances if we are to truly serve those that require our support.

As clinicians we have to thoroughly explore and question our own leanings and prejudices regarding various substances and expanded states of consciousness. If we have had personal experiences with expanded states, we should explore how we have made sense of them and whether there are any unresolved past experiences that require better understanding and tending to so that we can contain client material that might meet our own difficulties and wounds. It requires us as practitioners to have met our own appropriate edge with grief, loss of boundaries, and sometimes even madness and to have had the experience of reestablishing a solid sense of self so that we are able to facilitate safe and informed spaces for people to walk their path. Being aware of our own resistances to any aspect of this work will help us in how we meet our clients. When clients arrive at a raw and vulnerable place, they too come with enormous resistance to their own experience, and we have to make sure we don't match it. Time and time again, we will find ourselves trying to facilitate a safe space where our clients can sit with whatever is emerging, however painful and threatening. The deeper work with the experience starts when resistance is replaced by acceptance and a rising curiosity for what they might discover. But we won't always succeed in creating a safe enough container when people feel attacked on such a profound level.

Eva, a woman in her late twenties, came to therapy in a severely anxious state after two consecutive ayahuasca journeys in an inadequately held space. The first one was traumatic, but she was encouraged to work through the process in a ceremony the following evening. People arrive in these spaces sometimes with little knowledge of these substances and what to expect, as in Eva's case, and trust that the people holding such spaces are experts whom they can trust to keep them safe—which is not always the case. Eva was a survivor of childhood sexual abuse, and her ayahuasca journey took her to the epicenter of her wounding. The ayahuasca experience is very embodied for most people. At the point of onset, Eva felt the transition to an altered state, as if the medicine was "spreading through her body." The other embodied aspect of ayahuasca is the purging, which may be vomiting, diarrhea, tears, or sweat. In the indigenous traditions, this purging is an important aspect of the healing and cleansing process; however, for Eva, these overpowering embodied sensations brought up feelings of loss of control and of being trapped. Her innate knowing that she was not in a safe space brought to the surface her early unprocessed trauma of her abuse.

Eva arrived at the therapy space feeling intolerably anxious and rageful. She wanted me to relieve her from everything she felt, and it was not possible to contain the enormity of her experience. Two months later, despite continuous attempts to help her sit with her experiences and deter her from making rushed life decisions, Eva aborted therapy, left her job, moved back to her country of origin, and returned to a relationship she had had when she was fifteen years old.

Eva's unprepared mindset, which was met by an unempathic and unsupportive ceremonial setting, meant that the basic framework for her experience was severely compromised and inadequate. In addition, Eva's inability to sit and meaningfully engage with her inner experience meant that her projections could not be retrieved from the outside world and worked with in therapy. Eva acted out in every conceivable way in her attempts to fend off her inner world and the pain it carried. But invariably, if the process—and in her case, her whole current life structures—is aborted in such an incomplete way, what we try to defend against will affect us in ways that will continue to define our lives. Until we find ourselves further down the line in a place where we can resume what we hoped we had left behind.

When operating from a space in between spaces, we approach the work without any clear presuppositions about whether using these substances is useful or harmful. We have to occupy a middle ground from where we can explore each individual case as it presents itself. These journeys take people to the deeper layers of the psyche. For some, it might be the most useful experience they have ever had, and for others, it can create fractures they are not ready or sufficiently prepared and resourced to withstand and process.

MOVING TOWARD WHOLENESS

Beyond the aesthetics of the psychedelic state lies a world of meaning that is experienced and absorbed through the mind, the body, the psyche, and the soul. In working through a psychedelic experience, we have to weave our way through the mind-body-heart-psyche-soul-personal-collective continuum. A therapeutic space can offer a useful container for negotiating what belongs to the present and what belongs to the past, what belongs to the mythic and the mystical dimensions and what belongs to the earthy dimensions of everyday living, what belongs to the personal and what to the collective—and accommodate each where they belong. It can support newly acquired awareness to embed into everyday life and inform positive changes, for the individual and for the collective systems they are part of. Unless the insights from a psychedelic experience are sufficiently integrated, they can easily sink back into the unconscious, and in the case of material that has reactivated our deepest wounds, such unintegrated experiences can be deeply disruptive. It is in our wholeness that we meet with these experiences, it is in their wholeness that they need to be considered for integration, and it is our sense of wholeness that they carry forward and support. Wholeness emerges out of the complementary union of our conscious and unconscious Self. The new attitude toward one's Self, or the new attitude toward life that arises out of the tension between conscious and unconscious and supports their union, is what Jung called the transcendent function, and that is the ultimate postintegrated position.

5

Daimonic Experience and the Psyche's Archetypal Self-Care System

Scott Hill

I came to more fully appreciate the way past trauma emerges in psyche-delic experiences through Jungian analyst Donald Kalsched's book *The Inner World of Trauma: Archetypal Defenses of the Personal Spirit* in which Kalsched discusses the unconscious images revealed by adults who have suffered early childhood trauma. The dreams of Kalsched's patients consistently reveal disturbing images, such as powerful demonic figures, remarkably similar to images encountered by some people during psychedelic experiences. Kalsched's findings therefore support the suggestion that psychedelic experiences can release unconscious imagery and emotions associated with past trauma.

Kalsched defines trauma as any experience that causes "unbearable psychic pain or anxiety" (1996, 1). Even though trauma can occur under a wide variety of experiences, from physical injury and sexual abuse to the destructive psychological effects of unmet childhood needs, the distinguishing feature of trauma for Kalsched is what Heinz Kohut calls "disintegration anxiety," which stems from an event that threatens to dissolve the personality's coherence and is "the deepest anxiety [one] can experience" (Kohut, quoted in Kalsched 1996, 34). When such trauma occurs in early childhood, before strong ego defenses have developed, the psyche relies on more primitive and dissociative unconscious defenses to protect itself.

Although it is widely understood how destructive these archaic, or primitive, defenses can become in later life, Kalsched argues that we need to recognize their initial life-saving potential for the child. Kalsched suggests that the child's dissociative defenses protect him or her by ensuring that he or she will always remain on guard. We have to realize, Kalsched explains, that the defenses preventing the early trauma patient from trusting others and forming meaningful relationships as an adult "have literally saved the patient's life as a psychological being" (Kalsched 2003, 203). When trying to understand this paradoxical and initially bewildering dynamic, it helps to imagine parents who protect their children from life's dangers by keeping them locked up in the cellar: they protect destructively.

Kalsched's thinking about trauma-induced disorders developed out of Freud and Jung's early dialogue about the mythopoetic, daimonic, and uncanny imagery revealed by traumatized patients. And Kalsched's approach to trauma-induced disorders has clear parallels to Jung's approach to dissociation, which Jung described as a weakening of consciousness resulting from a splitting of psychological content that becomes increasingly independent from consciousness.

Kalsched's work highlights the way dramatic and bizarre dream images symbolize the psyche's fragmentation and defenses. When consciously faced in therapy, these dream images can promote healing. This insight brings to mind the work of Jungian analyst John Weir Perry, who in the 1970s advocated the transformative potential of acute psychotic episodes. Perry (1999) asserted that, with proper attention, even the apparently chaotic images expressed by a person suffering acute psychic upheaval may take on coherent form and reveal meaning. The therapeutic principles underlying Kalsched's and Perry's work support the value of carefully analyzing the bizarre and terrifying imagery associated with traumatic psychedelic experiences and psychedelic-induced psychotic states. Such analysis can reveal meaningful patterns that reflect the psyche's attempt to protect and heal itself.

KALSCHED'S MODEL OF
THE PSYCHE'S ARCHETYPAL SELF-CARE SYSTEM

Kalsched is concerned with what happens within the psyche of those who experience unbearable events in their lives, whether those traumatic events be physical or psychological. He has found that, in response to overwhelming pain, the vulnerable psyche creates persecutory figures that emerge in dreams and fantasies as archetypal daimonic images, such as a witch, a mad doctor, or the Devil. These daimonic images paradoxically attempt to protect the integrity of the personality by carrying out inhibiting attacks that split the psyche. Such inhibitory attacks thereby reduce the traumatized person's ability to form relationships in the external world, relationships that potentially expose the person to retraumatization. The damage caused by such "protection" can be severe and can understandably require painstaking therapeutic intervention.

In Kalsched's judgment, these daimonic persecutory images reflect the dynamics of the traumatized psyche's dissociative defenses, which divide the psyche in an attempt to protect the personality from further trauma in the external world. (The Greek word *daimonic,* a variant of *demonic,* comes from *daiomai,* which means "to divide.") More specifically, unconscious imagery that Kalsched's therapy patients have reported, in combination with clinical research, reveals that trauma often results in psychic fragmentation that manifests as personified dyads. This dyadic structure typically takes the form of a "progressed" part of the personality that adopts a "caretaking" relationship to a "regressed" part. The progressed caretaker part is often represented by a threatening figure, such as a murderer or a demon. The regressed part of the personality is usually expressed through images of vulnerability and innocence, such as a child or a fragile animal. These images of vulnerability and innocence represent, Kalsched suggests, the essence or core of the individual's personality, which he calls the "personal spirit" (Kalsched 1996, 1–3).

The progressed, or caretaking, part of the personality can be represented by "a powerful *benevolent or malevolent great being* who protects or persecutes its vulnerable partner," explains Kalsched (1996, 3). Sometimes the protector figure presents both benevolent and malevolent aspects, thereby representing a protector and persecutor in one. An excellent example of this complex protector-persecutor figure is the image of a threatening God.

Usually, however, the caretaking part is represented unambiguously, though ironically, as a terrifying figure. As such, it exhibits compelling parallels to Jung's concept of the Self's dark side, the archetype of evil. One of Jung's psychological characterizations of the Devil archetype is "the diabolical aspect of every psychic function that has broken loose from the hierarchy of the total psyche and now enjoys independence and absolute power" (Jung 1968, para. 88). Kalsched points out that the root meaning of the word *diabolical* is to throw (*ballein*) across or apart (*dia*), which is also the origin of the common meaning of "diabolos" as the Devil, "he who crosses, thwarts, or dis-integrates (dissociation)" (Kalsched 1996, 16–17).

The key principle underlying Kalsched's trauma theory is expressed in his hypothesis that violating the personality's inner core is untenable. If, therefore, other defense mechanisms fail, archetypal defenses will go to any length to protect the child's "personal spirit." As Kalsched conceives it, the dynamic of progressed versus regressed parts of the personality makes up what he calls *the psyche's archetypal self-care system.* As its name implies, this psychological system appears to emerge from the deepest layers of the unconscious because the imagery and emotions associated with it have the numinous qualities of the collective unconscious. "When the ego falls through the abyss of trauma into the darkness of the unconscious psyche," Kalsched points out, "it falls into an archetypal world which is experienced by the ego as numinous—dark or light. Unfortunately for the trauma victim, the numinous usually constellates negatively" (1996, 216).

The ultimate effect of the psyche's protector-prosecutor figures is to defend the trauma victim by becoming an anti-life force in which new situations and opportunities are experienced as threatening. The trauma victim thereby becomes isolated from reality through dissociation, addiction, depression, or schizoid withdrawal. As much as one wants to change, "something more powerful than the ego continually undermines progress and destroys hope," Kalsched says, "as if the individual were *possessed* by some diabolical power" (1996, 5).

I illustrate the relevance of these complex dynamics to psychedelic experiences with accounts from LSD-assisted psychotherapy. But first, what follows is an example from personal experience.

In 1967, at the age of nineteen—after several mild psychedelic trips on which I experienced, really for the first time in my life, the natural world's inherent beauty—my reckless use of LSD led me into the darkness of the unconscious.

I was initiated into those dark realms after taking what turned out to be a large dose of LSD one day on the Big Sur coast of California. In the woods at the base of a canyon there, I came upon a hallucinated image the size and shape of a full-length oval mirror on the trunk of a large tree. The area within its border was packed with the tear-shaped faces of old bearded men, each weeping with the same lamenting expression. Later, when I climbed out of the canyon, I became convinced that I had come up into another world. Although the vision of being in the wrong world came to an end as the effects of the LSD faded, it resumed and intensified during subsequent LSD trips until I was certain that this material world was only an illusion created to test me. At one point—despite the lack of any previous religious inclination—I became convinced that God was demanding that I prove my spiritual integrity by ending my life in this absurd and evil world to be with him in Heaven. Fearing divine punishment if I failed this test, I attempted to honor that command.

Looking back many years later on my mirrorlike hallucination, it occurred to me that when I entered the canyon that day on LSD, I had entered the unconscious sphere of my own sorrow, represented in symbolic form. Reflecting on Kalsched's insights, I have found it useful to consider the extent to which some of my LSD images and visions in 1967 were a psychedelic version—a kind of flashback experience—of the trauma I endured in connection with third-degree burns I suffered as a two-year-old boy. I have found it worth considering, for instance, the possibility that my being hit in the face by a cascade of scalding water and rolled on a gurney into a hospital's emergency room was so overwhelming and incomprehensible that I had the experience of coming into another world. It's also possible that the psychedelic-induced image of God demanding that I kill myself was a manifestation of the kind of persecutory-protective figures Kalsched has witnessed in the dreams of his trauma patients.

TRAUMA AND DISSOCIATION IN JUNG'S PSYCHOLOGY

The symbolic daimon figures Kalsched has seen so often in the dream images of his traumatized patients seem to personify the psyche's dissociative defenses against overwhelming events that his patients are unable to integrate. Yet, Kalsched asks, "How did the internal guardian figures of this [archetypal self-care] 'system' and their vulnerable child 'clients' get organized in the unconscious, and from whence did they derive their awesome power over the patient's well-intentioned ego?" (1996, 12). To start to answer these fundamental questions, Kalsched turns to Jung's approach to psychological dissociation.

Jung demonstrated that dissociation is the psyche's defense against the damaging impact of trauma. When withdrawal from injury is impossible, the psyche withdraws part of the personality by splitting itself into fragments. Memories and emotions associated with the unbearable experience are distributed to different parts of the person's body and mind, especially to the unconscious. This accounts for flashbacks of sensation, notes Kalsched, which are often disconnected from the context in which they occur. This resonates, of course, with the phenomenon of a psychedelic flashback, which often seems to come out of the blue.

Although the distribution of traumatic memories and emotions to the unconscious can initially help trauma victims go about their lives in the world, the psychological consequences can be severe. The effects of trauma can continue to haunt one in the form of what Jung called unconscious *feeling-toned complexes*, which manifest as images of frightening figures (Jung 1969b; Jung 1969e, para. 253; Kalsched 1996, 12–13). Jung observed that a trauma-induced complex can take on an independent quality that acts in tyrannical opposition to the conscious mind. "The explosion of affect is a complete invasion of the individual," says Jung. "It pounces upon him like an enemy or a wild animal" (Jung 1966, para. 267). Jung also notes that "the complex has an abnormal autonomy . . . and a tendency to an active separate existence, which reduces and replaces the constellating power of the ego-complex. In this way a new morbid personality is gradually created, the inclinations, judgments, and resolutions of which move only in the direction of the will to be ill. This second personality devours what is left of the normal ego and forces it into the role of [an oppressed] complex" (Jung 1973a, para. 861).

Kalsched presents extensive evidence of these attacking dissociative defenses from his therapy practice. He has observed repeatedly that, as his patients begin to consciously approach repressed trauma, "an intra-psychic [dream] figure or 'force'. . . violently intervenes and dissociates the psyche. This figure's diabolical 'purpose' seems to be to prevent the dream-ego from experiencing the 'unthinkable' affect associated with the trauma" by terrifying one into a new state of despair (Kalsched 1996, 14, 16). These attacking figures traumatize the patient's inner world to protect him or her from becoming traumatized again in the outer world (that is, with the therapist).

The intrapsychic figures from many of Kalsched's case-study descriptions resonate strongly with the persecutory images that can permeate difficult psychedelic experiences. It isn't unusual, explains Stanislav Grof, for threatening or demonic images to arise, or for the therapist to assume demonic form, when a person undergoes psychedelic psychotherapy for severe trauma (2001). The Jungian-oriented British psychiatrist Ronald Sandison, who pioneered LSD psychotherapy in the early 1950s, reports the case of a twenty-six-year-old woman suffering suicidal depression related to her psychopathic father and the death of her mother when the woman was twelve years old. During her first LSD therapy session, she "met the spider, a huge, ugly, terrifying and menacing animal, quite out of her control" (Sandison 1954, 512). In subsequent sessions, the woman had many encounters with the spider, as she reports: "Flashes of a woman's face, I think my mother's. Continuous pictures of the four eyes of the spider and complete spiders advancing upon me (colored green and black). . . . The spider never touches me but seems to want to enfold me and take me bodily" (1954, 512).

Margot Cutner, Sandison's Jungian associate, discusses the case of a woman in her early thirties suffering from severe depression and paranoid tendencies. As a child, this woman was severely neglected by her mother. Reporting on one of her LSD sessions, the woman says, "I saw my mother driving the sheep down the lane, and I saw a full-sized bear walking among the trees and peeping at me" (Cutner 1959, 740). Cutner notes that threatening archetypal figures such as a bear or a witch would appear to the woman when memories of her mother surfaced during her LSD sessions. Cutner reports, for instance, that "the witch was actually seen [by the patient] sitting on the chair in the clinic room. On another occasion, the image of the bear was projected directly onto the analyst after the patient had experienced 'deep longing' for her mother" (1959, 741).

The German psychiatrist Hanscarl Leuner, who also pioneered LSD psychotherapy in the 1950s, relays an LSD-induced vision by a twenty-three-year-old university assistant during psychedelic-enhanced therapy. The young woman had a history of traumatizing experiences during early childhood, and she suffered from recurrent depression, aggressive outbursts against her parents, and suicidal tendencies. "I saw Hitler several times. Then something very strange happened: Hitler became my father, drove our car and came into our house" (Leuner 1983, 180).

The key to understanding Kalsched's concept of daimonic persecutory-protective figures is to see that the daimonic figures that emerge in the psyche as a result of the original trauma protect the person from reexperiencing the pain of the original trauma by continually terrifying him anew. If therapy brings the person too close to reexperiencing the original pain, daimonic dream figures can disrupt therapy by terrifying him or her. I don't mean to suggest that every terrifying image arising in a psychedelic session should be interpreted in terms of Kalsched's archetypal self-care system. But when such terrifying imagery arises, this model provides a fruitful line of inquiry into the possibility of underlying trauma and a useful method of treating trauma that manifests in such imagery.

I think, for instance, that it is likely that this persecutory-protective dynamic played out in an MDMA-enhanced psychotherapy session dealing with my own LSD vision. Following an especially intense flashback experience in 2006 at the Burning Man festival, where I was working as a member of a psychedelic emergency response team, I accepted an invitation to work on my traumatic psychedelic experiences with an experienced guide and his assistant. The MDMA session went well until I started to describe the time in an LSD trip when I had attempted to violently sacrifice my life in this world. At this critical point in the session, as I struggled to recount that terrible moment, I perceived a man observing the session to be Satan, and I felt I had been lured into Satan's den. This shocking experience initiated a challenging process of working through my delusional vision and reestablishing trust for the two people supporting my session, a process that had benefits of its own. But in a way that is consistent with Kalsched's observations, the session was dramatically diverted from coming to terms with past trauma by the emergence of a persecutory-protective figure that seemed to be "protecting" me from reexperiencing the trauma of my suicide attempt and perhaps even the trauma of my third-degree burns. Reflecting later on my experience of Satan and his helpers in the light of Kalsched's insights, I wondered how a two-year-old boy would have experienced the doctors and nurses who were treating his burns.

Given Jung's view that a diabolical split-off psychic function can be perceived by a person only when that function becomes an objective entity such as a dream image, the kind of frightening images represented in these cases are potentially healing when brought to consciousness and worked through therapeutically. This healing potential was realized in each of the psychedelic psychotherapy cases I have cited, including my own MDMA session.

Trauma and Jung's Theory of the Complex

Through his word association studies, Jung came to understand that his subjects' associations were often blocked by emotions, which led to his theory of psychic dissociation and the idea of feeling-toned complexes, each with an archetypal core of images and emotions grounded in the collective unconscious. The numinous domain of the collective unconscious is potentially awe-inspiring and terrifying—and therefore potentially traumatic in its own right. For Jung, this realm of archetypal images and complexes became the source of trauma-induced unconscious anxiety and fantasy. "A situation threatening danger pushes aside the tranquil play of ideas and puts in their place a complex of other ideas with a very strong feeling-tone," explains Jung. "The new complex then crowds everything else into the background" (1972a, para. 84). For Jung, then, complexes originate in the shock of trauma (1969d, para. 204).

Jung's model of dissociative complexes is beautifully illustrated in the case of one of his patients, a nineteen-year-old woman who had become catatonically psychotic after she was sexually abused by her older brother when she was fifteen. She had withdrawn from the world into dissociative fantasies of an alienated life on the moon, which was ruled by an evil vampire who killed women and children. Having patiently coaxed the young woman into revealing the content of her psychosis, Jung recognized meaning in her psychotic fantasies. He realized that the insufferable nature of the young woman's trauma had given rise to a metaphorical form of representation in her psyche that he understood as ultimately redemptive. Jung's commitment to the young woman's struggle allowed her to overcome the daimonic power of her fantasy figure and relate meaningfully to another human being for the first time since her psychosis had broken out, whereupon she slowly came to recognize the necessity and value of living on Earth (Jung 1972b, paras. 571–72). Jung's understanding of the dynamics underlying this young woman's psychotic fantasies and his commitment to her treatment provide a model for how therapists can work with and treat a trauma underlying bizarre and bewildering imagery manifested in some psychedelic states.

In Kalsched's terms, the young woman's trauma had fragmented her psyche and given rise to the archaic, daimonic image of the moon vampire that paradoxically persecuted and protected her by drawing her vulnerable personality into a delusional isolation from the outer world; that is, the psychotic imagery of her primitive self-care system destructively protected her from injury by ensuring that she would never trust anyone again.

Jung's appreciation for the redemptive value of the psyche's symbolic form of representation brings to mind the relationship between trauma and religious imagery. In his book *God Is a Trauma,* Jungian analyst Greg Mogenson writes, "It is not just that God is unknowable and unimaginable; it is that we reach for 'God' most earnestly when imagination fails us. . . . To stand before an event for which we have no metaphors is to stand in the tabernacle of the Lord" (Mogenson, quoted in Kalsched 1996, 77; see also Mogenson 2005; Kalsched 2003). And, Mogenson suggests, the path to healing lies in slowly, painfully working and reworking the symbols that arise from the unconscious in response to trauma. This alludes to the creative work of integrating symbolic imagery from the unconscious into consciousness, which Jung calls *the transcendent function* (Jung 1969a; see also Hill 2019, 137–45).

As part of the psyche's symbol-generating nature, says Kalsched, a feeling-toned complex tends to take form in dreams, fantasies, and other manifestations of the unconscious as a personified image, or being, that interacts with the conscious ego (1996, 89–90). Jung speaks of such a complex-based image as an "image of a personified affect" (1969c, para. 628). Complexes constitute, then, according to this psychological interpretation, the people who populate our dreams, the hallucinatory voices that haunt schizophrenics, and the figures, demons, or spirits of our psychedelic visions.

More or less autonomous complexes exist in everyone, Jung maintains. Yet, he explains, "in those states where the complex temporarily replaces the ego, we see that a strong complex possesses all the characteristics of a separate personality . . . somewhat like a small secondary mind, which deliberately (though unknown to consciousness) drives at certain intentions which are contrary to the conscious intentions of the individual" (1973b, para. 1354; see also para. 1352). The extent to which these complexes disturb the ego depends on their autonomy, which is influenced by their emotional intensity. The superstition that insane people are possessed by demons has a certain validity, notes Jung, because these people are affected by autonomous complexes, which can behave independently of the ego and completely overpower the patient's self-control. Jung even refers to some forms of psychosis as a "complex disease" (1973b, para. 1353; see also para. 1352).

In his essay "The Psychological Foundation of Belief in Spirits," Jung explains that people confronted by a complex embedded in the archetypal psyche experience it as utterly foreign and irrational; and they can understandably perceive its influence as literally coming from outside themselves. Experiencing a complex arising out of the archetypal psyche "is felt as strange, uncanny, and . . . fascinating," says Jung, and "the conscious mind falls under its spell, either feeling it as something pathological, or else being alienated by it from normal life" (1969b, para. 590).

The eruption of such alien content from the unconscious, Jung notes, can be a symptom of mental illness, and in his judgment, this occurs "when something so devastating happens to the individual that his whole previous attitude to life breaks down" (1969b, para. 594). If, on the other hand, this alien content can be translated into the language of consciousness in some form, it can have "a redeeming effect," Jung says, suggesting the healing and even transformative potential of complexes (1969b, paras. 594–96). This also suggests the wisdom of appreciating the value of the alien images and visions that can arise in psychedelic experiences and working carefully to integrate them into consciousness, a process that is potentially healing and even transformative.

6

The Healing Potential of Challenging Psychedelic States

Tim Read

Expanded states of consciousness often hold deeply positive feelings of connection, compassion, and the sheer joy of being alive. Our concerns may be radically changed by new perspectives: our creative instincts are renewed, and we may gain insights into the essential nature of things.

But to get to this point, we may traverse some difficult territory involving the wounds that inevitably lie in the deeper parts of our psyche and the defenses that we have built over them. In an unsupported setting, these wounds may take the form of a challenging psychedelic experience that feels unwelcome. But in a supported setting, the aim is to welcome this unconscious material so that it can be made accessible to processing and thus lose its destructive power. This processing may happen in a number of ways, and it may take successive exposures before the wound is fully experienced and resolved. Some of these wounds may never entirely resolve; it is more a matter of ongoing management so that the dangers lurking in the dark recesses of our psyche become known quantities that have lost their charge. We no longer need to live our lives defined by the defenses we have constructed against them. Our deep wounds may even become our allies.

For this to occur, we need to go repeatedly to the deep well. We need the courage to surrender to those parts of ourselves that we have always defended ourselves against. We need to not only visit these places but immerse ourselves and fully reexperience them. The gift of psychedelics—and this is dose dependent—is that this layer of psyche, where our deepest wounds lie, becomes available. But when it does so, we do not touch it lightly. We feel it deeply; we go to its visceral depths. We need to have faith that the medicine that sometimes tastes so bitter is actually good for us if handled skillfully.

As therapists, guides, and sitters, we need to know this territory so we can support those who follow. The way in which we engage with our clients to prepare the set and setting needs to anticipate working with them in these challenging states where the healing opportunities are most precious. We need strategies to work with people in the deep so that their experiences can be usefully integrated after the psychedelic experience is concluded. In entering this archetypally charged territory with our clients, we may be triggered in ways that reopen our own wounds, and we need to have ways of working with this too.

Modern psychoanalytic models focus on the vicissitudes of the early relationship with the nursing mother and the importance of attachment patterns. Indeed, in any work with people in expanded states we need a quality of facilitator presence that is more like a mother tending her infant. The qualities required are of absolute compassion, attunement, and gentleness while rooted in strength and the ability to manage the safety of the setting. As facilitators, we need to hold those maternal qualities of holding and containment, where we can tolerate and metabolize any primitive material that is expressed, while providing the secure base that so often allows for corrective experiences around unresolved attachment issues.

OUR DEEPEST WOUNDS

In expanded states we may have experiences to which we cannot attach a narrative because they lie beyond conscious memory. These unconscious psychic residues, which often affect us powerfully in adult life, arise at the earliest stages of our development, and it is helpful to have some models of how such mental structures arise and how to work with them.

The idea of primitive traumas arising very early in our lives playing a formative role in adult personality and relationships is in tune with the key ideas from psychoanalysis. The object relations school developed by Melanie Klein (1959) found that the deepest roots of our personality development lay in infantile relationships with the primary object, the nursing mother. Here the traumas are more often psychological rather than physical, but the emotional world of an infant has an extraordinary visceral intensity, indeed an archetypal quality, that shapes the developing ego structures and leaves a powerful residue in the adult psyche.

Stanislav Grof, the pioneer of LSD psychotherapy, found that in therapeutic LSD sessions an even earlier layer of psyche was exposed and this led to the development of his influential perinatal model based on the short-lived but utterly traumatizing experience of our birth (1975). From the perspective of the baby, this process involves both a profound rejection by mother and a life-threatening journey through the birth canal. Not only is paradise lost as the primal unity of life in utero comes to an end, but it feels like a murderous attack as the uterus violently contracts. As the uterine existence dies, there follows the heroic journey toward a rebirth in an unimaginably new world. Grof described four distinct phases of this perinatal process:

The first basic perinatal matrix (BPM I) is the uterine state that lasts until the onset of labor. The baby develops peacefully in the amniotic sac with all her needs met by the encompassing and nourishing mother. Occasionally, this resting state becomes poisonous due to medication, metabolic toxins, or lack of oxygen. From an archetypal perspective, good-womb experiences would equate to oceanic feelings of bliss, connection, and cosmic unity. A toxic womb state will trigger toxic emotions, perhaps feeling drugged, poisoned, or paranoid.

The second perinatal matrix (BPM II) is the physical onset of labor where the uterus contracts against a closed cervix. There is no available exit, and the baby is being crushed, so this state involves an experience of constriction, entrapment, and fear; the paradise of the good womb is lost, and the baby faces death. Experientially, there is profound hopelessness and despair. This is thought to form the template of the futile position described below.

The third and fourth matrices form the basis of the death-rebirth dynamic. BPM III represents the physical process of movement from the contracting uterus through the opening cervix, followed by the "life or death struggle" through the birth canal. This is the archetypal hero's journey, the call to arms, the tumultuous and perilous struggle.

The fourth perinatal matrix (BPM IV) is the birth: the sudden dramatic emergence into a new life, the first intake of breath, and the recovery phase for mother and baby. The ordeal is over, and they can meet each other for the first time in the outside world. From an archetypal perspective, there may be themes of triumph and deliverance, new horizons, revolution, decompression and expansion of space, radiant light and color. For others it may be experienced more as a devastating loss of their fusion with mother and their emergence into an alien and threatening world.

Grof found in his clinical work with LSD and Holotropic Breathwork that our deepest root of trauma springs from this perinatal process, and this becomes the primary template around which we organize our subsequent development. If these formative traumas loom large in our psyche, then we unconsciously attract events and relationships that reenact the emotional tone of our formative traumas. The significance of the perinatal layer of psyche lies in its extraordinary duration, intensity, and violence both on an emotional and a physical level. Very few people will have experienced anything approaching this level of physical violence and annihilatory anxiety in the remainder of their lives. It is not surprising that opening to this layer of psyche in an expanded state is often experienced as torture or death.

To summarize Grof's conclusions:

- The birth process leaves its residue in adult psychological structures.
- The embodied memory of the birth process can be accessed in expanded states of consciousness.
- Working through perinatal issues can provide relief from a number of psychological and somatic ailments.
- These experiences have an archetypal quality.
- Accessing this perinatal layer in an expanded state can act as a portal to transpersonal experience.

THE FIVE CHALLENGING POSITIONS

The five challenging states or positions, described below, represent a synthesis of Grofian and psychoanalytic schools. Such a synthesis helps us understand the complex area of psyche beyond conscious memory that forms the foundation of our ego structures. I think that psychoanalysis is generally blind to the import of perinatal trauma while Grof underestimates the significance of postnatal events. The names of these states or positions highlight the meaning tone and the archetypal character of the mental experience that arises. The five states are the:

- Futile position
- Death-rebirth position
- Paranoid position
- Mourned position
- Transpersonal position

I want to underline the rooted and dynamic nature of these positions. Rooted because they are not caused by the psychedelic experience; they lie deep within us but are exposed by it. Dynamic because we flow between these positions, and each can be exposed to some extent by triggers.

The Futile Position

The futile position is characterized by pervasive feelings of alienation, despair, constriction, hopelessness, and disconnection. This is an existential depression, a dark night of the soul, a black hole where light does not penetrate. It is a stark contrast to the feelings of connection, compassion, and love that are the hallmarks of a deeply positive psychedelic experience. The futile position raises some special challenges around how to work with it: determining what strategies are likely to be helpful and how to manage risk if these feelings are not completely resolved is particularly important.

Grof developed his ideas about the formative role of perinatal trauma after a session with 300 mcg of LSD (Walsh and Grob 2005, 131). He describes entering a place of despair; he tried to find beacons of hope but without success. Surely knowledge was worthwhile? But what is the point of spending your life amassing knowledge when eventually you become so old you cannot even remember what you ate for dinner. Surely children are worthwhile? But they themselves simply grow old and die after living a pointless existence. While having these thoughts, he became aware of tremendous pressure on his head and jaws and difficulty breathing. He had a paradigm-changing realization that he was reexperiencing the physical sensations and emotions of his biological birth.

What followed was profound and underlies the importance of surrendering to and properly integrating such experiences, especially when they are as challenging as this. Grof came to a realization that, while his body had been born physically, there was still a part of his psyche that remained stuck in the birth process and was still trying to get out. He realized that some aspects of the way he lived his life had arisen as defenses against this sense of emotional entrapment. Grof's dark night of the soul transformed after three hours or so into a feeling that life was wonderful and meaningful. This psychological rebirth seems to be typical of the cathartic process: if the futile position can be fully experienced, the awakened place is right next door—if we can only find the way in.

Grof linked the desolation of the futile position with the second perinatal matrix, but in my clinical work I have also found a strong link with the fourth perinatal matrix associated with the devastating separation and dislocation of birth. My experience is that some people are more rooted in the futile position than others. Some people touch this place quickly and fruitfully, but for others, it is such a deep and profoundly formative part of the psyche that repeated exposure is required over a longer period of time—and this is difficult work. The futile position is an internal structure that strips meaning, so those who are rooted in that position have a greater requirement to find meaning in external structures, which makes them vulnerable to belief systems of whatever nature. I think that those who have successfully negotiated this position, either in early life or as a result of their own deep inner work, have a more reliable attunement with meaning that arises from within.

As facilitators we need to hold the hope when the situation seems hopeless. We may offer words of encouragement, such as "stay with it," "this is important work that you're doing," "this is your healing journey." We need to have built up a sufficiently strong and stable therapeutic relationship during the preparation to instill a sense of safety when a person feels in existential danger so we can support him or her to more fully surrender to the process, to go deeper, perhaps even make the feelings of hopelessness even bigger in the service of resolution. We may need to tolerate revisiting the futile position ourselves in the fused state that we often reach when working in such a tight emotional space. The futile position is often associated with powerful and constricting somatic sensations, and appropriate somatic release work may be highly effective. We need to have an aftercare strategy if this state has not resolved at the conclusion of the retreat; this may include risk management and psychological support in the short term and consideration of further work in expanded states to complete the work.

The Death-Rebirth Position

When Albert Hofmann took LSD intentionally for the first time, he thought he was dying. This led him through a paranoid state and the futile position as he realized the tragedy of the situation: he would leave his family fatherless, and he would leave his research unfinished. He settled after his family doctor, who became the world's first LSD sitter, attended him, reassuring him and staying with him for a while. The next day, he awoke refreshed with a sensation of well-being and renewed life. "In the garden everything glistened and shone with a fresh light—the world seemed as if newly created" (Hofmann 1979, 50).

Hofmann describes the classical death-rebirth sequence, which is characteristic of expanded states. The death-rebirth archetype is expressed in resurrection myths around the world and was the central part of the Eleusinian mysteries, the psychedelic ceremony that shaped the classical world and formed the basis of Western philosophy. Anyone working with psychedelics needs to be familiar with this sequence, its challenges and various manifestations.

Hofmann has some justification for his fear—this was a new and untested substance after all—but most journeyers know on a rational level that they are not in danger of physical death. However, this does not diminish the visceral fear that some feel when they access primitive anxiety around annihilation. Such fears lurk below the surface of our everyday lives, and I think they are often important determinants of our behavior as we find ways to distract ourselves from these subterranean anxieties. At the time of the coronavirus crisis, many became more familiar with anxieties around death, our innate annihilatory anxiety, and the defenses we construct against them. Such insights may give us an opportunity to change the way in which we choose to live our lives.

One of the hallmarks of the psychedelic state is the way in which such annihilatory anxiety becomes intensified. I suggest that there are two fundamental ideas that help us to understand this: first, that we re-reconnect with unresolved traumas arising in our early development; second, that our ego structures strongly resist attempts to relinquish them and the more acute the challenge the shriller the response. The dissolution effect of a high-dose experience is an existential threat to those ego structures that developed very early in our existence as coping mechanisms to protect us against primitive fears. So, when those defenses are dissolved, we are likely to encounter those formative psychological events.

Psychoanalytic thinkers have identified fear of annihilation as perhaps the deepest anxiety that we encounter in our formative years. Theories have linked it to Freud's death instinct, the failure of omnipotent ego defenses, and have emphasized the importance of the mother's ability to contain and metabolize this primitive anxiety so that it becomes less threatening. The physical support a mother can provide through skin contact with her infant (Bick 1968) seems to be of primary importance in containing infantile anxiety, and perhaps this links to the way physical support for someone in a psychedelic state, such as holding the person's hand, seems to enable the person to surrender to or deepen into the experience, which in turn increases the prospect of completing the sequence and achieving psychospiritual rebirth.

From the perinatal perspective, the death-rebirth position has very different characteristics to the futile position, although it may develop from it. Rather than passive and hopeless, the epic voyage through the birth canal has qualities of engagement. It is an active process with light at the end of the tunnel. The emotional tone holds fighting qualities, although the degree of suffering may feel more intense than anything previously experienced and the archetypal quality of the experience is perilous in the extreme. Grof (1975, 95) found with his LSD patients that in such states their deep realization of the frailty and impermanence of man as a biological creature is accompanied by an agonizing existential crisis that also has a high degree of transformational potential.

There may be sexual or scatological content, typically accompanied by shame. Other shame-filled events or emotions in our life journey may come to consciousness too. It may seem as though we are confronted with the most unspeakable parts of our personality, the darkest parts of our shadow. There may be sequences involving a titanic struggle, a battle with supernatural forces, or a purification by fire. There may be an experience of sexual excitement or of enormous energy pulsing through the body. There may be profound physical manifestations, such as writhing, shaking, feelings of pressure, experiences of pain or constriction. Support and encouragement are often helpful: the guide may offer words of encouragement, such as "keep going," "you're doing great." Intensification of the physical processes is often a useful strategy to deepen the process in the service of a more complete unfolding.

The rebirth experience may be subtle or dramatic. It may have the quality of a white light experience, a union with cosmic oneness. During his first LSD experience with Timothy Leary as a sitter, the writer and theologian John Huston Smith describes ascending step-by-step "to those things on which angels themselves long to gaze." Smith felt that if he took the last step and merged with the all-consuming limitless bliss, he would die, but there followed a sublime experience of union with cosmic consciousness that he had been seeking without success through Zen Buddhism for many years. Smith had no doubt that his experience of cosmic consciousness was an authentic religious experience, similar to that described by mystics and saints over the millennia (Smith 2005, 230).

After powerful states of expanded consciousness, it is of crucial importance to allow time for the experience to settle, with sufficient integration before people reengage with the everyday world. The group setting amplifies the grounding aspect of this. The image of birth implies a tender space, where the newborn requires care of a gentle and delicate nature. If this does not occur, there may be complications, such as an incomplete death or an unbounded rebirth.

In *Breaking Open: Finding a Way through Spiritual Emergencies* (2020), Jules Evans and Daniel Sherwen describe very different experiences after their ayahuasca retreats. Evans describes an abrupt transition from feeling deeply sensitized by the retreat to the noisy, dirty everyday reality of the outside world. He felt that he was either dead or in a dream; it felt as though he were in a computer game, and the next level had failed to load, as though he were in some ghastly afterlife. Sherwen's ayahuasca retreat culminated in a profound ego-dissolution experience, followed by pulsing energy flowing through every cell of his being and an identification with Jesus. He did not sleep for some days, and on his return home, developed a sudden fear that he was dying followed by a short-lived paranoid state. Both found it difficult to function during their post retreat crisis, requiring support from friends and family before making transformational recoveries.

The Paranoid Position

There is a close relationship between the annihilatory anxiety of the death-rebirth position and paranoid states, especially if the setting is suboptimal. During his historic LSD journey, Albert Hofmann projected his fear that he was dying onto the outside world. His furniture assumed grotesque threatening forms, and he saw his kindly neighbor as a malevolent witch (Hofmann 1979, 49).

We all have our paranoid places. From a psychoanalytic perspective, what lurks in the unconscious of the infant searches for meaning in relational terms. In this model, the paranoid position is a normal part of ego development as the infant projects intolerable discomfort, such as hunger, onto the mother, who then becomes a persecutory figure as the cause of the tormented feelings. From a perinatal viewpoint, the paranoid position arises as the expulsion process begins and we are attacked by the contracting womb.

Most of us only return briefly to the paranoid position at times of stress or with a particular trigger. Some of us may be more rooted in the paranoid position, with a tendency toward black-and-white thinking, fundamentalist perspectives, and belief in conspiracy theories. The paranoid position has an important defensive function, and if a psychedelic experience accesses an early wound, this defense may be deployed. This is particularly likely where there is:

- Failure of setting
- Dominance of paranoid position in ego structures
- Activation of early trauma

With appropriate selection, preparation, mindset, setting, and integration, a sustained paranoid state is rare. Any paranoid state is likely to be brief and responsive to the therapeutic relationship with the guide. The guide can invite the client to take the projection back into the inner world, to reorient his focus from the outside world, with a prompt, such as "this is part of your process; go back inside." Thus, the curious, healing-seeking mindset is encouraged. A person who habitually uses paranoid mechanisms, has prominent fundamentalist views, or a history of delusional states is high risk, even in a well-designed setting. Some people may be constitutionally vulnerable; a first-degree relative with a history of paranoid psychosis may be indicative.

Sustained paranoid reactions may arise when an inner experience is projected onto the external world. This occurs most frequently in a recreational setting but may occur if a person leaves a retreat with an unresolved process. In my psychiatric practice, I have had a number of referrals of people who had an acute paranoid reaction in ayahuasca ceremonies and were allowed to leave in this condition. Their paranoid state became entrenched with disastrous consequences. The paranoid participant who wants to leave is a challenging scenario, and every setting needs to have a range of strategies to manage this. The strategy should include screening and preparation, as well as aftercare provision. It is not acceptable to abdicate responsibility and simply let someone go.

Sometimes the setting is inherently high risk despite the best efforts and intentions of everyone involved. Toby Slater gives an account of a paranoid reaction while in an MRI machine after taking LSD in a research setting. His feelings of confinement and isolation combined with the threat of ego death and the revisiting of traumatic material were projected onto the external environment. The setting turned malignant, his guide seemed wolflike, and he tried to escape. Slater responded to a midazolam shot and was able to positively integrate his experience (Dickens and Read 2015).

Paranoid states may also arise as a delayed post-traumatic stress reaction to an event that occurred in childhood. The Jungian analyst Donald Kalsched (1996) describes how childhood trauma leads to the creation of internal persecutory figures that have an initial protective function. Expanded states can expose such persecutory scenarios in a way that is so vivid that people may feel driven to act on the feelings that arise. This may occur even with optimal set and setting. Scott Hill describes such a paranoid experience in a therapeutic MDMA session where he experienced his sitters as Satan's demonic helpers (see page 67 of this book). Hill links this to a severe burn injury he had at age two that required hospital treatment. How would a two-year-old experience the doctors and nurses who were trying to treat his burns?

The Mourned Position

A participant in a Holotropic Breathwork retreat described the following experience of mourning:

> *I cried and cried. I wept for myself, my family, and the world. I felt so deeply how we all hurt each other. I revisited the times in my life when I had been hurt and the life choices I made as a result of those hurts. I felt the deep wells of pain that I had never felt before, and then I realized that I didn't need the hurt any more. Like an old coat on a summer's day, it had served its purpose. I was grateful for its service, but now I could let it go.*

Mourning is essential for accommodation and growth. Freud's influential paper *Mourning and Melancholia* was the first to describe how failure in the mourning process predisposes a person to depression (1917). For Freud the melancholic is burdened with an internal object that cannot be relinquished whereas mourning allows a letting go and an ability to form new attachments. We know from bereavement studies how grief is a healthy healing process and that the blockage of this expression of grief may cause depression. Mourning is maturational. It promotes resilience; it makes space for a wider way of being in the world. The flowing, processing quality of mourning has a very different quality to the utter stasis of the futile position. One of the greatest fruits of a psychedelic experience is a deeply felt *moving through* to a position of acceptance that had previously seemed impossible. Such benefit may even be gained in one therapeutic session, although it may well require ongoing work for such gains to be maintained.

From a developmental perspective, Melanie Klein and the object relations school describe how the infant develops a more mature position with a movement from the paranoid position toward the establishment of good internal objects, acceptance, and love. The baby learns that the mother can be both the source of all that is good but also be capable of provoking bad feelings, so good and bad can be safely located in the same object. Earlier destructive, envious, and aggressive impulses become accommodated and no longer need to be split off and projected. People who are more rooted in the paranoid position have more difficulty with mourning and acceptance, but allowing themselves to stay with sadness in an expanded state can be deeply healing for them.

In practice, mourning can be a simple process. For others, it is hard-won and only accessible after successive experiences, chipping away at armorlike defenses, allowing sorrow to flow and learning the skill of self-compassion. Any professional working with expanded states needs to be able to not only tolerate people's sadness and their expression of it, but also to sometimes actively encourage people to stay with it, to allow themselves to really feel it, perhaps even move more deeply into their grief. Shame is an inhibitor of mourning, and the quality of the facilitator's presence, sometimes with physical support, can be a powerful factor allowing the easing of shame and the flowering of sorrow. A settling of the grief after the session, sitting quietly with the sadness, is important and will avoid a rapid rebound. Thoughtful integration decreases the risk of rapid reversion to previous entrenched perspectives.

The Transpersonal Position

Transpersonal experiences take us beyond the personal. Any of the previous positions can develop an archetypal quality that transcends our sense of who we think we are. We may identify with another person, an animal, a plant, a life lived in a different period in history or even in a different universe. We may experience a succession of deaths or visit periods before birth or after death. We may perceive that the cosmos is essentially composed of love, or we may have a numinous experience of union with the Divine.

In a profound transpersonal experience, the tectonic plates of the psyche move. Persons who have been on a spiritual development path may experience this as an acceleration of their growth process. But persons who are heavily identified with their ego may experience this movement as an earthquake. In Jungian terminology, we may develop a new internal structure where ego combines with the archetypal Self, or to use a phrase from psychoanalysis, our internal object relationships are enhanced and restructured as we form an adaptive new understanding of our place in the scheme of things. We see a bigger picture; a larger framework is revealed. We may agree with Jim Fadiman that "the universe is larger than I thought and my identity is smaller than I thought" (Walsh and Grob 2005, 26).

If safely negotiated, the spiritual emergence that often flows from such awakenings is beautiful to experience and to witness. The risk of problematic manifestations is minimized if people fully and completely emerge from their expanded state and engage in an integrative process before they rejoin everyday life. The deeper and more prolonged the immersion and the more profound the experience, the greater the importance of this integration. What follows are some adverse effects of the transpersonal experience.

- **Spiritual or psychedelic bypass.** The individual uses emergent spirituality as a lofty defense to avoid dealing with psychological issues and unfinished developmental tasks.
- **Amplification of the shadow.** This typically arises in association with bypass. In the afterglow of the expanded state, the sharp edges of personality may soften so that the individual becomes gentler and more loveable. Integration and readiness of personality may allow a permanent transformation. But sometimes as the high tide of the experience itself recedes, the unfolding process serves to energize the individual's problematic personality traits, which then reassert themselves with renewed force.
- **Ego inflation.** The power and energy of the transpersonal becomes introjected into narcissistic ego structures. At its most extreme, this can lead to the guru syndrome or cult structures.
- **Identification with belief systems.** As the individual relinquishes historic ego structures, alternate structures to replace the ones lost are needed, and the individual may cling to such structures to the detriment of further growth. The individual may be particularly vulnerable to the belief systems of the group within which the mutative experience was had, especially in the immediate aftermath.
- **Confusion of levels.** The inner experience loses its symbolic quality and the individual projects it onto the everyday world, sometimes with delusional intensity.
- **Boundary violations.** The individual may project an experience of universal love onto another person or a feeling of emotional connection onto an inappropriate physical connection.

CONCLUSION

Early developmental trauma is of crucial importance because of the way it shapes and impacts us. The significance of such early events is easily overlooked precisely because these lie so deep in our unconscious, but they profoundly affect the development of our emergent ego structures, our relationship patterns, our neural networks, and our relationship with our bodies. Often, work with psychedelics tends to use brief integrative strategies, using the skills of a guide rather than a psychotherapist. Longer term therapy using successive exposure to expanded states is a more complex process than brief work with psychedelics or traditional psychotherapy. Such work requires an understanding of how to allow transformative and integrated expressions of deep psyche so that exposing these deep wounds engages a healing process, rather than simply a traumatic encounter with shadow—and this understanding can only be gained by doing our own deep inner work. Expanded states allow us to access and work therapeutically with these formative structures and the defenses that we build around them, and this is where much of the transformative potential of this work truly lies.

7

The Weekend Workshop

Group Therapy with Psychedelics

Friederike Meckel Fischer

I decided to train as a psychotherapist after going through my own psychological crisis, which had developed without any obvious cause in my personal life or in my professional life as a doctor. But my talking therapy and group analysis did not resolve my issues or bring back joy into my life. My first Holotropic Breathwork session at a workshop with Stanislav Grof opened up my unconscious and allowed a glimpse of the work I needed to do on myself, so I signed up for the training and eventually was certified as a Holotropic Breathwork facilitator in 1991. At this time in Switzerland, Dr. Samuel Widmer was conducting legal training in psychedelic psychotherapy, and I began my training with him in spring 1992. In fall 1993, permission for the therapeutic use of MDMA and LSD in Switzerland was withdrawn, so when I finished my training in 1995, half of the training had been legal, but the second half had been outside the legal framework.

As a psychotherapist, I found that some clients simply did not respond to conventional talking therapy, and I decided to offer some of them psychedelic therapy. From my personal experience and my training, I felt that the potential benefits to them outweighed the consequences of working outside contemporary legality. I worked with around one hundred carefully selected patients over a ten-year period in a group setting in weekend workshops until my work was brought to an end by my arrest, after a former client informed the police of my work. The full story is told in *Therapy with Substance* (Meckel Fischer 2015), but in this chapter, I will focus on how I developed the format of the weekend workshops and how I worked with clients in the medicine sessions to fully support their experience.

PREPARATION

After I selected a client for this work, we always started with an individual medicine session before progressing to the group weekend workshop. The therapeutic process was supported throughout by ongoing conventional psychotherapy sessions and various integrative activities.

A first session with a psychedelic substance is always unique and overwhelming. I always started with MDMA for this first individual session. I found that the empathogenic effects of the MDMA, with the warmth and loving feelings that come up, strongly supported my emotional connection with the client and boosted the therapeutic rapport. The strength of this initial therapeutic relationship provided a platform for some of the more difficult work that inevitably lay ahead. This preliminary session provided a valuable opportunity to observe the client's reaction and behavior to a first experience with a psychoactive substance. I had to be aware of possible adverse reactions or the potential for dissociation. It also gave the client a "test drive" and an opportunity to decline further psychedelic work at this point, before they were introduced to the group. Sometimes I offered a second session before we made a decision.

We began the workshop on a Friday evening as a group of twelve to sixteen people. I knew each of the participants well from previous therapy sessions I had hosted. After a welcome dinner, we met in a circle where each reported on what had happened since the last session and carefully expressed an intention for the session of the following day. I found that this statement of intention for the session was a very important precondition for progress in this type of therapy. The intention engages the energy of the unconscious processes and provides a focus for material to emerge in the medicine session. To underline its importance to the clients, I used to say: "If you do not know where you want to go, then each path will be the wrong one."

The intention question was critically investigated by myself and the group members: Did it really meet the topic? Was the wording adequate? Was the intention itself useful? This careful treatment of the intention statement helped to crystalize it clearly and deepened its imprint. However, during the medicine session at the point where the substance starts to take effect, the instruction is to let the intention go and simply work with whatever wants to emerge.

CHOOSING THE MEDICINE

The decision as to which substances to take and at what dose was made by the group. One of the advantages of the careful discussion of doses was that we were able to prepare all the various dosages before the medicine session.

We varied in how we took the medicine, either taking MDMA alone, LSD alone, or combining the two. We discussed the sequence, and we experimented with the effect of taking the two substances together at the same time or taking them one after the other. Mostly we decided to take one substance first and then ingest the second after three hours or so. After ingestion of the second substance, we would lie down again and very silently move through the ascent until the second substance had unfolded its full effect.

We found that combining substances deepened the experience, providing an opportunity to look at the same topic from two different perspectives. Sometimes the second substance completed the insights or the work of the first segment of the session or led further and deeper into the subject matter. Also, the length of the session increased, sometimes up to ten hours.

We usually decided on MDMA if the majority of those present were addressing relationship issues or childhood memories and when it was felt to be important to revisit an event without fear. In a first individual MDMA session, the dose was 90 to 100 mg to allow a relatively gentle first acquaintance. In the group setting, the usual dose was 120 mg, occasionally 130 mg for men with very rigid defenses.

I initially used LSD as an adjunct by adding a low dose of 50 mcg some two and a half hours after taking the MDMA. This has a number of advantages; the MDMA process is lengthened, allowing a longer period for material to emerge, the perceptual disturbances of the LSD are less likely to occur, the sweetness of the MDMA is reduced, and the LSD adds an element of clarity and sharpness of thinking. I found that many people are afraid of LSD, and combining it with MDMA in this way was a gentle introduction to the drug. The use of MDMA as an adjunct to an initial dose of LSD is different. The impact of the MDMA is less emotional, but it gives a greater emotional range to the LSD, which can then become more authentic and sustaining. We always thought about the dose for the second substance from a very individual perspective. For sensitive people, we would suggest taking no more than half a dose of MDMA after LSD, while others were able to work with a full dose of MDMA after taking 150 mcg of LSD.

If the intention was for a more general exploration or to solve a problem, we would often begin with LSD. I would only allow a session with LSD taken alone after a client had completed a session of LSD taken as an adjunct with MDMA. I would always start with a moderate dose of 75 to 100 mcg of LSD, which tended to find the sweet spot between overcoming resistance and preventing the client from entering a trauma-induced state of dissociation found with higher doses. I generally found that this was a dose sufficient to do the inner work required while retaining the ability to be self-reflective. Over time, I could raise the amount to a maximum of 200 to 250 mcg if necessary. It was not necessary to go beyond this dose because as people became more experienced, they became more adept at navigating their inner territory.

Taking a second substance is challenging as the first substance is still active. When the second substance starts to unfold, there comes a moment when the two meet. At this intersection, one has to be very still and quiet. Then the second substance takes over, sometimes more powerfully than it would be if taken alone as it arrives on the crest of the wave of the first substance.

We sometimes used 2-CB, a psychedelic phenethylamine, if the intention was to work on ambivalence or resistance. 2-CB seems to combine some of the empathogenic qualities of MDMA with the clear insights of LSD and the visual changes of mescaline, but the 2-CB experience has a different quality compared to the combination of LSD and MDMA taken together. The heart opening is less intense than MDMA, and 2-CB has the awkward but useful quality of facilitating content with the shadow: it relentlessly brings to light the issues one does not want to look at. 2-CB also seems to go to the heart of psychosomatic issues. If one resists the opening, it can induce feelings of nausea or feeling blurred, so one has to stay focused and surrender to the substance. The ascent can have several steps. After forty-five minutes or so, it can feel that the opening is over, and then one has to remain very still and silent so that the next step can be taken. This may happen two or three times. 2-CB is said to be an aphrodisiac, but this is not my experience in the setting of the weekend workshop. The dose range of 2-CB was from 10 to 30 mg; 30 mg was reported to be almost toxic, and I found that 22 mg seemed to produce outstanding experiences. The substance is short acting; after 20 mg the session is over in about four hours. The descent with 2-CB is often unpleasant. We found that the addition of 50 mcg of LSD made the descent both longer and gentler.

WORKING WITH SUBSTANCE

We began the session with a ritual that included promises of confidentiality, not harming oneself or others, and taking responsibility for the work that we do. Then everyone took the substance at the same time and lay down on their mats. At this point, I invite the participants to let go of their intention and rely on their unconscious to let the relevant material emerge.

Each substance has its intrinsic four phases of ascent, peak, plateau, and descent. We started the ascent phase in an introspective, lying-down setting. During ascent, the only goal was to let the substance unfold and surrender as best we can. Eyes were kept closed or covered with eyeshades; there was no or very little movement and no speaking, just centering on what was going on internally.

With beginners, I guided this initial stage, saying: "Let all your thoughts go . . . just listen . . . just observe . . . stay in the present . . . don't react." I coordinated these instructions with the unfolding effect of the substance and also supported it in line with individual pieces of music that were seven to ten minutes long. In between, there would be periods of silence. I found this guidance was helpful in teaching the participants how to deal with a psychoactive substance: watching without judgment, listening without reacting, being still and staying in the moment. Learning these skills was important so that when material emerged in the session, they reacted in a different manner compared to how they would react to emotional triggers in everyday life. It also provided them with a skill set for the task of going deeper and reaching the core of their issues in subsequent sessions.

The quantity and the choice of music depended on the experience of the participants. I found that beginners easily got lost in their thoughts and feelings without music and were better off with mildly evocative music. With people who were more advanced in the work, I played less music and played pieces that evoked challenging feelings, if that is deemed appropriate. I would play the music pieces according to the unfolding of the substance. With MDMA, I used carefully selected pieces, which gradually became more harmonious and touching. The piece for the peak was usually a melodic, very simple instrumental solo or just a gong.

About ten minutes after intake, I would play a piece with a distinct rhythm that gives a sense of forward motion, of being on a journey. This more energetic music generally eases resistance or stress, directs attention away from the everyday thoughts, and protects against anxious thoughts about what may lie ahead. About thirty to thirty-five minutes after intake, sensing the atmosphere in the room, I would introduce a piece of music with a character of dissonance; some people may even find it irritating. This facilitates the emergence of more challenging emotions. If I were to play gentle, loving music too early, then these more difficult emotions or thoughts would not have a chance to emerge.

When we reached the peak after ninety minutes, I interrupted the music set so the plateau phase began with a silent period of around twenty minutes, in which each person could examine what had come up and reorient around their original intention question.

We then sat up in a circle and began the expression and process-oriented part of the session. Some people shared their insights and realizations, or someone asked to work on an issue. Often participants requested assistance with an insight or a body sensation they were experiencing or an issue that they could not grasp or fully understand. A person could describe a vision or sequence and ask for some help in interpreting the meaning. A person could be in a difficult emotional state needing support. In each case, the work was determined by what had presented itself.

THE ITERATIVE INTEGRATION PROCESS

During and after the plateau phase, I worked with each participant. These individual work sessions constitute what I term the *iterative integration process*. Iteration describes the process of repeatedly processing material so that each successive pass brings you closer to your goal. In retrospect, we see that the knowledge gained from each session and the integration steps that follow guides the inner focus to the next step and the next intention question. But the path of development from one intention to the next is not linear; it tends to be circular, although the circle never closes—hence the term *iterative*. Each sequence of steps forms the path, which progressively provides a basis from which the client can embark on new paths. Thus, iteration embodies the principle that the path is the true destination.

My method of working with individuals during the session likely differs the most from those therapists who prefer a more silent and introspective approach during the session, with participants lying down. Their perspective emphasizes that the whole process should be experienced internally, and processing and integration should happen afterward. I agree that inappropriate interventions present obvious risks, potentially interrupting the participant's evolving inner process or inadvertently manipulating the client. Indeed, when I began this work, we used the silent nonintervention setting with participants lying down throughout.

But my clients had the same experience as I had had when I was a client: they felt stuck in their thoughts and feelings; they sometimes did not know how to pilot themselves through difficult emotions; they went to difficult sad places and once again felt helpless and alone. So, in visiting their traumas, they were just reexperiencing them rather than resolving them. If a person had been left alone in a frightening moment as a child, it is crucial to avoid a retraumatization, a repetition of the abandonment in the moment of reexperiencing the trauma. If left alone, the same conclusions would be confirmed and drawn anew: "There is never anyone by my side; I am always alone. No one takes care of me; I have to do everything on my own." It felt as though they needed more help. We found that simple interventions such as "I am here with you" or physical support such as hand holding would allow the client to go through the experience while feeling protected. This then builds resilience by providing a psychological template for how to navigate similar experiences in the future.

WORK IN DEEP PLACES

The therapeutic work with individuals is different each time and is difficult to describe in words. The main goal is to accompany and guide the client's process, avoiding interpretations and our view as to what may be a desirable outcome. It is always only about the ongoing process of the client. I find that the best place to start is with basic questions, such as: Where are you? What is going on within you right now? What sensations are coming up in your body? Where in your body do you feel this? This teaches the client to be aware of his body as a reference point to feelings and sensations. I might offer an invitation to stay with that sensation and just observe it, waiting for whatever comes up. I encourage the client to describe what he perceives or what situation he finds himself in.

With these questions, he focuses exactly on the moment of his experience. I try to accurately follow his own words and use his expressions. He stays with the feeling or the sensation, while at the same time searching for the meaning behind it. For example, if he reports a strange feeling in the stomach, I ask, "Where do you feel this exactly?" He searches for the exact point. I invite him to only focus on that point and wait for his descriptive remarks. With each answer I try to deepen the process. I may repeat his answer and ask for other sensations: "What else do you hear, see, smell?" The longer he lingers in that state, the more feelings or memories come up, very often something that has been hidden and lost from conscious memory.

To go deeper, I may enquire about atmospheres, sounds, or smells. Very often then the client reaches the causative event directly, regressing to the age when it happened, dropping into the location and the circumstances—actually reexperiencing the event. Then I may hold or touch him, keeping eye and voice contact while maintaining contact with the trauma. At this point he is in two places at once, with me here and also back there then. In many cases, the client may be reexperiencing something on a deeply physical level, perhaps adopting a posture. I encourage the body to express itself, to move, to do whatever it needs to do, and I offer whatever support is helpful to allow the process to proceed to its natural conclusion.

Throughout the process I encourage him to stay with his feelings while reminding him that this event lies in the past and that he is just resolving a memory. "Look me in the eye! Do you see me? Are you with me?" The goal is to work through the event and fully feel the emotions that go with it in order to assign it to the past so that the emotions and the event are separated.

FORMING THE CIRCLE

The setting for the group and the manner in which we worked together developed organically. In the early workshops as the participants settled into the work, I was called for help increasingly often, and when this happened, I talked sotto voce with the participant. Afterward, group members reported that they felt disturbed by this, or some would sit up because they were interested and their own process became engaged. We evolved from lying down all the time to sitting up for a designated period when we worked together and then lying down again. When sitting, we mostly formed a circle where I would sit next to the person I was working with. As the group developed, the sitting up time increased so that the group sat up for several periods and would then lie down and go inside again, until another participant would ask for attention. Sometimes it became apparent in the subsequent integration that an earlier intervention would have been more helpful.

Sometimes a client declared that she was not feeling anything, even accusing me of having given her a placebo. Usually, this indicated that the client was in a dissociative state and needed support to help her make contact with her experience. Again, it was often helpful to focus on what was arising in the body. I found it best not to wait too long before intervening.

I think that psychotherapeutic work of this nature during the session is extremely important and indeed necessary. The verbal expression of new insights and feelings in the psychedelic session, often linked to body sensations and reflections about self-limiting beliefs in the past, can give powerful momentum to change. This new corrective path needs to be reinforced by repetition after the session; otherwise, it may get lost. Thus, the content of the session sinks in more deeply, and the effects are more likely to endure. Seen from a neurophysiological perspective, perhaps new neural circuits start developing in the brain at this very moment.

INTEGRATION IN THE GROUP

After breakfast on Sunday morning, we gathered in a circle for the sharing. This work cannot be rushed, and we gave ourselves plenty of time. This group lasted from 9 a.m. to 2 p.m., with a short break for lunch. Here each participant gave an account of personal highlights and the important insights gained. We recapitulated the session and what we had learned in the pieces of individual work, and this helped me to understand what they had learned and what they would take home. We sometimes rehearsed some of the implementations by repeating a sequence, or we added a resource to stabilize the new experience. We would discuss future steps and sometimes practiced and embodied new attitudes, like giving the boss or the partner an important message. The group members could give or ask for feedback. We would discuss topics such as disturbances in relationships. We found that the combination of group process and the psychedelic space is particularly powerful. The role and the assistance of the group became progressively more important as the group matured and we deepened into the work.

In therapy, a group provides all the available options for interpersonal projections, and we explored, expressed, and corrected these. We practiced to sustain proximity and intimacy and also to accept confrontation and criticism as part of a normal relationship. We philosophized about general themes, such as encounters with shadow aspects, our conditioning, and our attitudes to our parents and how these factors have influenced our processes and the development of our belief systems. The group presents a vessel for the individual, in which her own process is supported and can be reflected, and this approach to difficult issues also can be taken into everyday life. Before we parted, I reminded all the participants to send me, as a final integration exercise, a piece of writing around their experiences within two weeks.

SUMMARY

The weekend workshops that I have described were important milestones in the ongoing therapy of my clients. Looking back at this work with the advantage of hindsight, I am firmly of the opinion that that the work we did during the drug-assisted sessions was the most powerful component of the therapeutic process. The individual work that I have described above was amplified by the deep connectedness and the trust within the group. This enabled an opening and a depth of exploration in the knowledge that the group would be supportive but not judgmental. I have arrived at the view that the therapeutic work in the session itself forms a platform for a more complete integration later and that such an integrative process is more likely to be retained and lead to lasting change. But the most important element is the caring support, the trusting relationship between the clients and the therapist, which provides a container for the iterative integration process.

8

Underground Psychedelic Psychotherapy

Lisa Marie Jones

You have to learn to how to open a container, keep a container and close a container.

ANONYMOUS

I came to this work unintentionally. I knew that I was damaged when I started medical school. I felt existential loneliness and despair and had obsessive compulsive disorder (OCD) and intimacy issues (commitment, vulnerability, and trust). But combined with this was a deep desire to be whole, to heal, and (initially) to escape my family legacy and upbringing. I embarked on personal psychotherapy for fifteen years, which built my ability to trust another person and helped me overcome my OCD, but it did not address my deeper issues, and I knew that I needed more. During my therapy, I chanced upon a book by Stanislav Grof, which led to my first Holotropic Breathwork session. This opened me to an important array of experiences and aspects of myself that were not accessible through talking therapy, giving me the hope of deeper change. With more Holotropic Breathwork sessions, my enthusiasm and yearning for transformation flourished, and as I integrated these experiences into my life, I could see myself transforming.

A chance encounter led me to my first psychedelic therapy session with MDMA, which was utterly transformative. It seemed to be a culmination of all the previous work I had done on myself over a twenty-year period. It took me to a deeper level of myself in a way that I could not have understood or predicted, even with my previous Breathwork experience. I was witnessed and accepted in an internal place that I had not known that I needed to be seen in. In that session, unexpectedly, I asked to be trained as a therapist in this work.

Since then, I have experienced a range of psychedelic settings. The majority have been formal, well structured, therapeutically directed sessions. Others were shamanically oriented with people trained traditionally in their land (mostly South America) or with others who have woven together their experience and training in psychedelics with their conventional psychotherapy background. Most were well held, but some were not. Very little of my experience has been what may be termed recreational.

I have now completed a formal underground training as a psychedelic psychotherapist. This involved seven modules over two and a half years and covered multiple aspects, including pharmacology, law, music, bodywork, transference, resistance, systemic constellations, and pre- and perinatal psychology, as well as fourteen therapeutic group sessions with a range of substances. While this work currently stands outside the legal framework, for me the therapeutic benefits outweigh by far the legal risks, and I have felt others deserve the opportunity to experience the healing and change these experiences can offer, if they so wish.

QUALITIES REQUIRED IN A THERAPIST: SELF-WORK, DEPTH, WIDTH, AND HONESTY

Psychedelic therapy is deep work, deeper work than most people have ever previously experienced, involving a much wider internal landscape than we routinely encounter in regular therapy. To work at such depths with others, we need a more developed skill set than standard psycho-therapeutic training. To support our training, additional skill sets are required to equip ourselves to be of greater service to those we guide through these realms. This skill set begins with our own inner work and this self-work with psychedelics in a well-held therapeutic context naturally leads to the development of greater depth, width, and, hope-fully, integrity. It is not enough to have a singular psychedelic experience in order to be trained.

The requirement of inner work and self-development is widely accepted in all psychotherapeutic trainings, and it is no different for psychedelic psychotherapy. What does differ is the content and range of this inner work. It is arduous and heart breaking, requires courage, curiosity, and an ability to ask difficult questions of oneself with hon-esty, and relies on good support.

As psychedelic therapists, we have to be comfortable with our own significant experiences: our ancestral history, our prebirth and birth experiences, the family and culture we grew up in. We need to engage and work through our corresponding feelings, reactions, and beliefs. This means really experiencing and expressing our feelings of grief, loss, sadness, anger, rage, hatred, vindictiveness, powerlessness, terror, shame, guilt, hopelessness, and nothingness, as well as love, joy, hap-piness, ecstasy, laughter, peace, and acceptance. In short, to have fully experienced our own personal hells and heavens to be able to not only tolerate ourselves but to also be present to the full spectrum of another.

FAMILIARITY WITH SUBSTANCES

Various substances are used: commonly MDMA, LSD, and psilocy-bin (mushrooms); more rarely mescaline, ayahuasca, iboga, peyote, San Pedro cactus, and 2-CB. Some can be taken in combination, like MDMA and LSD or sometimes LSD and psilocybin. Others absolutely cannot: for example, MDMA and ayahuasca is a dangerous and poten-tially life-threatening combination. For some substances, a follow-up supplemental dose or boost can be taken within the same session (e.g.,

MDMA, psilocybin, and ayahuasca), whereas for others, follow-up doses cannot be taken (e.g., mescaline and LSD). On a basic level, the therapist needs to know about the pharmacology, dosing, and interactions of each substance with other medicines.

On an experiential level, the substances have different characteristics, different emotional and physical aspects, and different trajectories, which the therapist needs to have an intimate and thorough knowledge of. For example, with MDMA, one will experience sweating and a racing heart, whereas psilocybin is visual. The therapist needs to know that psilocybin takes the lead in an inner journey and will direct things, whereas it is possible to be more directive with MDMA. The role of the therapist here is similar to that of an experienced mountain guide who is familiar with many different paths leading to the mountaintop.

The type and dose of medicine used and the ability of a client to cope with the material brought forward is of utmost importance. Although the material brought up arises from our own innate healing intelligence, the amount and extent of its intensity is directly influenced by the dosage as well as the set and setting. While MDMA is not dissociative, psilocybin or LSD can be, or they can bring up material that can overwhelm an inexperienced client. This needs discernment and is discussed below in aspects of the work. If we misjudge this, we may encounter more than we feel we can handle.

I have been taught to always start with MDMA, as it is not a dissociative substance and it gives the experience of being safely in one's heart; this can be a useful positive anchoring experience that can equip the client to face a more challenging set of emotions later on. After this initial session, it is always useful to change the vehicle regularly. This means not using the same substance repeatedly in a row. This allows different perspectives on an issue and can allow the opportunity to see, explore, and move past a resistance to a feeling.

During the course of our training, we generally used doses that could be termed psycholytic rather than psychedelic. I remember when I started out, I wanted a big experience, thinking that just one ego death would bring me the peace I sought. Wisdom and some very difficult sessions where I reached my limit taught me this needs to be measured, and time taught me that change is a process that needs to be integrated. As such, I am less enthused by very large doses of psychedelics as it seems much harder to bring something useful back that can actually be integrated into everyday life, and there is a greater risk of having unresolved difficult material, resulting in what is mistakenly labeled a bad trip.

BODYWORK AND EXPRESSION

We are not accustomed to witnessing or supporting the full depth of our feelings. As a consequence, the arc of an experience or feeling and its resolution is not familiar to most of us. This process can be both surprising and intimidating when first encountered.

One central tenet of this work is that the full experience and expression of a feeling leads to its resolution. To put it simply, if we wish to heal, we need to feel, and the facilitator needs to fully support and enable this. It's not catharsis for the sake of catharsis; it's a journey to follow a bodily held feeling, sensation, or emotion and see what story it holds and wants to tell. This approach includes allowing and following the bodily reaction to a trauma alongside the emotional one. The bodily reaction may include shaking, sweating, and twitching, as well as a need for some sort of bodily support in the affected area.

Working with these deep feelings requires trust, acceptance, openness (see below), and a willingness to feel a feeling completely. A central tenet for this process is the ability to be a compassionate witness of oneself and one's experience. Without this ability to hold presence to the experience (perhaps with the support of the therapist), the experience may well be retraumatizing.

I cannot stress enough how important it is to follow a process and to really allow it to unfold. It may be the first time the client completely experiences and accepts the completeness of her feeling (and in turn herself). At this point, if the therapist is inclined to turn away, limit, or somehow change what is present for the client, the therapist may not truly mirror the unfolding, which is what the client needs, and the process will be aborted or stalled. If the process is supported, however, the client may at first experience a subtle body effect, such as a slight tension in the head or back, which then could lead to a full birth or rape experience—merely by following the body's impulses and expressing what is there and trusting what comes up without knowing beforehand what it is or where it may lead.

This order of work—body, feeling, emotion, insight, knowing, talking—is often the reverse process of traditional talking psychotherapy, and it requires a great deal of trust from the client. What also grows with time is a recognition that the heart and the body go first in this. This means we don't know what will show up in a session before we start but trust that what we are being shown will lead to an answer. Even if it is an answer we may not like, it is an answer that we have indeed already survived.

This process, with whatever feelings may be involved, is often noisy and may be very physical. We have immense reservoirs of energy and potential feelings that may need expression. This needs trust from the therapist (in turn communicated to the client) that while the therapist does not know the outcome, he will follow the client's process, with encouragement and acceptance of what is present. The therapist may also offer a form of physical presence, such as therapeutic touch or holding, or some help with intensification of a bodily feeling. A training in working with the body, such as in Holotropic Breathwork, is very useful in such work. While in traditional psychotherapeutic approaches, touch is a taboo, work with altered states requires that we are able to skillfully use touch to support the client's unfolding process. The guide has to discern how and when to do so; failing to provide the necessary physical holding can prove countertherapeutic and retraumatizing.

CONSTELLATION
AND ANCESTRAL WORK

The webs of relationships in which we exist include a genetic element. Part of us was physically present in our grandmothers (your life as an egg started in your mother's developing ovary, as it developed within your grandmother's womb) and all of our mitochondrial DNA is maternal. Through our DNA, our ancestral experiences are born with us. Epigenetics is adding a scientific perspective to the experiential aspects that those familiar with constellation work and psychedelics already know. We inherit not just physical tendencies but behaviors, feelings, and loyalties from our ancestors, be they alive or dead.

I recognize this may strain credulity, but work with these substances repeatedly brings us to the realization that we belong not just to our immediate family but are also part of an entire extended family going back many generations. Very often there is a previously hidden thread that is revealed in the psychedelic experience that often relates to the client's intent and unconscious feelings. We can see and feel what it was like to be a parent that was abused, or feel what the cold rejection of a great-grandparent did to our father, as well as find ourselves carrying forward our ancestor's experiences, like migration, war, slavery, and genocide. We learn that our ancestors pass on to us what they could not themselves resolve, and we can find ourselves carrying their feelings, generations down the line. These ancestral currents, in addition to their own biographical feelings, add depth, width, and context to their circumstance and, most importantly, does not replace the need for their own feelings to be expressed.

As a therapist one not only needs to be familiar that this can happen but also be able to facilitate the various aspects of the family constellation. Family constellations can map out the wider systemic picture of a client's story and explore the hidden influences through loyalties and systemic pulls that might have shaped their lives. Our need for belonging is where these loyalties emerge from, but once we unearth their true cost in our current lives, we can begin to ask ourselves whether we are prepared to continue to pay the price. This awareness allows us to have, perhaps for the first time, the possibility to make a more fully informed choice.

Once we recognize that our life experiences can be influenced by the experiences of our ancestors, we are able to understand our lives in greater depth. With this aspect of ancestral work, we come to witness ourselves within the wider network of our families (or even wider), and this experience opens us up to greater compassion for ourselves and others in our life.

SELF-INTAKE

Psychedelic therapy in clinical and research settings does not involve the therapists taking a dose of the medicine alongside the clients. But this is not the only way of doing this work. There are multiple examples of shamans leading medicine groups in traditional cultures—in South America with the use of ayahuasca, and in the Native American Church with peyote—where the person holding space also takes some of the same medicine that the participants take. They have demonstrated for generations that it is possible to be under the influence of a substance and still effectively hold the space.

When this is discussed in the psychedelic community, concerns are often raised. I often detect both fear and an intellectual and racial elitism in not exposing oneself to the same medicine at the same time as the client. Some of this is based on a Western assumption that we can do things our own way, selectively taking the medicine without its wider context. While this may be appropriate in some contexts, we could learn something from the traditional and indigenous ways of working with altered states, acknowledging the lineage and wisdom they carry through their practices. This is an area that requires a lot of discernment from the guide.

In self-intake the therapist usually takes a smaller dose than the client. Taking a smaller dose of MDMA is less necessary, but for every other substance, the therapist will need to take less. I know that I cannot hold space if I use over 60 to 75 mcg of LSD, for instance, but the client may have taken 125 to 175 mcg. The therapist has to have significant experience with all the substances she intends to use.

There are multiple advantages for the client when the therapist takes the substance alongside the client. It becomes easier to follow the client's story, remain deeply attuned, and mirror a situation back to the client. The enhanced perception gained by the therapist makes it easier to support the client as needed by exploring a constellation or with bodywork. I am not saying this cannot be done when the therapist doesn't take the substance, but I am saying the work can be augmented, with potentially greater therapeutic value to the client. I have experienced holding space both with and without taking a substance. In my experience, without self-intake I find it harder to follow someone's process, and I am more likely to misunderstand a situation. A number of times, important details were missed by me but picked up by the other therapist who had taken the substance. In group work, we generally work in male-female pairs; this is preferable for clients as it mirrors the mother-father dyad and supports deep work through the therapeutic use of projections and transference. While using a psychedelic, a therapist can much more easily perceive the other people present in a person's experience and emerging stories and reflect some of the feelings present for the client. This constellation work with expanded perception and intuition has to be experienced to be fully appreciated.

With self-intake, I find it easier to not only understand the client's spoken intention or meaning, but also to feel emotions, to perceive where that person is and what else is present—perhaps also what is being avoided. This can offer the client more effective mirroring, and it can be immensely healing when a client realizes that another person not only understands him from the inside but can also feel what it is like to have a particular feeling and not turn away from the experience. This provides an anchor or a hand to hold as the client goes through an experience, perhaps fully for the first time.

There are many fears often cited in discussion at this point, primarily seemingly centered around the safety of the client and to an extent the therapist. To be clear, we have to have worked with substances enough to have found our own center in order to support a client in such depth. We have to have had enough experience to know the difference between different substances and their dosages and their effects on us. If we have not done that work ourselves, we have not prepared sufficiently for holding space for someone else.

Some may argue it is possible to do all this just as well from a normal state. To them I would ask, Have you experienced a well-held psychedelic therapy session where the therapist intakes? It is a different qualitative experience most importantly for the client but also for the therapist. It would be an interesting and important area to research: outcomes from psychedelic therapy with a sober versus a partaking therapist.

The expanded perception allows a feel for what is next and an ability to follow the felt process in the client much more carefully. It is also possible to an extent to look ahead and see what is present in front of a client and look at the next steps in his or her process. This can be very helpful when the client is dissociated. As a therapist, you can perhaps feel and sense a range of the experience that's present in the client, and then by checking with the client, it is possible to go through the experience, ever so slowly. If a feeling is too much and the client dissociates, you come back to the moment just before it became overwhelming and explore what happens in the client in the next moment. It is essential that as a guide we constantly check the client's ability to stay in balance with the material that emerges. This can be deeply healing when done well but needs good training, experience, plenty of patience, and often supervision.

When we mirror an experience in a psychedelic state, we are exposed to the full, amplified feeling of that experience as the client moves through it. This can mean being exposed to some very difficult emotions—rage, hatred, disgust, sadness, to name a few. To offer effective mirroring, we must be willing to experience parts of the client's story to a similar depth. Mirroring means bringing witness and presence to the feeling of the client. It is very often less about words and more about a felt expressed process by the client, which the therapist supports. This support may involve therapeutic touch. This takes courage and energy on the part of the therapist, and it can be exactly what a client needs to feel validated, witnessed, and seen. After an experience, that their story is worth feeling by another being present alongside to witness it can demonstrate a fundamental worthiness in the client that he or she doesn't have to go it alone (as was so often the case).

As there are advantages, there are also some disadvantages to self-intake by a psychedelic therapist. These sessions are more intense physically and emotionally. They open up the therapist more and can make them more vulnerable, and there are limits to how frequently one can take a substance. These sessions are potentially more fulfilling for the client but more draining for the therapist.

The therapist who works in expanded states by taking a substance should be experienced with them and with how to work with them and the client. They must also have a greater commitment to self-care and accepting the limits this type of work brings. The aftereffects of sessions with substances usually need greater rest, different food, and exercise, as well as an acceptance that when the work is done this way it cannot be done often. How often this work can be done varies with different substances; for example, it is advisable to take MDMA no more than once a month or less frequently if possible.

There are many ways to work with substances as a psychedelic therapist, and self-intake is one of these. It is not for everyone, and neither should it be. Its promise and potential should not be denied but explored with the same passion and determination as the initial psychedelic renaissance has been, for we all need a space to share and be seen, and budding psychedelic therapists need the option of being able to choose to explore this rich and fertile area of therapy.

The psychedelic therapist needs to be familiar with the arc of the experience, the physical and emotional effects at various time points, as well as the particular characteristics of each medicine or combination. This is a whole set of experiential learning, with all the personal lessons learned from these experiences, as well as understanding how to use them with clients. The therapist has to know how to weave experience, training, and ability to be present alongside the expanded consciousness that comes with this terrain and all its possibilities.

In closing, psychedelic therapy holds much promise for healing and resolution for the client and potentially a revolution in psychotherapy. It is not an easy or a simple solution, and it requires much courage and determination on the part of the client as well as the therapist. For therapists, this is a new frontier that demands a different and more demanding experiential and open-hearted skill set than we have had before. It holds the promise of being able to witness real change and growth within people and, in turn, the resolution, fulfillment, and peace this brings. It offers a different way of being of service to those that come to us in hope of being helped and in hope of finding a way to heal.

9

Preparation and Integration in Holotropic Breathwork

Marianne Murray

Stanislav Grof's work during the 1960s and early 1970s, first at the Psychedelic Institute in Prague and then at Johns Hopkins University and the Maryland Psychiatric Research Center, is now legendary in the field of psychedelic research. Perhaps less well known is his ground-breaking theoretical work in relation to the nature of consciousness arising from his many years of accompanying patients in psychedelic sessions, as well as through his own direct experience. Grof's expanded view of consciousness, along with his recognition of the healing potential of nonordinary or holotropic* (2010, 9) states of consciousness, led to his central role in the founding of transpersonal psychology.

With the closing of the psychedelic research program in Maryland in 1973, Grof was invited to Esalen Institute in Big Sur, California, as a scholar in residence. There, he and his wife, Christina, explored

---

*The word *holotropic* is a neologism coined by Grof that means "moving toward wholeness": the Greek word *holos,* meaning "wholeness," is joined with the word *trapein,* meaning "moving toward."

alternative ways through which to offer people access to expanded states of consciousness. Drawing upon his extensive experience facilitating psychedelic sessions, and gleaning insight from traditional practices used by indigenous, spiritual, and religious cultures around the world, Stan and Christina developed a method for working with groups that incorporated the catalytic power of the breath along with music and physical support. They named their method Holotropic Breathwork.

Over time, and through the experience of several generations of practitioners working around the world, the form and practice of Holotropic Breathwork has matured. Yet the fundamental model remains true to what Grof came to understand through his many years accompanying patients in psychedelic sessions: the healing and transformative potential of work in expanded states of consciousness lives not only in the session itself but also in the continuum of preparation, session, and integration. Holotropic Breathwork, as a method, embodies this principle.

What follows is a description of *preparation* and *integration* within the context of a Holotropic Breathwork workshop. The effectiveness of this model increasingly is being recognized within the reemerging field of psychedelic therapy and research.

PREPARATION AND CONNECTION

There is an adage among many who facilitate Holotropic Breathwork that the participant's experience begins with the decision to attend the workshop. The act of registering stirs up anticipation and often apprehension. From that moment of first connection, our presence as organizers and facilitators will have an impact upon the participant's unfolding experience. The establishment of the set and the setting begins at this point.

Participation in a Holotropic Breathwork workshop involves a rigorous application process, including a review of any medical issues that may prove contraindicative for the work. Facilitators may request information about prior experience, what is drawing the participant to the workshop, and any concerns or questions held by the participant. Some facilitators conduct phone or in-person conversations with participants who have not previously experienced Holotropic Breathwork, and they may supply information for the participant to read before coming to the workshop.

As facilitators, we want participants to understand as much as possible what it is they are signing up for physically and emotionally. For example, participants should understand that the length of each Breathwork session is approximately three hours, and during the session, they will be lying on a mat or sitting on a cushion or in a BackJack floor chair during their partner's session. It is important to explain that Holotropic Breathwork is an internal experience in which challenging feelings, sensations, emotions, and memories may come up during a session. We need to ascertain that the participant can approach inner experiences with interest and tolerance and has the capacity and resources to integrate these experiences following the workshop. As facilitators, we want to be as prepared and well informed as possible to meet and support our participants.

The ground for each participant's experience of the workshop is laid in these preliminary communications. We want participants to feel our presence as they go through the application process, to have access to any information they need, and to feel invited into the workshop. We can learn a lot about participants through the questions they ask and the degree of support they need leading up to the workshop, and equally, we can be curious about them if there is no communication beyond the basic application. Participants, whether they are new to Holotropic Breathwork or not, are taking a step into the unknown—how they do so and how we meet them will shape their experience.

Environment

The venue in which a Breathwork session is held is determined by many factors including location and the aesthetic taste of the workshop organizer, as well as logistics such as budget, number of participants, and availability of facilities. Workshop venues vary greatly. Examples include retreat centers, hotel conference rooms, yoga studios, or facilitators' living rooms. Whatever the location, attention to the environment in which the work will take place is essential in preparation for the workshop, and there should be space for quietness and privacy as well as community sharing. The images, objects, and furnishings that are predominant in the room have an impact upon participants from first impressions as they arrive and throughout the unfolding of the workshop. Many facilitators will place flowers and a candle on a beautiful cloth to create a centerpiece for the opening and closing circles. During the session, this can be moved aside to create an altar where participants place objects that hold special significance for them. Even the most spartan of environments can serve well if we bring intentionality and care to the setup and introduce the group to the space in an inviting manner.

The Opening Circle

The Holotropic Breathwork workshop begins formally when the group gathers and is welcomed by the facilitators. During this opening circle, participants are invited to share something about themselves and what brings them to the workshop. The guidance for this introductory round sets the stage for a culture of deep listening and elevates the potency of being witnessed as a speaker. This somewhat ritualized form for starting the workshop serves a number of purposes: it invites a group culture of receptivity, activates the process of connection among group members, and begins to establish the group field or container that is an essential holding energy for the workshop.

At the end of the opening circle, each participant is guided to find a partner with whom they will work for the duration of the workshop, alternating sessions as breather and sitter. The Grofs introduced this form of working in dyads early on in the development of Holotropic Breathwork, recognizing that it creates an additional layer of safety and support during the course of the Breathwork session (1988, 199). The breather-sitter pairing also can play an important role in the integrative process following the session.

Information and Orientation

Integral to any Holotropic Breathwork event is the orientation talk, held before the Breathwork session, in which the facilitators describe the setup, the overall Breathwork process, what to expect during a session, and offer guidance for both the breathers and the sitters. Usually, this talk includes a short overview of Grof's work and the theory behind this form of breathwork, including an introduction to Grof's map of consciousness.

Practical information includes a description of how the session begins and the length and trajectory of the session. Basic guidance is given for the breather including how to orient to the breathing not as a specific technique but rather as an increase in the pace and depth of their normal breathing. Guidance includes options for moving, making sounds, and general encouragement to explore and bring curiosity to the experience. The facilitators cover functional aspects such as the role of the sitter in support of the breather, how the facilitators work with the group, ways in which a participant can ask for and receive support, and considerations about safety and confidentiality.

New participants often are not aware that music is an active component of Holotropic Breathwork, so a brief introduction to the use of music and the theory behind it is helpful. While not intended to direct the Breathwork session, music does play a role in enhancing the expansion of consciousness. The music for Holotropic Breathwork creates a carrier wave that helps the activation and opening of internal experience as well as supporting participants to move through challenging moments in the session. In addition, because it is played quite loudly, the music helps to mask sounds and activities in the room that might otherwise be distracting.

The design of a music set follows an arc that reflects the typical internal trajectory of a holotropic session. During the first part of the session, the music is dynamic and rhythmic with a driving pace. During the second hour, the pace shifts, and the music becomes more expansive, layered, and emotionally evocative, increasing in intensity toward the end of the hour. During the third hour, the music softens, becoming more spacious, soothing, and meditative. While individual taste is always a factor in designing music sets, it is important to consider the impact of sound on a breather and avoid using music that might be frightening or threatening or pieces that are overfamiliar. The human voice can be a powerfully evocative element in music, but when using vocal music, we ensure that the language is unfamiliar to participants. In essence, the music is intended to be inviting and supportive for breathers as they each navigate their unique journey during the session.

Perhaps the single most important point to convey during the orientation is that this work in nonordinary or expanded states of consciousness is for the most part an internal process, and the content and experience of each person's Breathwork session arises from personal and intrinsic healing intelligence rather than from any external guidance or an objective directive. Frequently, participants look to group leaders as experts and defer to them to understand what arises during a session. It is our work as facilitators to support and encourage each participant to discover their own way and follow their own inner healer and not to impose ourselves upon their experience.

It can be helpful to seed the idea that in these states we can open to and gain insight through a much-expanded array of awareness: somatic, emotional, energetic, visionary, and so forth. We encourage receptivity toward and engagement with whatever arises during the course of the session, considering everything as an offering of information. Rather than being like a cat with our attention riveted singularly and solely upon the bird, we can soften and open so that our awareness receives input from the whole matrix of our inner landscape.

Lastly, in relation to preparation, there is the paradox of attempting to prepare for what is unknowable. When we open to expanded states of consciousness, we embark on an inner journey beyond the structures and boundaries defined by our everyday awareness, and our assumptions about *self, truth,* and *reality* may be stretched and challenged to a significant degree. Our job as facilitators is to help a participant feel safe enough to experience freely the feeling of being unsafe, afraid, or disoriented if that is what arises in the session. We want to create conditions in which the participant's psyche—consciously or unconsciously—can soften, expand, and surrender to whatever is within them that wants to become known.

Through the process of preparation—our communications, the physical environment, the structure of the workshop, and the information that we share—we hope to engender enough confidence in the participant so that she has a sense of being held with intention and benevolence. The concentric circles of support provided by the group, the breathing partners, and the facilitation team create a strong and dynamic container with capacity to attend well and consistently to all the participants for the duration of the workshop.

Checking in before the Session

As the participants prepare for the start of the Breathwork session, the facilitators check in with each of the breathers. This last-minute connection allows facilitators to respond to any lingering questions or concerns and to bring support if a participant experiences anxiety or strong emotion. Most often, the check-in is a simple warm contact and an offering of well wishes for the breather's inner journey. At times, the presence of the facilitator provides an opportunity for a participant to acknowledge a fear or to talk through some issue that has previously been unexpressed. Rarely, but occasionally, a facilitator will provide extended reassurance for a participant, remaining present through the guided relaxation that marks the beginning of the Breathwork session.

INTEGRATION

As the Grofs refined Holotropic Breathwork, they began to experiment with and incorporate ways to support participants following the Breathwork session. Some of these processes are now formalized as integral parts of any Holotropic Breathwork workshop; others are more emergent and occur naturally within the context of the group setting.

Entered into with intention, these early integrative steps set a trajectory for the participant to further integrate the experience following the end of the workshop.

At the end of the Breathwork session, a facilitator checks in with each of the breathers. Often this is a short but unhurried conversation in which the facilitator ensures that the breather feels steady and grounded and ready to leave the room. The facilitator attends to the quality of each breather's presence: noticing whether each can make eye contact, is aware of his or her own physicality, and can communicate easily and coherently. If there is any discomfort—emotional or physical—the facilitator will explore this with the breather and, if the breather wishes, may engage with energy release work or offer support in some other form such as a hug or light contact, helping the breather open to whatever is emerging and allowing that impulse to come to completion.

At times, a breather takes quite a long time to come out of the Breathwork experience. There can be many reasons for this, and it may be necessary to do some extended work with the participant so he or she can complete the session. More frequently, the breather simply needs a little space and time to reconnect with himself and with the facilitator and his sitter. Like coming out of a deep sleep, there is a process of reorientation that has to happen. For the facilitator, this involves simply being with the breather and, at some point, slowly encouraging connection, to speak a bit about any feelings or sensations or about the experience, and to remember and piece together various moments in the session. For the most part, the facilitator simply listens, focusing on the quality of engagement and gently helping the breather find his or her way back into contact. Often the facilitator may sit close to the breather during this time and may make a gentle physical connection, such as placing a hand on the breather's shoulder. Quite frequently, a breather may ask to be held or may lean into the facilitator for connection and support. For many participants, these intimate, quiet times of connection are an essential and healing first step in the integration process.

Creative Expression

Following the session, we encourage breathers—and sitters if they wish—to draw or paint a mandala, taking time to capture something of their experience while still in a somewhat expanded state of consciousness before the felt sense of the session dissipates, and before getting caught up in conversations or other activities. (See chapter 19 for a comprehensive discussion of mandalas.)

Writing is an option for those who are averse to working visually and can be an effective addition to the creation of a mandala. We encourage participants to explore stream-of-consciousness or free writing rather than trying to analyze their experience at this point.

Sharing with the Group

Usually at the end of the day, when participants have transitioned out of the session and have had some time for personal reflection, quiet conversation, or reconnecting with others over a meal, the group reconvenes to share experiences from that day's Breathwork. This sharing group represents an important moment in the integration process in which each breather reflects upon the most essential aspects of their individual session along with any insights that may be evolving. Depending on the size of the group, this may be a brief summary or a lengthier description of the session. In some cases, we may divide a large group into small subgroups to give time and space for a more in-depth sharing.

During the sharing group, we ask participants to hold an open, nonjudgmental attitude as listeners and not to offer crosstalk, advice, or interpretation to those speaking. For the participant, the potency of this sharing circle lies in speaking about the impact of the Breathwork session, in being listened to and received by the group, in hearing the experiences of others often with recognition or deepening of their own insights, and in a sense of connection with the group's shared experience.

Some of what the participants bring to these sharing groups may already have been spoken about in informal conversations in the group or with their sitting partner. However, the formal structure of the sharing group and the attention and validation of the group presence potentizes and amplifies the impact of the participant's telling. The act of speaking about what arose in the session and of being witnessed and received with compassion and friendship makes it difficult to diminish or dismiss the experience later when the participant leaves the workshop.

The Closing Circle
Just as the workshop began with an opening circle and the creation of the group container, so the workshop ends with a final closing circle. The form of this closing may vary somewhat; however, the usual invitation is for each participant to say something about what he or she is taking away from the overall experience in the Breathwork workshop, as well as any words of closure offered to the group.

There is an art to the closing of a workshop. It takes a clear holding of form and intention to bring the workshop experience to completion in a manner that is empowering for participants and supportive of them as they take leave of the group and move back into their lives. The closing circle is an ending, and at the same time, it can be seen as a beginning. For participants, the ending of the workshop is an opening or reentry into their ongoing journey of self-discovery.

Before the end of the closing circle, we share information about self-care and integration. Self-care is necessary as an immediate support for the process of integration, and good guidance can help to alleviate concern during the days following the workshop. Here are some examples of self-care guidance given to participants:

- After leaving the workshop, be careful when traveling. For example, it is important not to play music if you are driving as it may reactivate the process.
- Get enough rest; this is essential, especially as you may experience emotional highs and lows for some time following the workshop.
- Engage in physical care, such as light exercise, yoga, or massage.

- Spend time in nature.
- Be mindful when tempted to suppress intense feelings, sensations, and thoughts, even if they are uncomfortable.
- Make good choices around food, alcohol, drugs, using electronic media, or participating in social activities.
- Be discerning when speaking about the workshop: respect your own experience.
- Go slowly, especially before acting upon insights that are potentially life changing. Give them space and time to mature.

A useful way to think about integration is as an experiential learning cycle. There are many variations on this model, but at its simplest, it can be described as follows: (1) we have an experience, (2) we reflect on that experience, (3) through an iterative process of reflection we begin to find meaning in the experience and see how this impacts who and how we are, and (4) we begin to apply and experiment with what we are learning.

Many participants will leave a workshop clear about what they are taking away from their session and with the resources and capacity to integrate the experiences into their lives. For others, it may not be so easy or clear. A powerful session can be deeply disorienting and may lead a participant to question beliefs and assumptions that had previously seemed part of their personal identity and understanding of how life works. When this happens, there may be waves of grief, strong emotions, or confusion. As each participant leaves the group, they need assurance that this is not an unusual response to a deep dive into the process of self-exploration. Self-care and using integrative resources can slow and stabilize the intensity of the experience without shutting it down. Each participant must find his or her own pace for digesting what is being learned and healing what needs to be healed.

While we, as facilitators, may offer some follow-up support, in addition to encouraging connection between peers in the Breathwork group, the onus for integration lies with each participant. Offering coherent and substantive guidelines for integration is, therefore, an essential component in the closing of any Holotropic Breathwork event.

Integration can be an ongoing and iterative life practice. While it may take time to find meaning in a specific Breathwork experience, from a larger perspective we might see the experience as just one event in a continuously unfolding journey. As facilitators, we encourage participants to keep the process of integration alive by incorporating practices that support ongoing insight and self-discovery. These practices could include:

- Contemplative practices such as mindfulness meditation
- Expressive practices such as journaling, creating artwork, chanting, or singing
- Physical practices such as walking in nature, dancing, or swimming
- Intellectual or analytical practices such as reading and researching
- Therapeutic practices such as actively inquiring into the experience with the support of a therapist or counsellor or within a sharing group of like-minded friends

CONCLUSION

As a methodology for transformation and healing, Holotropic Breathwork has taken root in many countries around the world. Participants are motivated to attend Holotropic Breathwork events for many and widely varied reasons, including the desire by a growing number of people to understand more about facilitation and support for expanded states of consciousness. In the past decade, there has been an increasing interest in Holotropic Breathwork as a model for alternative and emergent therapeutic practices, especially in the rapidly growing field of psychedelic therapy. The principles inherent in this way of working, including the dedicated attention to preparation and integration as essential aspects of the healing and transformative experience,

Preparation and Integration in Holotropic Breathwork 125

offer a perspective grounded in more than half a century of practice and refinement of theory.

Yet the principles are only as good as the practitioners. The facilitation of Holotropic Breathwork requires a personal, embodied understanding of these principles. We have to practice and integrate our own deep inner work in order to be trustworthy and respectful facilitators. We need each other as colleagues, holding one another accountable and true to the sacred task of facilitating healing and transformation in expanded states of consciousness.

10

Set and Setting, Facilitator Presence, and Bodywork

Holly Harman

The idea that the power to transform comes from within lies at the heart of this work. That we all have an organic wisdom, an inner healing wisdom, and if we create a safe set and setting, our innate wisdom scans our body and psyche and brings to the surface whatever has the most psychodynamic charge at that time. Whether physical, emotional, biographical, perinatal, or transpersonal, this material emerges from our unconscious into consciousness, offering the possibility of transformation and healing.

What can we learn from the holotropic perspective? And how is it applicable to psychotherapeutic use of psychedelics? In this chapter, we'll touch on three areas of fundamental importance: set and setting, facilitator presence, and bodywork.

SET AND SETTING

In the context of Holotropic Breathwork and applicable to all work in expanded states of consciousness, a safe set and setting is both simple

126

and complex. At the forefront of safe set and setting is safety itself. Ethics, support, and respect are also constants in the setting.

What do we mean by safety? On a practical level, it means a space that is dedicated for the duration of the session, in which participants see, know on an intellectual level, and feel within themselves that the environment is a protected and sacred space set aside for the experiences that lie ahead. A space where the participant can get comfortable and where there is *enough*. Enough mats, enough blankets, enough pillows, enough support. Where noise can be made without raising concern and where no one will stop by to see what's happening. Soft lighting, appropriate music, eye masks (optional), and the absence of external distractions (phones, books) all lend themselves to safe set and setting, to this intentionally created journey space in which the participants can open to the deeper, wider realms of consciousness and where sitters and facilitators remain present and available witnesses. This space is a physical space and a metaphysical space. On a meta level, safety has to do with presence, support, and nonjudgment. Safe set and setting are brought to life by the intention we bring to creating this dedicated space with attention to detail, with care, with love, and with respect. So the space has both a tangible physical comfort and on a metaphysical level is steady, gentle, and kind.

For the purpose of these inner journeys, safety also means agreement and understanding about boundaries. In all work in expanded states of consciousness, there are important agreements about the way in which we work. We ask for agreement from all for confidentiality and nonjudgment. We emphasize that each aspect of the way the workshop or experience is set up is a part of the safe set and setting and that preparation, session, and integration are all essential components of the work. In Holotropic Breathwork we also discuss boundaries relating to safety and ethics and use of the word stop.

In this safe set and setting, whether in the context of Holotropic Breathwork or of psychedelic sessions, the participants know both on a cognitive level and from the core of their being that the environment is safe and they are absolutely and fully protected. This external fact of safety and internal sense of safety allow the possibility of connection with our inner landscape and beyond. In Holotropic Breathwork we use our breath and music to connect to these other dimensions within ourselves. When our session begins (and sometimes before), our innate wisdom—our inner healing intelligence—scans our body and psyche and begins to make available whatever has the most psychodynamic charge. Safe set and setting do not mean that sessions will always begin with a sense of calm. What it means is that there is room for calm, room for fear, room for excitement, trepidation, anger, and sadness. The knowledge that the setting is safely held allows a deeper opening to psyche. There is room for the expression of the complete range of the human experience and beyond. Neither does the safe set and setting predict or induce a comfortable or easy inner journey. The inner journey will be whatever it is. The adventure of self-discovery is not for the fainthearted; it is for the courageous.

FACILITATOR AND SITTER PRESENCE

Fundamental to safe set and setting is sitter and facilitator presence, full presence. What do we mean by presence? Physical presence of course, mindful movement in the room, open body language, soft steps, and careful choice of language. Awareness of the breathers' hypersensitivity to sound, to language, and to body language. But there is a depth to presence that extends beyond the physical. Tav Sparks describes this as our *individual atmosphere*. Presence is our ability to show up in mind, body, and soul, free from any agenda other than *being* or *being with*. We can't fake this presence; we can't *do* it. We have to embody it, to *be* it.

The sitters' role is to be a guardian for the duration of the session—present and available. To support the breather to go to the bathroom, to pass them a drink of water or a tissue, to offer them a hand to hold. Sitters respond to their partners' requests; there is no other intervention unless safety or ethics come in to play. The facilitators' role is much the same as that of a sitter, with a few additional layers. In Holotropic

Breathwork sessions, a facilitator will check in with each of the breathers at the beginning and at the end of each session (this could be a chapter in itself!). During the sessions, facilitators are available for support if a breather asks for help or is stuck or needs support to keep from bumping the floor or a wall or bumping into anyone else. Facilitators work with and alongside sitters, respecting their role as guardian.

So, as sitters and facilitators, we are simply present and available for psychological, emotional, or physical support and for safety. That is all. We are not experts, healers, fixers, or doers in these sessions, even if we are any of those things in our lives outside the sessions. We leave our professional trainings outside the journey room and we show up, free from any agenda other than being present and available. Our role is to be there with a presence that is nondirective, without judgment and without prescription. We will have absolutely no idea what is happening for the breather during a session—ever. The facilitator is a supporter, an ally, available to be with whatever emerges from the seeker's session. We have to let go of ego, of any desire to be the director of the breathers' experience. Letting go of any agenda we have other than keeping the breathers safe, being present and available and trusting in the intrinsic wisdom of each individual in the room. Trusting in the power *within*. It cannot be overstated that in this context, in this perspective, the only people we are ever *working on* is ourselves. Whether we are participating in a journey session or whether we are sitting for or facilitating a session.

In the sessions, there is no limit to what breathers may experience. Anyone who has been in a share group after Holotropic Breathwork can testify to the fact that the range of experiences available to us is beyond extraordinary. Biographical, perinatal, transpersonal, archetypal, mythological, numinous, visual, sensory, physical, with story, without story. Many Holotropic Breathwork sessions and psychedelic sessions will be a deep inner journey, requiring nothing from the sitter or facilitators other than a steady and available presence. There may also be sessions where support is requested. In these moments as facilitators, it is essential that we are free of any perception of our own expertise, of any need to be the healer, the fixer, the doer, the rescuer—whatever it is we think we are or could or should be. These are the moments when we check in with ourselves to make certain we have put aside any agenda other than meeting each breather where he or she is and keeping each participant safe. There is simply no other way of being truly present.

If we are to be truly present, mind, body, and soul, we have to be willing to look at our own material; this is what we mean when we talk about working on ourselves. To hold awareness of what is our own process, our need, our history, and our story. To hold awareness and to leave all those parts of us to one side, to put them on the back burner. To know that the desire we suddenly have to cover someone's cold-looking bare toes in a session is our desire, not asked for by the breather. The work required of us here is to notice the desire, notice what is triggered in us, bring awareness to it, and let it go. We might notice that we want to dab away someone's tears that we see as a sign of suffering or pain. We see the tears through our own lenses of perception, but we truly don't have the faintest idea of what the person is experiencing inside. Again, we watch our own need and bring awareness to the situation, acknowledging that something inside us is touched, triggered, or moved. Acknowledging that whatever that is, whatever is happening inside us, is inside *us* and has nothing to do with the breather. It's our work to not act on the impulse, to do *not doing*. This practice of presence is an art, not a science. It's not possible to read about presence and then *do* it. There is no technical manual available that can teach embodying the art of being present. We learn it from the inside, through the experiences of journeying ourselves, through having an honest and rigorous practice of working on our own material and growing the muscle of self-awareness.

BODYWORK

The same can be said for the nuance and subtlety of supporting bodywork. We can read about it, but we simply can't learn it by rote or intellectually. We learn through the experience of expanded states of consciousness, as participants, as sitters, as facilitators. It is another octave in the adventure of self-discovery and is a journey without end.

In Holotropic Breathwork, working with the body, with energy, is known as *focused energy release work.* This aspect of Holotropic Breathwork is a supportive component only. We, as facilitators, are not making an assessment of what the breather needs and then prescribing some form of bodywork based on our perception of the situation— we have no idea what they need. And if we think we do, we have to free ourselves from the illusion so that we can be really present. In the Holotropic Breathwork facilitator training, much of the training is about our own inner travels, our experience of expanded states as a breather, sitter, or facilitator. In addition, there is a module dedicated to the practice of bodywork, and most of us who work in this field have attended the module many times. The teaching is a deep experiential dive into the practice of Holotropic Breathwork with demonstrations and discussion around working with the body. Enough material is always covered, and there is always the sense that we could discuss more.

There are some practical guidelines with bodywork that are quickly and easily taught in the Holotropic Breathwork training. Such as be safe and ethical at all times, protect the head, and follow the breather. There is also the idea that in Holotropic Breathwork, healing can happen through the intensification of symptoms. Breathers may be able to intensify a symptom themselves. If a breather's toe or foot is moving, for example, then intensification of the symptom could be to really let it move more and still more. There are also times where a breather may ask for support, perhaps asking us to press here or push there. We may encourage, in the moment, a fuller expression of whatever is there, whatever is emerging. We can offer support in the form of contact, perhaps asking the breather, "Show me where." We might ask the breather to do something to intensify whatever is happening, to follow the cues given by the body.

Remember, we are not working on anyone, so in the example given here, we would offer support in the form of equal and opposite force where the breather asked us to press or push, really encouraging the breather to intensify from the inside. The breather is leading the process and doing the work. We are following, supporting the breather with a practice of not being the doer, with a practice of doing *not doing.* We are with the breather, present and available, offering support, support, support. The art of facilitator or sitter presence in the context of bodywork is simply about being with the breather and supporting the emergence of whatever is there without the need for intellectual understanding or framework. Supporting the emergence of whatever comes, no matter how simple or bizarre it seems. The following scenario is just one example of how we might support working with energy intensification or release.

> *In a Holotropic Breathwork workshop, a breather, let's call him Richard, asked for some support with his body during the session. Richard had been working on his own body during the session—holding his foot for a while, pressing here and there on his body, shaking, making sounds, and occasionally shouting. When he first asked for support, he placed my hands here and there, seemingly where he had earlier been working on his own body. He continued to make sounds while I was supporting him, sometimes shouting, sometimes saying words that were intelligible, sometimes saying words that weren't. Periodically, he would move my hands to a different spot—his shoulder, his eyebrow—or would tell me where he wanted some support. After some time, he sat up, still with his eyeshade on, and asked me to sit beside him with my arm around his shoulder. I followed his request, and not even a moment later, he pulled me around to his back so that I was holding him from behind. He clasped my hands in his and rested them on his belly. And he became very quiet and very still. We stayed in this position for a while, until he eventually let go of my hands, nodded his head, gave me a thumb's up, and lay back down. All the while, his sitter had been available and present without being intrusive. I moved away from Richard and sat quietly for a while until it seemed clear that, for now at least, no more support was needed from the outside. At the end*

of the session, I checked in with him to see how he was doing both physically and emotionally. He had a long and beautiful story to share about his experience, a part of which was that in his daily life he had never had the experience of "having someone at my back." He described how having this physical experience of someone at his back in his session had led to important insights about his early life, what he described as an enlightened perspective.

In a Holotropic Breathwork session, there is also the possibility of gentle, physical contact. Perhaps in this scenario the breather simply reaches out for a hand to hold and then finds that their body wants a little more contact or simply to be held. There may be a story that the breather is aware of, such as earlier traumas, or there may be no known story at all. Facilitator and sitter presence in this situation is gentle, ethical (as always), kind, and patient. Any body movements on the part of the facilitator or sitter would be gentle and slow. This space can feel intensely sensitive for the breather: our breath near the breather's face can feel like a hurricane; a gentle adjustment to get ourselves comfortable can feel like a huge disturbance or wave of energy. We are mindful with our bodies, gentle with our presence, soft if using our voice. As facilitators, we get our bodies as comfortable as we possibly can and hunker down for the long haul. We may be there for minutes or for much longer. We have absolutely no idea. We're simply meeting each breather where he or she is, meeting the call for contact and staying until the breather gives an indication otherwise either verbally or with a gesture. It may be that the breather has a sitter in contact on one side and a facilitator on the other. And when that happens, we may check in softly, gently with words as simple as, "How are you doing?"

This type of contact is illustrated with an example from a session I was facilitating.

A breather, let's call her Alice, began her session by rolling gently from side to side. Alice's sitter was seated beside her with his body close enough for her to feel if she moved much beyond her mat but far enough away not to interrupt or direct her experience in any way.

After a while, the rolling became more active, and I sat down, very gently, on the other side of Alice, still allowing her the space to move but ready to offer support or cushions for her body to meet if needed. As I sat close, Alice started to move much more energetically, and keeping in mind the golden rule—protect the head—I moved a soft cushion to the space beside her mat where her head would land if it came off her mat and onto the floor. In the second that I was placing the cushion there beside her, Alice flipped her head from side to side in a strong movement and her head came to rest in the palm of my hand. Alice nestled her head further onto my hand and moved her body closer to mine so that much of our bodies were in contact, and there we stayed, still as can be, for the remaining two or three hours of the session. When the music stopped, we all stayed exactly as we were. In Holotropic Breathwork sessions, music plays an important support role; the music coming to an end is an indication that the session is coming to an end, but some people will complete a session before the music stops, some as the music stops, and some may remain in process for longer.

Some time after the music stopped, Alice moved her body, very slightly, and started talking. Slowly. Softly. She asked why we (her sitter and I) had stayed with her all that time and went on to talk about having a sense that in her life she was always the caregiver, both for her family and for her friends. She talked about having a sense that no one really noticed how she was doing. She was surprised that we had noticed her body moving and were there to support her and even more surprised that we stayed. Alice described having the sense that this experience was the first time in her adult life that she felt she mattered enough. She tracked back through her adult life, all the way back through her adolescence to her childhood, describing major events and her sense of experiencing them alone. Not mattering enough to those around her. She wept as she spoke. Her sitter and I stayed close, saying very little, just listening and acknowledging what she was saying with the occasional nonverbal sound mmm or an encouraging, open question. Following her, supporting her, with respect, respect, respect.

After some time, perhaps another hour or so, Alice wanted to move her body. She sat up, had a sip of water, and lifted her eyeshade. Alice looked us both in the eyes, one at a time, each time holding our gaze for a while. She wept some more, talked some more about her life, and eventually felt it was time to close the session. We spent some time checking in with her about how her body was doing and how she felt emotionally. She took her time to move from lying down, to sitting, to standing up and went, with her sitter, to draw a mandala. Her sharing in the group that evening was deeply moving.

There is an ocean to be explored and discussed in the domain of bodywork or focused energy release work. These short and simple examples are just the very the tip of an enormous iceberg. There are as many possible scenarios as there are grains of sand in a desert, and there are as many styles of facilitation as there are facilitators. In the holotropic perspective, there is emphasis again and again on the importance of being fully present and available, of only ever working on ourselves. We could describe the three most important things after presence, safety, and ethics as support, support, support. And the next three most important things as respect, respect, respect.

EXPERIENCING
THE HOLOTROPIC SPACE

What is the difference between Holotropic Breathwork and therapy? Holotropic Breathwork is without doubt therapeutic, but it is not, in and of itself, a therapy. In Holotropic Breathwork, the breathers are their own experts; the breath, the music, the set and setting create a space in which each individual's organic wisdom directs his experience from within. It is empowering. There is a distinct differentiation between a prescriptive model, such as the medical model or an expert-client relationship, and the holotropic perspective, in which we trust in the inner healing wisdom of each individual.

There are many similarities between the experience of Holotropic Breathwork and the experience of psychedelics, and there are some distinct differences. Holotropic Breathwork sessions are typically around three hours long. Each breather has a sitter, and in addition, certified facilitators are present and available. Psychedelic sessions can be much longer than three hours, and this is an important consideration when thinking about sitting or facilitating a psychedelic session. How long can one person sit for, and be present for, the experiencer? There will be times during a long session when a sitter needs food, to go to the bathroom, or simply to take a break. So, it is essential to consider how many people journey with a substance and how many sit or facilitate the session. In Holotropic Breathwork sessions, facilitators switch out with sitters who need a bathroom break so that breathers are never alone. In psychedelic sessions, there may be a different setup with ratios of available presence, but the same principle would apply: that the seeker or experiencer is never left alone; a supportive presence is always available.

In my experience of psychedelic sessions in a clinical trial, bodywork was very rarely required. Beyond help with eating, drinking, and going to the bathroom, occasionally a participant would ask for a hand to hold or for reassurance that support was available, but there was not the intensity of physical activity that we often encounter in Holotropic Breathwork.

Another obvious difference between Holotropic Breathwork and psychedelics is that during a Holotropic Breathwork session there is the possibility of the breather stopping the session at any time if the experience becomes overwhelming. In fact, this scenario seems to be extremely rare. There are times where a breather may say, "I can't do this. It's too much!" The facilitator would then offer, "Remember, you can say stop," and invariably the breather will respond with something like, "No, no, I have to do this." In Holotropic Breathwork sessions, the way out very often seems to be through, and this is something that seems to be innately understood. But if the process ever is too much, and the breather does want to stop, she can open her eyes and can soon reorient to a more familiar state of consciousness. There may be intense emotions or a sense of confusion for a while, but it is possible to return to ordinary consciousness within a relatively short space of time. This contrasts with a psychedelic session where there is no natural way of terminating the experience before its natural conclusion.

What can we learn from the Holotropic Breathwork perspective? Preparation is very important, as is establishing a safe set and setting. Preparation before the session followed by integration after the session forms the container for the work. But it is the facilitator or sitter presence—true embodied *presence,* free from any agenda other than *being* or *being with*—that is one of the greatest gifts of the holotropic perspective.

11

Holotropic Breathwork and MDMA-Assisted Psychotherapy with Trauma Survivors

Ingrid Pacey

As a psychiatrist who is also a woman, I stumbled into a practice that focused on female trauma survivors early in my forty-year career, mainly because they were the patients referred to me. These women arrived in my office with all sorts of diagnoses, but as we went deeper into their personal histories, sexual abuse kept coming up, something for which my psychiatric training had not prepared me.

Talk therapy certainly helped, but unless they were able to process their trauma, their healing could only progress so far. Symptoms might be managed for some time, but they recurred or new symptoms emerged. Talk therapy eventually brought these women to the edge of overwhelming fear, and transcending these barriers could take many years. Healing seemed inaccessible through the usual Western mind-based psychiatric approaches, and trauma continued to limit the ability of these clients to live life fully, without chronic anxiety.

No one came to me saying they wished to heal their PTSD or

process the lingering impact of childhood abuse. Instead, they came to my practice with depression, in the throes of marital breakdown, or with anxiety disorders. Many had already seen other psychiatrists or psychologists or both. In other words, the effects of trauma were chronically misdiagnosed. This continues to be true today, despite the now widespread recognition within the psychiatric community that much of psychiatric illness is trauma based. This reality should serve as a warning to therapists who begin to offer expanded state treatments: it is impossible to predict what will emerge.

A safe, supportive environment, thorough assessment and preparation, and ongoing therapeutic follow-up are critical. Offered in conjunction with long-term, one-on-one psychotherapy, therapy involving the use of nonordinary states of consciousness opens up new realms of possibility for healing. But these sessions cannot take the place of long-term work. On their own, without integration, these sessions can be dangerous, leaving the client destabilized and even suicidal. This is especially true for individuals who have experienced early trauma.

A WAY FORWARD

In 1986, I participated in a five-day Holotropic Breathwork workshop with Stanislav and Christina Grof. The enormity and depth of my own experience, along with the tremendous healing power I could sense in this method, changed the arc of my career. I completed the Grof Transpersonal Training between 1987 and 1990 and began to lead monthly Breathwork groups with my partner, Wendy Barrett, a psychotherapist who focused on body-based treatments. These trauma groups had between sixteen and twenty-four participants, almost all women. Some groups were limited to participants committed to attending over an extended period; some were open so new people could also attend. We facilitated groups from 1990 to 2004.

Wendy and I offered Holotropic Breathwork sessions as part of our treatment of psychiatric patients, most with complex trauma. Between monthly group sessions, I saw my clients, and Wendy saw hers. Some of the women saw other therapists, and we were all in communication. The Breathwork group became part of the ongoing process of therapy, and each session an individual took part deepened her process. The love, mutual support, and healing in these sessions were so powerful it was easy to sense that a fundamentally transformative process was underway for participants. In a conversation I had with the Buddhist mindfulness teacher Jack Kornfield, he said that he saw providing Holotropic Breathwork as a calling. It felt that way to both Wendy and me.

During the sessions, the women paired off, with one being the sitter and the other the breather. Then they'd swap roles, so both had the experience of being the regressed and needy breather and of being the sitter, who used her awareness, strength, and warmth to sense what was wanted or needed by the breather and gave it to her in a way that respected the other's boundaries. The learning was phenomenal and could translate into everyday life in relationships, such as sitting with a distressed friend or with someone who is very ill or dying.

For many of these women, the Breathwork group was their first experience of safety and support in a group and of the one-on-one experience of working with a safe partner. In the sessions, the two women, sitter and breather, were often holding each other by the third hour—this physical warmth that could be provided safely in this setting but usually not during individual therapy in an office. There is so much healing in that simple, body-to-body holding—an out-in-the-open, safe physical connection that is not sexualized. The energy of the group is a significant element in the intensity of the experience, often catalyzing the participant's experience.

Organically, women felt the benefits, and some began to come each time we offered a group session. Others came at varying intervals that were appropriate for them. Most were between thirty and sixty years old, had had some psychotherapy before, and had struggled with their symptoms for years. They were all psychologically aware and had the language to talk about what was going on for them. About half were aware of their histories of sexual abuse when they began the groups; for the rest, these memories emerged over the course of their treatment.

It's vital for Holotropic Breathwork facilitators with little previous experience of working experientially with trauma survivors to know how to approach someone who is screaming or cringing under a blanket; knowing what to do can bring the traumatic event fully into the present moment. Similarly, trauma can be relived fully with MDMA-assisted psychotherapy. Physically, the participant may enact the extent of the terror, torture, or abuse she experienced. As therapists, the challenge is knowing how to be sensitive to her experience and to realize that the terror emerging is real to that person's experience. It's critical to be cautious and to give the person freedom to express and yet remain supportive emotionally and physically, with attention to boundaries.

Under any circumstances, Holotropic Breathwork is a psychospiritual experience. Having a single Breathwork experience can also be remarkable and important and needs to be integrated afterward. People in an expanded state must be treated with respect and delicacy. One group participant, a man who had been a minister, said that the Breathwork session was probably the most religious experience he'd ever had. It's therefore crucial that therapists who work with clients in expanded states have personal experience in these states themselves.

RELEASING TRAUMA FROM THE BODY

In the following stories, two women had profound experiences of releasing trauma through their bodies.

Bess, a woman in her thirties, came from a small town in northern Canada. She was referred to me as she was struggling after leaving an abusive relationship. She lived alone with her five-year-old son.

Bess's mother had had an affair and became pregnant with a man who was black, a conductor on the railway. Bess was born with dark skin, dark eyes, and black hair, yet her mother denied that she was any different from her other children, who were white skinned, blue eyed, and fair haired. She insisted that everyone deny that Bess was a child of a different color. She was cruel and abusive to Bess, harshly scrubbing her skin to make it "clean," leaving her outside in the cold of the harsh winter, and locking her in her room for hours.

In the Breathwork groups, as these experiences started emerging, Bess had an intense sensation of being cold. We wrapped her in blankets, and her sitters held her. She would warm up briefly, but when she came to the next group, she was colder still. We probably had four groups where, in each of them, she became icy cold. No matter how many blankets she had or how much her sitters held her or rubbed her feet—everything a mother would do to help a child feel warm—nothing was shifting. Finally, during a session, I said, "Bess, I don't think this is just about physical coldness. I think it's the emotional coldness you grew up with as well." She burst into tears and felt the deep emotional pain of rejection and abandonment. The next group was quite different, and Bess was able to go on and process how her family had treated her.

Bess had memories of being left in a stroller out in the northern winter and of being cold, but without emotion or physical sensation. In Breathwork, once she got the actual feeling of the cold, she was able to shift into the bigger pain, the emotional coldness in which she grew up. We had talked about it in the office setting, but there was no way there for it to shift. In Breathwork, because we knew her and were able to track her experiences through consecutive sessions, this awareness could evolve.

Bess's story is an example of one of the tenets of Holotropic Breathwork: trust the process and the wisdom of the inner healer. For many women, the beginning of an issue, experience, or memory would emerge initially in Breathwork or traditional psychotherapy. There would be feelings and body sensations that occurred without explanation. It required an expanded state of consciousness in the safety of the group to be able to get to such painful memories.

Tracy, a librarian in her fifties, knew that she'd been sexually abused. She had been in therapy for a long time but had remained very depressed. During the first two years of the Breathwork process, she relived her birth process and infancy. All she wanted to do was get onto her hands and knees and bang her head against a pillow. Sometimes she wanted comfort; sometimes she didn't. However, as time went on, she felt lighter, less depressed. She felt better. She functioned better. She started new relationships. Although it looked like she was doing the same thing all the time without being able to verbalize what it was about, life improved for her. Because she was able to relive her early life in a safe, supported environment, she could incorporate that experience. We had been confused by her process, wondering if we should interfere in some way in her repetitive actions. Fortunately, we did not, and her life changed.

These Breathwork participants made gargantuan leaps as they came to understand themselves and their trauma in a far greater context. Our experience has been that both healers and participants who have experienced Breathwork find that a deep, intrinsic healing force is activated. Whatever the content of the experience, going to deeper realms of the personal and collective unconscious leads to healing and transformation.

EXPANDED STATES AS PATHWAYS FOR TRANSFORMATIVE HEALING

It is estimated that 30 to 50 percent of women and 10 to 20 percent of men have experienced sexual abuse. Holotropic Breathwork and MDMA treatment, used as part of ongoing, one-on-one psychotherapy, have been and continue to be a way forward for these individuals. Trauma survivors are supported in processing the original experiences and moving on toward a place of openness, grace, and acceptance.

For a lot of people, Breathwork, which entails overbreathing, is very physical. As dissociation begins to break down, the individual may first get a picture, a smell, an emotion, or a body posture. During Breathwork, one woman first smelled leather and eventually realized that the abuse she experienced as a child happened in a stable where saddles were mended. Another saw herself as an infant lying terrified in a cot, with a curtain blowing in front of a window beside her. Later, her mother told her that a drunken man leaving a pub next door had climbed into her room through an open window and abused her. Sometimes a movement that makes no sense initially, such as feeling one's arm being pulled, leads to the memory of being grabbed and abused.

Breathwork can bring awareness to places of physical tension in the body; sometimes the breather has an overwhelming sensation of being completely constrained. These sensations of tension and constraint may be specific to early events and abuse, or they may relate to unconscious memories of the birth process itself. Traditional psychotherapy is a verbal, intellectual process, with the client sitting across from the therapist. For someone in the throes of strong emotion, it's an environment that often leads to feeling unsupported, which leads to reined-in feelings and emotional shutdown. In Breathwork, on the other hand, clients are invited to be as physical and emotional as they want to be.

Anne, age forty, came to me because, although she was professionally and socially successful, she was often anxious. She was inwardly unhappy and uncomfortable. Extremely bright and personable, she was respected and rapidly promoted in her field. At the same time, the men with whom she formed relationships were often demeaning to her, and one was physically violent. Her outer persona was vibrant and successful; inside, her self-esteem was low. Her initial focus was healing from the constraints, oppression, and shaming she had experienced with her parents and their religious order. Her mother had been emotionally cold and limited by her severe arthritis in how much she could hold her children. Anne remembered being beaten by her father and sitting in religious services where, even as a very small child, she was pinched and shamed if she moved. She made progress in our work together, but it was slow, and she continued to struggle.

A lot of Anne's initial Breathwork was without a storyline: just hitting, pounding, pushing, and weeping. During the sessions, she had vivid memories of being beaten by her father, hiding from him, being found. But, slowly, a whole new sense of aliveness started to awaken in her body. While her sessions still began with intensely physical experiences of pushing off oppressors, at a certain point in the work, after about a year, she would emerge into a beautiful, spiritual state. She felt ecstatic. She reported being filled with light and would reach up as if the whole universe were opening to her. It was enormously healing. Soon, Anne changed her work and started her own consulting firm. Her life was moving in a positive direction, and her therapy ended for a while.

Many years later, Anne came back to therapy. She was in a new relationship, and she and her partner were locked in power struggles. She felt that things still weren't right.

By this time, I was the lead investigator in a research study into the potential of MDMA-assisted psychotherapy for the treatment of trauma survivors. Through MAPS (Multidisciplinary Association for Psychedelic Science), I became the principal investigator and therapist for the Phase 2 MDMA-assisted psychotherapy research study for treatment resistant PTSD in Vancouver. The preparation for this started in 2009; we began working with subjects in 2013. I could immediately see the potential benefits and also that my experience in Holotropic Breathwork with trauma survivors was an excellent training ground for MDMA therapy. As an empathogen, MDMA increases levels of trust and feelings of safety, which is especially powerful in individuals who have been traumatized by other people. It also diminishes fear and allows ongoing exploration of traumatic events without the person being overwhelmed.

Alongside her psychotherapy with me, Anne participated in three sessions of MDMA-assisted psychotherapy. After Breathwork sessions, everyone in the group drew mandala art. Years before, Anne had drawn an infant with a terrified, open mouth and a severe rash on its cheek. In the expanded state created by MDMA, Anne's mind could safely access and confront deeply buried memories of being sexually abused by her grandfather when she was an infant. (He died when she was six.) The specific memory she first recalled had to do with oral rape, which connected to the picture she had drawn of an infant with a rash on her cheek. During the earlier Breathwork, the image had come to her, but fear prevented her from going deeper and completing the memory. With MDMA, the full experience came to her. As in the Breathwork experience, Anne engaged in a lot of physical expression, pushing away her abuser and screaming at him. With the aid of the MDMA, Anne accessed the rest of the story.

Today, after processing those deeply dissociated memories in therapy, Anne feels more settled and peaceful. Until the MDMA sessions, she experienced ongoing jaw pain and periods in which her chin spontaneously started to tremble. Jaw tension had cracked her teeth, and she had to have restorative dental work. All of her intense facial tension has now disappeared. Breathwork and MDMA sessions enabled Anne to progressively recover and process early abuse memories that, although walled off from her consciousness, had influenced her emotions, choices, and health.

ONGOING SUPPORT FOR PARTICIPANTS

We found that, for most of the women, staying with the group for about three years allowed them to work through their fear, shame, and depression and to a considerable resolution of their PTSD. Insomnia and other symptoms slowly resolved. They required ongoing follow-up for a time, but afterward, their symptoms were minimal and easily managed. They were able to live full lives.

Because the groups were ongoing, the women got to know one another well. We were able to create an atmosphere in which people stayed kind and sensitive to each other. They understood their vulnerability and learned a lot from it; their ability to trust grew and was supported. In their lives outside the group, they gradually became less anxious. By the end of the three years, most of them felt much more grounded and positive. They had much more confidence in knowing their own feelings and were better able to tolerate discomfort. If they were triggered, they knew what the trigger was and that they were having a flashback. They didn't go into an anxiety state or dissociate. We had three cohorts of women who completed this cycle.

Breathwork empowers participants, revealing the ability of the psyche to self-heal and putting suffering into a much larger, universal context. Many of the women in the groups knew no one else who had been sexually abused as a child, whereas in the groups they were surrounded and supported by other women who had undergone similar trauma. They learned they were not alone, and the shame they felt shifted to the perpetrator. Their perception changed from "Why did that happen to me? What did I do?" to "I was only a child; it was not my fault. Now I understand why my life has been so difficult."

Participants reported a greater range of emotion. Anne, for example, was kind but emotionally very guarded. Afterward, it was as if she filled an inner void so that her personality was grounded in a feeling of being a solid, able person. The kindness and generosity that she felt was then transmitted to others as warmth. First, with Holotropic Breathwork and then with MDMA, as she resolved deeper levels of fear, body shame, self-hatred, and doubt, she became more open and less guarded.

BREATHWORK VERSUS MDMA SESSIONS

In Breathwork, the body and the breath are the anchors for the experience. Overbreathing and powerful music start the process, as the participants lie on mats and go inward to follow their own inner compasses. Participants know that if they stop breathing fast, open their eyes, and sit up, they can move out of the expanded state of consciousness. Integration starts with mandala drawing followed by a group sharing session.

In MDMA sessions, the medicine is the agent creating the expanded state; the facilitators are the anchors who can direct the participant back toward the current reality of where she is and what is happening, if necessary. As Albert Hofmann and Stanislav Grof realized with their first LSD experiences, they were along for the "ride" for the duration of the medicine's effect. The expanded state of consciousness continues until the medicine is metabolized and inactive.

MDMA sessions can be difficult and painful for a trauma survivor, but there are times when her psyche shifts and she becomes aware that she is safe in the moment and that she survived it all, then and now. There might be periods of openness in which she can trust the therapists more than she has ever trusted anyone in her life before. Two of my clients reached places of extreme terror in Breathwork and years later had the opportunity to have three sessions with MDMA. During Breathwork, one moved into spiritual experiences, while the other ran out of the room and avoided further Breathwork altogether. MDMA diminished the fears of both clients, and they were able to tolerate learning the rest of their abuse history and processing it.

In the group room after Holotropic Breathwork sessions, the environment becomes informal as people draw and quietly chat. There is laughter, warmth, cups of tea, juice. In the MDMA session, the participant is lying down with the therapists close beside her or on either side. Again, there is an informality as we listen, comfort, move closer at times to hold the client or do bodywork. Transference is directed toward the therapists and is powerful because of the increased sense of trust induced by MDMA. The client often requires holding, whether it's for two minutes or an hour. Holding also occurs in Breathwork, but the sitter usually provides this care, and it takes place in the open, in the group. With MDMA, it is the therapists doing the holding in a private context. Best practice in the research so far has been to have cotherapists in the MDMA session, usually a woman and a man but not necessarily. Therapy builds an intimacy, but a different kind of transference develops with the sensations of love and openness engendered by MDMA and by the physical contact. Because of this intense level of transference, MDMA therapy demands a context and structure where therapists understand transference. Boundaries need to be clear and not violated, especially sexual boundaries.

PREPARING THE THERAPIST

By the time Wendy and I came to expanded consciousness therapy, we were mature therapists in our forties. We had both done therapeutic work ourselves. Together, we knew a lot about what bodies can go through in working through trauma and the role of the body in healing. Through the three years of training with Grof, I had about forty sessions myself and had led some groups. I think it was clear to our clients that we weren't going to be horrified by or judgmental about anything they told us; we were totally there to support them through all the aspects of their stories as they knew them and as they emerged.

I believe therapists have to have that level of nonjudging, nonshaming acceptance as each client sorts out her story as different parts of her story emerge and the client comes to understand the events with more perspective over time. Being willing to listen, accept the process, and accept all of the emerging content is critical.

The Duty of Care

The opening up of traumatic memories underlines the importance of immediate follow-up. You can't say, "Come back in a week." Daily follow-up by telephone, or in person if necessary, should start the next day. Ongoing integration and further learning go on for some time and need to be supported in therapy depending on the needs of the client.

The emergence of traumatic material can be very powerful and sudden, e.g., unsuspected sadistic abuse, in expanded consciousness therapy. There needs to be close attention and support to avoid retraumatization or acting-out.

Expanded Consciousness and the Body

It is of vital importance that the therapist has an understanding of the role of the body in holding the trauma history and in healing physical and emotional symptoms. Training and personal experience with bodywork are necessary for therapists doing this work. Not everyone undergoing MDMA or Breathwork has a physical process, but when it arises, the therapist must know how to work with it to move the process forward.

A therapist without some knowledge of healing on a body level might not understand that release can come with violent shaking, a release similar to that experienced after the body has "frozen" during a terrifying experience. With training, one learns methods of helping the person get through this experience; remaining calm oneself while reassuring the client that the shaking is safe and part of the healing and suggesting ways to work with it. The client may be encouraged to amplify the movements, even hitting and kicking into cushions—taking some control of what her body is doing and no longer feeling victimized by it.

In both Holotropic Breathwork and MDMA therapy, participants are empowered through realizing their true history, processing shame and guilt, and releasing pain and anxiety from the body and psyche. These modalities where expanded states of consciousness are integrated with psychotherapy offer trauma survivors a powerful way to work through the painful and terrifying events of their childhoods at the hands of those who should have loved and protected them. They also offer a reparative experience of safety and love.

Both modalities, Holotropic Breathwork and MDMA-assisted psychotherapy, offer similar and different aspects of expended consciousness therapy. Hopefully one day we will have therapeutic settings where both can be offered for different stages of therapy.

12

Cultivating Inner Healing Intelligence through MDMA-Assisted Psychotherapy

Shannon Carlin

INNER HEALING INTELLIGENCE

Just as a seed has within it the knowledge to grow, humans have an innate capacity to heal. Both healing and growth are supported by environmental conditions that promote safety and nourishment. When help is needed to create such an environment, psychotherapy, like the shelter of a greenhouse, provides a container conducive to healing.

Inner healing intelligence refers to the knowledge and power within oneself to move toward wholeness and well-being. The term stems from a concept described by Carl Jung and later adopted by Stanislav Grof:

> Jung saw the task of the therapist in helping to establish a dynamic interaction between the client's conscious ego and the Self, a higher aspect of the client's personality; this interaction takes the form of a dialectic exchange using the language of symbols. The healing then comes from the collective unconscious and it is guided by an inner

intelligence whose immense wisdom surpasses the knowledge of any individual therapist or therapeutic school. This is the essence of what Jung called the individuation process (Grof 1996, 516).

There are many terms that could be used to describe an inner source of healing. Various cultures and paradigms articulate these concepts in different ways: some might reference spirit, truth, unity, or source, and there are many other terms that carry similar meaning. I once heard a participant call it the inner champion, as she grappled with its destructive counterpart, the inner critic. In the Multidisciplinary Association for Psychedelic Studies (MAPS) modality of MDMA-assisted psychotherapy, we adopt the phrase *inner healing intelligence* and similar terms such as *inner healer, deep knowing, innate wisdom*. If you connect with the concept of an intrinsic ability to heal and grow yourself, I encourage you to consider any other name you like and to think of that name as you read on.

Given a nourishing environment, rich soil, water, air, and light, a seed will naturally develop into a mature and thriving plant. It will develop roots, establishing the ability to take in nutrients and water from the soil and stay grounded in the midst of erosion. Leaves develop to absorb energy from sunlight and carbon dioxide from air so that the plant can initiate photosynthesis and transform these ingredients into food. So long as the plant continues to receive what it needs from the environment, it will grow to full capacity, expressing its intrinsic qualities.

When the environment does not provide what is necessary, a plant demonstrates signs of poor health: wilting leaves, pale color, or blossom rot. If the conditions aren't adjusted, the plant's health continues to deteriorate as it strives for survival. If the outside environment is unable to provide what the plant needs, a greenhouse can offer shelter—respite from extreme temperatures and protection from the elements. The conditions inside the greenhouse are set specifically for the plant it intends to serve. The sanctuary of the greenhouse demonstrates the importance of the setting, analogous to the care put into creating a therapeutic environment for healing trauma.

MDMA-ASSISTED PSYCHOTHERAPY

MDMA-assisted psychotherapy aims to establish a sanctuary for healing, with conditions that empower a person in deepening connection with their own inner healing intelligence. Participants in an MDMA-assisted psychotherapy protocol are cared for by two therapists who work together as a cotherapy team throughout the treatment program. The therapeutic relationship is co-created among participant and therapists. The therapeutic container is built upon alliance, safety, and support and customized to the unique identity and needs of the participant. The course of treatment is designed to provide the time and space necessary to engage in a deep healing process: the MDMA sessions are eight hours long, preceded by a preparation phase and followed by several integration sessions. The MDMA molecule itself serves as an incredible resource and catalyst as it acts to promote self-empathy and self-compassion and reduces fear. Together, these elements make up the greenhouse for healing and growth in the modality of MDMA-assisted psychotherapy.

Therapists and participant collaborate to identify and engage resources and support systems that will assist the participant in moving through the trauma healing process. Throughout the treatment, therapists prompt the participant to reach for internal resources, validating the participant's strengths and capability while reinforcing that the therapists are there to support the developing process. There are infinite resources available, internal and external, such as connection with the breath, spiritual beliefs, ancestors, a role model, asking for and receiving help, visualization, imagining a healed and whole self, music, art, therapeutic relationship, respectful attentiveness from the therapists, asking to hold the therapist's hand during the session, anxiolytic and prosocial effects of MDMA, self-compassion, empathy, and hope.

The inner healing intelligence is at the forefront of the impetus for change, and the therapists encourage the participant to consider, in ways and words that make sense to her, that she has within her the wisdom and ability to heal. Sadly, we don't all know our own ability and strength; faith in ourselves must be cultivated. Traumatic experiences can further erode belief in oneself, trust in others, and faith in humanity. So it is important that therapists express a belief in and commitment to the participant's innate wisdom and ability to heal. Therapists inquire about the participant's beliefs and interpretations and explore ways they can connect with her inner healing intelligence. For example, she may locate a place in her body where she experiences inner wisdom, listen for different voices and perspectives internally and be curious about them, make an art piece that represents her inner healing wisdom, write a letter to the inner healer, or from the inner healer.

The process of MDMA-assisted psychotherapy is described as inner directed, meaning that the content, focus, pace, and direction of the session is informed primarily by the participant's inner healing intelligence. The participant is encouraged to do what feels right. In any given moment that may be: talking, not talking, moving their body, lying down, sitting up, singing, allowing tears to come, yelling, turning toward traumatic memory, talking about something happy, taking a break. The therapists invite the participant to notice if there is anything he is avoiding and to be curious about that, without judgment. There is no pressure to talk about the trauma at any particular time or order. However, therapists *do* obtain the participant's permission in advance to check in during the MDMA session if several hours have passed and he hasn't brought up the trauma already, with the intention of supporting the participant in addressing the trauma so that he can experience healing from it. This is rarely necessary. Almost always the participant brings up the trauma during the session when he is ready.

In communicating about trusting the process, therapists may say something like:

> We are here to support you and help you when you need it. We trust your process and encourage you to do the same. You are resilient, motivated, and wise. If you come to a place of confusion or feel overwhelmed, please let us know; we are here with you. At that point, we encourage you to take a few breaths, slow down if possible, and

see if you can get in touch with the part of you connected to insight and clarity. In this work, you may find that, more often than not, deep down and with a little support and patience, it will become clear what to do or to allow to happen, and you will find many of the answers you seek. A large part of this work is connecting to that place of inner knowing; it's not easy and there's no one right way to do it. We are here to navigate the process with you.

Therapists practice beginner's mind, a stance of open curiosity. They do not guide the session in a particular direction; they work to set aside any agendas they may have. Likewise, therapists support the participant in cultivating open curiosity and trust in the process, connection with internal sources of wisdom, and, when needed, assistance in navigating and processing experiences as they arise. Therapists validate the participant's experience as it unfolds. This nondirective openness is counterbalanced with the active support therapists provide when ensuring participant safety and well-being. It can be challenging for a therapist to be nondirective. Typically, we want to *do* something to help, but an overly active therapist could inadvertently bypass or overpower the participant's own inner healing intelligence, robbing her of the experience of becoming empowered herself. Therapists who help their clients establish a deep connection with their inner guide offer a tremendous gift, one that endures as they become increasingly able to apply their own wisdom to life's myriad challenges.

A Specific MDMA-Assisted Psychotherapy Treatment Program

In the MAPS MDMA-assisted psychotherapy protocols, the two cotherapists are supported by a larger treatment team, comprised of medical doctors, attendants, and a coordinator. The protocol affords substantial time for participants to work through trauma. The protocol begins with three ninety-minute preparation sessions; the MDMA-assisted psychotherapy sessions last eight hours, each followed by three ninety-minute integration sessions. During the preparation phase, the cotherapists and the participant discuss the participant's experience of trauma and orient to the process of the upcoming MDMA-assisted psychotherapy session. Emphasis is placed on the participant's autonomy, choice, and direction. While there are pieces of information and questions the therapists are required to review, especially in the preparation phase, the participant determines what level of detail he shares about his trauma and generally what he would like to focus on during open discussion.

On the morning of the MDMA-assisted psychotherapy session, a designated friend or family member brings the participant to the treatment site. Therapy rooms are set up to be warm and welcoming; decorated with art, soft lighting, and a couch or futon made up with blankets and pillows for sitting or reclining. Music is played during the session to support the process. Therapists have hydrating beverages and snacks available for the participant. The intention is that the participant can experience this setting as a haven, a retreat space prepared for the healing process.

MDMA-assisted psychotherapy sessions are designed to allow sufficient time for the MDMA to take full effect and eventually subside. An optional supplemental dose, 50 percent of the original dose, is offered an hour and a half into the therapy session. The supplemental dose acts to prolong the effects of MDMA and is offered to support further processing, though it is not always necessary and the decision to take the supplemental dose is up to the participant. Many participants do choose to take the supplemental dose, although some do not. The duration of the MDMA session allows the participant to move through her process free from pressure to rush; it takes time to do deep healing work. It is powerful to communicate "There's time for you, there's time now for your healing process."

In the clinical trials, participants usually stay overnight at the treatment site following each MDMA-assisted psychotherapy session. They are cared for by a night attendant, who delivers dinner, stays on site, and is available for conversation if the participant wants that. The participant has an opportunity to vet the person who will be her night attendant and to be introduced in advance. Therapists remain on call overnight in case additional support is needed. The participant is encouraged to rest and invited to browse the collection of books, make use of the art supplies, journal, or listen to music. The next morning the night attendant delivers breakfast and the therapists return to the site for the first of three integration sessions before the participant's friend or family member takes her home. A full course of treatment includes three MDMA-assisted psychotherapy sessions, and forty-two hours of psychotherapy in total. The protocol is designed to provide participants with the space and time they need for healing.

The results of MAPS's six Phase 2 clinical trials of MDMA-assisted psychotherapy for chronic, treatment-resistant PTSD show that one to two months after two experimental sessions, 54.2 percent of participants in the active group (n = 72) no longer met the PTSD diagnostic criteria, compared to 22.6 percent in the placebo group (n = 31). These outcomes signify high efficacy rates not only in the active group but also in the placebo group, which had response rates approximately equivalent to other evidence-based trauma treatments. Though the active group receiving MDMA had more than double the response rate, it seems that the therapeutic modality itself, with its focus on the participant's inner healing intelligence, has a meaningful effect in addressing trauma.

SAFETY

Deep trauma processing can only occur when the conditions are safe enough to do so, and participant safety is the first priority in MDMA-assisted psychotherapy protocols. Therapists work with medical professionals to assess participant eligibility for MDMA-assisted psychotherapy. Each candidate's medical and psychiatric history is reviewed and assessed for any contraindications or risk factors, such as uncontrolled hypertension. Psychiatric risk factors include conditions that have a significant potential for destabilizing psychological distress, such as bipolar I disorder, psychotic disorders, and current serious suicide risk. Responsible screening is an obligation to participant safety.

In addition to screening, medical professionals monitor participant safety throughout the course of treatment, and the therapy team checks the participant's heart rate, blood pressure, and temperature at designated time points during the MDMA-assisted psychotherapy session. While this may sound odd or intrusive for a therapy session, the process has been well tolerated by participants and generally accepted as a normal part of the session. In some cases, participants have reported positive reactions to the vital checks, stating that it promoted their sense of safety and trust that the therapists were looking out for them. Another participant reported that the blood pressure cuff felt like a loving squeeze, the sensation of being held, a reminder that his heart is indeed beating and he is alive.

Just as the participant's physical safety is carefully tended to, psychological safety and well-being must also be prioritized. Emphasis is placed on establishing therapeutic alliance and building trust in the therapeutic relationship. Engaging in trauma therapy is a vulnerable process. Revisiting traumatic memories can bring up intense emotional and somatic responses, experiencing again the suffering and terror of the past. Doing so in the presence of another person, asking for assistance and giving an invitation into the process, also takes vulnerable courage. In this process, safety can be established through ample preparation, resourcing, and therapeutic alliance.

MDMA-assisted psychotherapy introduces an added layer of vulnerability and the need for special considerations of safety, ethical care, and trust. Nonordinary states of consciousness, including those induced by MDMA, can result in an amplification of transference and countertransference and participants may be especially open to suggestion. Therapists can appropriately respond by maintaining open communication, upholding clear professional boundaries, practicing self-reflection and examination, processing countertransference outside the session, practicing right use of power, obtaining supervision, and acting with respect for the participant's autonomy (Mithoefer 2019).

PREPARATION

During preparation, therapists gain familiarity with the participant's biographical narrative, the impact trauma has had on him, and his core beliefs and cultural identity. The preparation process also identifies resources that will support the participant through the course of treatment and beyond. Together, the therapists and the participant identify stress-reduction techniques and grounding practices that work for the participant. If they are not already seeing a regular therapist, participants are encouraged to consider regular ongoing psychotherapy to support long-term integration and care beyond the length of the MDMA-assisted psychotherapy treatment.

Finally, therapists orient the participant to the therapeutic approach and logistics of the MDMA-assisted psychotherapy session. They review the effects of MDMA, which can be felt as waves of experience, with various states of consciousness, empathy, amplified emotion, somatic sensations. Therapists describe how the processing of trauma happens during the session, that the participant will inform the pace of the session and when she chooses to direct her focus on the trauma. Inner healing intelligence is defined and discussed, with guidance on how the participant can connect with her inner healing intelligence and how the therapists will support her in doing so.

By directly stating the intention to be physically present and provide support throughout the session, the therapists send a powerful message that sets the tone for deep healing work. This affirms the container of safety, defining the growing conditions of the greenhouse. Below is an example of how therapists may articulate some of the ways they will be supportive and ensure participant safety.

We are here to support you and your process; this day is for you. We will be here with you. We encourage you to ask for what you need and will also do our best to anticipate your needs. There are no silly questions. We invite you to express yourself in any way that feels right, whether that's using your voice or moving your body. This can actually help the process unfold as things come up during the session. We are here to ensure your safety and will monitor your vital signs and hydration. When you stand up or move, we will protect you from falling or hurting yourself, such as helping you walk to the bathroom or using a pillow to keep you from hitting the wall or the floor if you are moving your body.

We want to do whatever we can to be most helpful to you; please let us know if there is ever anything we can do more or less of. You won't hurt our feelings. You don't have to take care of us. Each of us will take a short break for lunch; one of us will always be with you. We want to know about your experience and encourage you to share your internal process by talking with us when it feels right but not to feel any pressure to talk to us before the time is right for you. We will also check in with you regularly during the session to see what's happening so that we can best support you. If at any point you feel stuck, overwhelmed, or confused, let us know; we will help. That is what we are here to do. As you work through aspects of trauma, you may experience difficult, scary, or seemingly overwhelming thoughts, feelings, or images: we will be with you to support you in staying with them as much as you can to process and move through them. We are honored to be a part of your process.

FELT SENSE OF SAFETY

Peter Levine found from observations of animals in the wild that when prey survive attack by a predator their bodies often shake and tremble, a natural release of energy. Within a few minutes, animals return to their resting state and resume normal activity. Levine proposes that by mobilizing stuck energy and completing the body's natural response to a traumatic event, the body is able to return to a relaxed state (Levine and Frederick 1997). Levine's work was influenced by Eugene Gendlin's concept of *felt sense,* a physical experience of a situation, "a body-sense of meaning" (Gendlin 1981, 10).

When a person who has been burdened with trauma has an internal experience of safety, a *felt* sense of it, he or she has retrieved something precious: a reference point for healing. If we can find a mental and physical state of refuge—our greenhouse—we will have found a place to do our healing work. Beyond practical techniques to prevent injury or harm, a *felt* sense of safety is the internal experience of absolutely *knowing* we are safe and secure and feeling it in our body.

Many people experiencing post-traumatic stress aren't able to access this feeling of safety because their symptoms, such as hyperarousal, hypervigilance, and flashbacks, perpetuate a lasting sense of danger and high alert. When a person is exposed to a reminder of a traumatic situation, her body may respond automatically, as if there were a real and present danger, even when there is not. This hyperarousal is characterized by heightened activity, which occurs throughout the body, including the amygdala, which serves as the brain's fear response center. When the brain and body engage this stress response, it becomes difficult to differentiate between actual and perceived danger. The experience of hyperarousal and other symptoms of traumatic stress make it challenging to establish a true sense of safety. The neurobiological effects of MDMA on the amygdala and prefrontal cortex contribute to increased compassion, introspection, sense of well-being, and decreased fear. These anxiolytic and prosocial effects counteract hyperarousal and expand capacity to confront difficult experiences.

As a therapist who has worked with participants in MDMA-assisted psychotherapy trials, I have witnessed how MDMA seems to give participants the ability to revisit traumatic memories with great clarity, while simultaneously experiencing connection with present reality, in which they know they are safe.

One participant I worked with commented frequently during the process that she was amazed by her ability to feel completely connected to her body on the couch in the therapy room, in the presence of her two therapists, while also feeling as though she were actually present in the scene of the traumatic event she was recounting. She had access to emotional responses, somatic sensations, and thoughts—both of how she did respond to the situation in the past and also how she was choosing to respond to the situation as she was revisiting it during the therapy session. She described in great detail features of the setting of the trauma and the impact specific moments had on her, the thoughts going through her head at the time, and the ingrained beliefs in response to the trauma. For example, she spoke aloud the belief: "My value to others is in how much I please them," and then immediately said, "That's not true." She proceeded through the rest of the scene in slow motion, being able to observe, recount, and respond to each aspect of the traumatic situation. She came to completion with that scene, rested for a period, and then began reflecting on what she had experienced, noticing where her sense of self began to fray. She was now able to extract and replace the harmful and untrue beliefs that were ingrained in the trauma with the truth of her wisdom and power. This person was able to reclaim her own power through the experience of embodied safety.

To this participant who shared her journey with me, and to all MDMA-assisted psychotherapy participants who contribute their life stories to this body of work, I express reverence and gratitude. Like a loving and attentive gardener, therapists can best support people working with MDMA by dedicating themselves to the safe and nourishing conditions of the container, and then mostly get out of the way!

It takes great courage to heal from deep trauma. I am hopeful that there are increasingly more effective treatment options to make this difficult journey worth the effort. Let's strive for a world where all people can access resources and opportunities that allow them to know, to remember, their intrinsic wisdom, value, and capacity for healing.

13

Therapeutic Use of MDMA for Post-Traumatic Stress Disorder

Recovering the Lost Good Objects

Jo O'Reilly and Tim Read

The future may teach us to exercise a direct influence on the mind by means of particular chemical substances. . . . and there may be still other undreamt of possibilities for therapy as a result.

SIGMUND FREUD, 1938

In keeping with Freud's suggestion, evidence is emerging for the efficacy of MDMA as a catalyst for therapeutic change, and we will discuss this process of change from a psychiatric and psychoanalytic perspective. The MDMA-assisted psychotherapy program developed by MAPS is a relational treatment: the MDMA acting as a catalyst for change within the container of the relationship provided by the parental dyad of the two cotherapists. We will describe how the MDMA treatment not only allows a processing of a previously indigestible trauma but also how the relational aspects of this treatment allow a profound reshaping of psychic structures and perhaps some repair of early attachment difficulties. We suggest this occurs through the summative effect of a number of factors:

- The empathogenic effects of MDMA, which increases the ability to trust
- The availability of previously unthinkable experiences for processing
- The quality of therapist attunement at the moment of greatest helplessness when trauma resurfaces
- The parental dyad of the cotherapy team throughout the therapy program
- The increase of self-compassion and forgiveness while self-punitive feelings decrease
- The duration, intensity, and trajectory of the therapeutic relationship
- The reparation of previous traumas and abandonments
- Healthy mourning: a coming to terms with the terrible events that have happened and mourning for the pretraumatized self

As clinicians in the British National Health Service, we see many patients for whom traumatic experience underpins their mental health difficulties. The trauma may have arisen developmentally through abuse or loss or later in life through a discrete event or a series of events. Later trauma may also reactivate longstanding fractures and vulnerabilities in the psyche. The range of therapies available are not always effective, and some patients are simply too severely traumatized to be able to engage in therapeutic work. They cannot bear to talk about the trauma or its consequences due to their reexperiencing symptoms, their physiological hyperarousal, and the psychological avoidance that develops as a result. Their behaviors and lifestyles often become organized around their symptoms; relationships break down and their condition becomes entrenched.

The MAPS research program led by Rick Doblin and delivered by

Michael and Annie Mithoefer as cotherapists has produced promising evidence for the effectiveness of MDMA-assisted psychotherapy for post-traumatic stress disorder (PTSD). This has led to the training of large numbers of psychedelic therapists and a new paradigm for psychotherapeutic change that is rapidly moving from fringe to mainstream. This has major implications for these vulnerable people with mental health problems who are not able to benefit from existing treatments.

MDMA-assisted psychotherapy involves complex mechanisms. The effect of the MDMA on the brain and the therapeutic relationship between the participant and the two cotherapists are mutually reinforcing—acting together in synergistic fashion. There are effects on brain function that seem to have a direct effect on some of the core symptoms of PTSD but at least as important are the relational aspects. The manner in which the MDMA allows a sharing of terrifying material from the deep psyche with the cotherapists catalyzes a profound process of change of the inner world and its *internal objects*. By internal objects we are referring to the internalized formative relationships from which the developing psyche perceives the world and finds meaning in its experience. These include primitive, persecutory fantasies from infancy and their more mature counterparts developed through early experiences of nurture and care. These internal structures are largely unconscious and form the basis of how we relate to the external world.

TRAUMA AND THE MIND

The word *trauma* is derived from the Greek verb *titrosko,* which means "to pierce, to damage, to defeat." Freud wrote that in trauma our defenses become overwhelmed, meaning that the mind's protective shield can no longer screen out excessively stimulating and terrifying experiences. Trauma also confirms our worst unconscious fantasies about being utterly helpless, annihilated, abandoned, and subject to unrelenting sadism. The mind becomes flooded with terror and is rendered unable to think and process what has happened. In psychoanalytic terms, this is called a failure to *symbolize;* if you cannot think about what has happened, it becomes impossible to distinguish between something that stands for a potential danger or the danger itself.

In severe trauma we have not been protected in two fundamental ways: first, by those who are meant to keep us safe (in reality and/or fantasy); and second, by our own internal capacities and resources. This leads to a profound loss of our own sense of self or trust. Any reminder of the trauma becomes the trauma itself.

In psychoanalytic terminology, after trauma our supportive internal psychic structures—known as our good objects—become exposed as inadequate, appearing neglectful, weak, or malign. So, the trauma triggers a terrifying and life-changing realignment of crucial psychological internal structures. This immediately raises two major challenges for treatment. First, if you cannot symbolize, you can't use words to describe what happened without returning to the trauma itself. Second, if you have experienced your good objects as woefully lacking in their basic tasks of keeping you safe, how can you develop a trusting relationship with another?

TRAUMA IN THE BODY

Trauma is linked with excessive and prolonged states of physiological hyperarousal, the fight-flight response in which the body becomes excessively adrenalized. This is mediated by our sympathetic and parasympathetic nervous systems and in particular the vagus nerve, linking many of our viscera with the brain. Our heart, brain, and gut are intimately connected; we ourselves use terms such as *gut wrenching* and *heart breaking* to register our awareness that our bodily organs are affected by our states of mind. This helps explain the link between trauma and a range of health conditions, such as fibromyalgia, chronic fatigue syndrome, and medically unexplained symptoms. There is also evidence of trauma affecting the immune system as Bessel Van der Kolk (2014) describes in *The Body Keeps the Score.*

The Adverse Childhood Experience (ACE) study, which followed up the effects of childhood trauma on over seventeen thousand members of the public (Felitti et al. 1998), showed that in addition to the psychological and social damaging effects of childhood abuse and trauma, there were serious physical health problems, the risks of which increase with the severity of the trauma. High-risk behaviors, including smoking, alcohol, and substance abuse, predispose survivors of childhood trauma to chronic diseases and negative health outcomes in adulthood such as bronchitis, emphysema, diabetes, and heart disease. Health professionals are often dealing with the effects of trauma that occurred decades earlier.

TRAUMA AND THE BRAIN

Advances in neuroscience show how trauma affects the brain and how the world is experienced through a different nervous system after severe trauma. In brief, the amygdala, the area of the brain tasked with the recognition of threat and triggering the fight-or-flight response, becomes excessively activated while the prefrontal cortex and hippocampus, areas where the brain contextualizes and assesses threat, impulse control, organization of memory, and empathic understanding of others, show reduced activity. So, the brain is in a state of constant sensory overload, and the ability to process, contextualize, think, and organize memory is impaired. There is no capacity and no place for an appraisal of warning signals. Any warning signal triggers a response that is equated with the trauma itself.

The effects of MDMA on the brain are complex and not completely understood (Feduccia and Mithoefer 2018), but MDMA enhances release of various neurotransmitters including serotonin and noradrenaline, increases secretions of hormones such as oxytocin and cortisol, and appears to enhance brain development neurotrophic factor (BDNF), which increases neuroplasticity and synaptic connections. MDMA reduces activity in brain areas involved in fear and anxiety such as the amygdala and insula while increasing connectivity between the amygdala and the hippocampus. The point to be made is that there is a substantial biological effect that paves the way for the relational work of psychotherapy.

WHAT IS POST-TRAUMATIC STRESS DISORDER?

We will describe the clinical features of PTSD in some detail to assist an understanding of the complexity and disability of this condition and the challenges involved in treatment. PTSD is a condition with a constellation of symptoms, the most prominent of which are:

- Reenactment symptoms
- Avoidance
- Hyperarousal

The reenactment symptoms involve a repeated reliving of the trauma in the form of nightmares, flashbacks, or intrusive memories. Traumatized individuals may awake from a nightmare in a panic attack, feeling as though they are back in the trauma in a way that is visceral and terrifying. People with PTSD live their lives avoiding anything that reminds them of their trauma and anything that might trigger reenactment symptoms or anxiety. Their emotional range becomes blunted, with low mood, numbness, and detachment. Avoidance and hyperarousal are common barriers to accessing psychotherapy; it is simply too difficult to bear.

Hyperarousal refers to the way in which emotional and physiological responses rapidly escalate to panic attacks and overwhelming anger. Irritability is corrosive to relationships, and traumatized individuals tend to isolate themselves. Some people develop severe forms of depression and suicide, which is a major risk in PTSD. People may also self-medicate with alcohol or substances to the point where their addictions may need attention as a first priority.

To make matters more complicated, a new term, *complex PTSD*, has been introduced, where there is a history of childhood trauma, often with multiple abuses over a period of time. Many patients that we see in clinical practice, with their histories of childhood abuse, loss, disturbed attachments, and trauma, have complex PTSD. Their difficult history affects their personality development with emotionally unstable characteristics that hinders their relationship patterns, including with therapists.

Some people who initially appear to have developed PTSD after a single trauma, perhaps as a result of military service, turn out to have complex PTSD. It may be that this person had childhood trauma that led to the decision to join the military and thus contributed to the battle trauma. Or there may be racial trauma, which may have profound implications for the way in which a person is able to engage with treatment and develop a trusting relationship with therapists. So, it is necessary not simply to treat the adult trauma but also the underlying traumas that have reemerged and may now be available for healing.

The deeply ingrained patterns of behavior and thinking characteristic of PTSD are unlikely to be permanently modified by even the most intense experience with MDMA taken alone. It is not enough to simply provide a supportive environment in the hope that the medicine will produce lasting effects. A condition-specific psychological treatment is required that addresses the trauma itself, any underlying vulnerability factors, and how the patient's behavior and lifestyle has become organized around the condition.

So, recovery from trauma involves two major shifts:

- The client revisits the trauma while being anchored in the present so he or she can deeply know that the terrible events belong in the past (Van der Kolk 2014).
- The client goes through the core experiences of trauma (helplessness, loss of control, and isolation) and of recovery (empowerment and reconnection) (Herman 1992).

DISSOCIATION

The term *dissociation* describes the splitting off and isolation of traumatic memories. The neurologist Pierre Janet who first described dissociation found that unless the patient became aware of the split-off elements and integrated them into a narrative that had happened in the past but was now over, they would experience a slow decline in their personal and professional functioning.

Traumatic dissociation is a universal, instinctual, adaptive means to manage something unbearable. It allows escape and survival by splitting off the horror of what is happening so that the overwhelming experience is fragmented and disowned. Dissociation prevents the trauma from becoming integrated within autobiographical memory. In PTSD, the flashbacks and nightmares repeat what has been dissociated, being experienced as uncontrolled traumatic reenactments that are not amenable to conscious thought and processing.

In severe trauma people may literally experience themselves as being fragmented so that different parts of themselves have different natures. Thus, a child can still love the father who abuses her, as the abused child is in a different part. A related problem to these isolated pieces of unthought experience is that they find ways to exert their effects through repetition. Freud described how we repeat what we cannot remember and termed this *repetition compulsion*. An example that is commonly found in clinical practice is the child who experienced violence growing up and develops a series of abusive relationships in adult life.

MDMA-ASSISTED PSYCHOTHERAPY

The MAPS therapy program extends over three months. Three preparation sessions precede the first eight-hour MDMA session. Each of the three MDMA sessions are followed by three integration sessions. We suggest that the therapeutic elements of the treatment have the following qualities:

Empathogenic. A state of positive affect with increased trust and self-compassion. This emerges in a state of clear consciousness and is reality based, not an overly emotional or reality-distorting state of mind. The therapist couple, with their containing and nondirectional receptive stance, support the process during which the traumatic material almost inevitably emerges. Hence, the MDMA facilitates the revisiting in the present of the terrible events in the past, in a containing therapeutic relationship, in a way that can be remembered and is available for further processing afterward.

Recall. The relative lack of dissociation on therapeutic doses of MDMA means that the experience remains available to conscious processing and subsequent integration. Alexander "Sasha" Shulgin, the chemist who first synthesized MDMA, found that with a moderate dose, he was able to be attentive and hear and respond to other people's comments, and he had total and accurate recall of the entire experience (Shulgin and Shulgin 2005, 73).

Attunement. The extent of the bond that develops with the therapists and the duration of the MDMA session with its unfolding inner experience and extended contact with the therapists are likely to be powerful therapeutic factors. The combination of the strong sense of attunement with the therapist while simultaneously revisiting the trauma is a strong inducer of positive transference that is rekindled in the integration sessions, which in turn amplifies the overall therapeutic effect.

Holding and containment. Holding refers to the process where a mother is able to tolerate primitive states of affect that are unbearable to the infant. Containment describes the manner in which the mother is able to metabolize the baby's raw emotions and pass them back to the infant in digestible form, and this is how the infant learns to manage the range of emotions. A similar process of transformation occurs in the therapeutic relationship where the therapists are able to adequately contain primitive and terrified states of affect. The ability to provide physical support if required probably amplifies this effect—as it does in early life.

Overcoming resistance and defenses. This is an ongoing process during the treatment program. The Mithoefers highlight the importance of the inner healing intelligence, the idea that the mind, like the body, knows how to heal itself and that this process fails when there are obstacles to the healing process. Such obstacles can be referred to as resistance, envy, or death instinct. The MDMA sessions not only make the obstacles more available to the conscious mind but also provide favorable conditions for the healing process. MDMA decisively tilts the balance in the battle between surrender and resistance.

Compassion toward self. MDMA's empathogenic qualities allow a profound emotional connection, both to others and to oneself. Anne Shulgin found that "MDMA allows the participant insight into himself, while putting him in a state of peaceful acceptance with what he might unearth. . . . There is usually a strong sense of appreciation, even love, for himself as a total human being, warts and all, and often a deep compassion for his helpless, traumatized childhood" (Shulgin and Shulgin 2005, 77). The compassion toward one's younger self and the sense of forgiveness that arises in the MDMA session needs to be retained through integration. The links with guilt and shame, which may be unconscious but often so emotionally disabling for survivors of trauma, can be reassessed from this new perspective.

Engage and retain good objects. MDMA acts as a catalyst for the development of a positive transference to the therapists and for the restoration of an internal good object, which is key to recovery. The participant feels held and absolutely witnessed by the therapists while revisiting the trauma. So instead of the trauma being associated with abandonment by the good objects with all the feelings of desolation that follow, the participant feels nurtured and accompanied in his or her moment of greatest distress and need. This becomes reinforced and internalized during integration and subsequent MDMA sessions.

The transference balance. Freud (1938) observed that the balance between the positive and negative transference is important in determining the likelihood of being able to change in therapy. With the support of two therapists and other pharmacological effects of MDMA (serotonin and oxytocin), the positive transference predominates with a relative absence of negative transference. The power of the positive transference is enhanced as it occurs in the context of reexperiencing trauma when parental care is most needed.

Corrective experience of early attachment problems. It is known that the quality of early caregiving is critically important as a vulnerability factor for future mental health problems. We suggest that the heart of the transformative process lies in the meeting between the sensitized state of mind of the participant and the highly attuned responses of the therapists alongside the positive affect state allowing the visceral and embodied rediscovery of trust. Treatment needs to address not only the imprints of specific traumatic events but also the consequences of not having been mirrored, attuned to, and given consistent care and affection. Relationship maps are implicit, etched onto the emotional brain; they are not reversible by understanding only, and healing occurs by finding new ways to form emotionally intimate connections.

Recovery of symbolization. In PTSD, traumatic events are almost impossible to put into words. As the trauma becomes available for processing through treatment, a narrative develops to give it context and meaning. This allows a recovery of the ability to symbolize and invest events with meaning, leading to enhanced creativity and ability to think.

Mourning. The loss of the pretraumatized self can now be mourned. The participant acknowledges that he or she was not protected and that there are things in the world that one cannot be protected from. The consistent empathic containing that the

therapists provide allows the presence of good objects as supportive internal psychic structures, so that previously unthinkable
realities can finally be accepted as something that really happened but now lies in the past.

Somatic. Memories of physical helplessness can be stored in body
areas with numbing, lack of connection, and tension. Bodily sensations are explicitly worked with in MDMA therapy through
touch, active encouragement to focus on the body, breathwork,
amplifying movements, and with the use of aids, such as stress
balls, towels, or cushions.

Spiritual. Some report mystical experiences, which may add a
deeper order of meaning that may develop into a protective internal object relationship. There is no evidence linking such numinous experiences to clinical recovery from PTSD.

TRANSFERENCE AND COUNTERTRANSFERENCE REENACTMENTS

Transference is heightened in MDMA sessions. Because of the unconscious pull to re-create what cannot be remembered, there are some
characteristic transference reenactments that may occur in therapy with
traumatized patients, especially when the experiences are dissociative in
nature. These reenactments operate at an unconscious level and despite
the best of intentions. They are more likely to occur when therapists
are not adequately trained or supervised, but they can also happen with
experienced therapists, as the unconscious pressures can be so powerful.
The empathogenic effect of MDMA may increase the risk of such reenactments. Common patterns seen when working with adults who have
been abused as children include:

Neglected child and uninvolved parent. The therapist unconsciously reenacts previous failures of caregiving by inadequately
addressing the client's neglect and abuse.

Omnipotent rescuer and entitled child. A client who demands to be saved combined with a therapist or a mental health service that believes they are the only ones with the expertise or special understanding to help.

Sadistic abuser and helpless enraged child. A therapist who becomes intrusively drawn into an overinvolved relationship with the client with the potential for boundary violations.

Seducer and seduced. An excited state that can develop between therapist and client.

INTEGRATION AND LONG-TERM CHANGE

The development and working through of the negative transference is a fundamental aspect of psychoanalytic treatment. The ways in which the mother was not attuned, the blind spots of attachment figures, the unmet care needs, and the abandonments all become alive in the therapeutic relationship. These developmental edges are amplified by the intensity of the analytic setting and are projected onto the therapist. The analyst needs to tolerate the projections and allow them to fully manifest themselves in the transference so that they become available to consciousness. In time, the tectonic plates of the psyche undergo a fundamental shift as the problematic relational templates arising in early life become modified by the empathic attunement of the therapist. In psychoanalytic terms, the internal object relations undergo a restructuring. But this takes some years.

The mechanism of change in MDMA-assisted psychotherapy appears entirely different. Rather than draw out and examine the negative transference, the empathogenic effect of the MDMA generates momentum more through positive transference: an ideal experience of attunement by a parental dyad in the time of greatest need—when powerful trauma is present. The holding and containment effect may be further amplified by physical support, in the way that a mother may soothe a baby.

The three integration sessions after each MDMA session, with both cotherapists, enable a careful unpacking of the experience. The first integration session may have elements of idealization of the experience and the therapists. In subsequent sessions, there may be more discussion of the participant's fundamental relationship patterns, how he or she has influenced the trajectory through life and the perspectival shifts as a result of treatment. The positive transference needs to be worked through to some extent so that the therapists are not in an idealized position by the end of treatment.

We suggest that the way in which MDMA acts as a catalyst for the development of a positive transference to the therapists leading to the restoration of an internal good object is fundamental to recovery. However, there are risks; the positive transference can be easily misused, especially where there is poor maintenance of therapeutic boundaries. Evangelical enthusiasm is likely to be an indication of incompletely resolved positive transference to therapist or substance, an imbalance that may cause vulnerability for future relational traumas.

We simply do not know whether MDMA-assisted psychotherapy can facilitate sustained shifts in internal psychological structures and the extent to which this can be applied to clinical practice with the myriad manifestations of trauma. But we suggest that this treatment has the potential to inoculate the brain with trust in a way that overrides, at least to some extent, the early environmental failures that cause complex PTSD with its associated effect on personality development.

14
Cannabis-Assisted Psychedelic Therapy

Path of Gentle Power

Daniel McQueen

C annabis is psychedelic. Until recently, however, it wasn't grown with the quality, potency, and unique characteristics required to actualize as a reliable psychedelic medicine. The War on Drugs grossly distorted our understanding of it, even within the psychedelic therapy community, and this has limited our perception of what we thought possible. However, due to cannabis legalization, prohibition as a constraint is no longer a reality in many places, and people are waking up to the incredible potential of this plant and using it accordingly.

Not everyone has access to the type of cannabis I am referring to here, so I would like to briefly describe the quality of the medicine I work with. The psychoactive components of cannabis are unique in that they originate in the nectar of its flower. Many of us are only familiar with the stale, skunky, pungent, low-quality, low-THC-producing (less than 5 percent) "brick weed" that is full of chemicals and poisons. Clean, well-grown, organic cannabis has evolved today to be exceptionally potent (25 to 30 percent or more THC content), and depending on the terpene profile, it can smell like lemons, mangoes, oranges, peppers, candy, or spices, reminiscent of rich fertile soil and trees, or strong and soft like rose and other flowers. Inhaling modern cannabis can elicit the freshness of a beautiful spring day, be invigorating like lightning, or soft and relaxing like lavender and sage. Modern cannabis is beautiful, earthy, and uplifting, facilitating a sense of liberation and well-being.

The psychoactive components in *Cannabis sativa,* notably THC, CBD, CBN, CBG, and CBC, as well as the terpene profile, when combined together in a particular way through blending specific strains of the medicine, elicit deep psychedelic states identical to other classic psychedelics. Two primary differences in the experience between cannabis and other psychedelics, and what makes it unique as a medicine, are a greater sense of agency during the experience, even during episodes of ego loss, and a significant amount of inherent emotional support akin to MDMA.

At the Center for Medicinal Mindfulness, we use special blends of different high-quality cannabis strains to elicit therapeutic psychedelic experiences in groups and individual settings (McQueen 2021). With the right blends, it is possible to use cannabis skillfully in a way that minimizes undesirable effects such as anxiety and paranoia, while maximizing the positive effects such as deep physical relaxation, enhanced insight, and an activation of our imagination and innate healing intelligence. When skillfully and intentionally used, cannabis can mimic other psychedelic medicines, even different medicines at different stages in the same session, to elicit profound transformation and healing.

At the time of writing, *Cannabis sativa* is the only psychedelic plant medicine available for legal use in psychedelic therapy and psychotherapy settings in the United States, Canada, and an increasing number of countries across the world. MDMA and psilocybin legalization in a therapeutic context is still several years away, so cannabis has an enormous untapped potential for therapeutic use by large numbers of people before these other medicines become readily available. In the United States, cannabis is already available and requires no expensive FDA approval processes to create a large-scale psychedelic therapy protocol. Jeremy Wolff, in *The Pot Book*, describes cannabis as the "people's psychedelic" (2010). Cannabis used in this way addresses many of the significant issues facing the psychedelic community regarding accessibility, social justice, and privilege. The vast majority of people looking for psychedelic therapy are unable to legally access it or afford it, but cannabis is readily available to millions of people and can be effectively and affordably used for this purpose right now.

Colorado, alongside Oregon, instituted legalized cannabis for adult use in 2014, and my organization, the Center for Medicinal Mindfulness, was the first to implement legal psychedelic cannabis therapy in the United States at that time. We have since facilitated sessions for thousands of people in individual and group psychedelic therapy settings. These experiences gave us an opportunity to further develop the potential of using cannabis as a psychedelic in clinical settings. We now use cannabis in individual and small-group settings to treat trauma, post-traumatic stress disorder (PTSD), and other common disorders such as depression, anxiety, grief, and feelings of meaninglessness. What we have learned is that by combining skillful cannabis consumption (meaning the right dose and type of cannabis taken with intention) with the right therapeutic healing modalities in a safely guided setting, it is possible to reliably elicit profound psychedelic experiences for clinical purposes. This can be accomplished while fully complying with the legal regulations of adult recreational and medical cannabis use, as well as the professional code of ethical requirements of mental health professionals. Cannabis used intentionally as a psychedelic creates a valuable opportunity to gain experience as a legal psychedelic therapist, so that when other medicines become available, they can be easily integrated into an already existing clinical structure.

Unlike the therapeutic use of other psychedelic compounds, which require significant time between sessions for integration and physical well-being, psychedelic cannabis can be used safely and on an ongoing basis for therapeutic healing, even weekly within the appropriate therapeutic protocol. Cannabis sessions can be scaled from individual sessions to couples and groups. While most of our practice involves individual intensive sessions, we have also developed an eight-person small group trauma-resolution protocol, and we regularly host large psychedelic events for our community.

Clients often return from a psychedelic cannabis experience surprised by the intensity of their journey, and it is not uncommon for seasoned psychonauts to report having the most intense psychedelic journey they have ever experienced when using cannabis in this context. Ayahuasca and DMT practitioners regularly say the experience is equivalent to these medicines, finding cannabis to be an extraordinarily versatile, intelligent, and kind ally. Personally, I have had and seen psychedelic cannabis experiences that were indistinguishable from those elicited by MDMA, psilocybin, LSD, peyote, ayahuasca, N, N-DMT, and even 5-MeO-DMT, notably morphing between the varying types of medicine within the same experience. I am still regularly surprised by the intensity of psychedelic cannabis, both for myself and while witnessing my clients' journeys.

The Medicinal Mindfulness orientation actively implements safe-use strategies and psychedelic therapy techniques from all four primary contexts in which people use psychedelics: spiritual and religious contexts, psychological and therapeutic contexts, celebratory and creative contexts, and for intellectual curiosity and creative problem solving (McQueen 2021). Working within this multiparadigm approach increases the intensity and effectiveness of the psychedelic cannabis experience by creating a gestaltlike *entourage effect* within the experience itself that goes beyond, yet amplifies the effect of the medicine. The entourage effect describes how cannabis compounds other than THC act synergistically with it, thus amplifying the effect.

The Medicinal Mindfulness orientation subscribes to commonly held principles of psychedelic therapy, most notably LSD researcher

Stanislav Grof's concept of the *holotropic nature* of the human psyche—that given the right circumstances, we naturally move toward healing and self-actualization. We also subscribe to Grof's idea that a *symptom* in a psychedelic journey experience is something *halfway out* and that if we can accept the symptom, whatever it may be, relax around it, and allow it to move through us, then healing and understanding are a natural by-product of this process. In this vein, we tell our clients that "awareness with acceptance *is* the healing process."

Similar to MDMA-assisted psychotherapy, clients will often experience physical, emotional, and energetic releases through the body as we encourage them to stay in direct contact with their spontaneously unfolding inner journey. We invite acceptance and physical relaxation while gently inviting them to go deeper into their awareness of their experience. These somatic releases occur through trembling, shaking, and sometimes even cramping and appearing to convulse. They appear to be physical manifestations of the release of deeply held traumatic experiences. These releases are often accompanied by big emotions, as the client remembers and comes to terms with what had happened.

Since cannabis isn't generally considered to be psychedelic, my preference is to use the term *Cannabis-Assisted Psychedelic Therapy* as an umbrella for the use of cannabis as a potent psychedelic within the contexts of therapy, personal exploration, and creative problem-solving practices. Psychedelic cannabis sessions can be three to five hours in length, about half the length of other psychedelic psychotherapy sessions. Due to its shorter duration, a psychedelic cannabis experience is often easier to integrate into daily life than other psychedelic medicines.

The term *Cannabis-Assisted Psychotherapy* describes a subset of sessions that are generally shorter in duration (two to three hours) and have a specific clinical purpose. The content of the psychotherapy sessions is generally more psycholytic in nature compared to the longer psychedelic therapy cannabis experiences. This is because there is a natural cycle in the psychedelic cannabis journey that deepens and lengthens when more medicine is taken.

Cannabis can also be used in very small doses to enhance the psychotherapeutic process within a regular hour-long therapy session. It is not uncommon for clients to self-medicate with cannabis before a psychotherapy session in many people's practices. Bringing this behavior into the session is a skillful way to reduce the ingrained shame felt by a client for smoking secretively, by honoring the medicine as a legitimate tool for therapeutic release.

PSYCHEDELIC CANNABIS FOR TRAUMA RESOLUTION

Cannabis sativa is a safe and sacred medicinal tool that supports clients in turning inward, resolving tensions stored deep within the body, tracking inner sensations, and releasing traumas from the nervous system and fascia (McQueen 2021). When used in a particular therapeutic context with a professionally trained psychedelic therapist, this modality deepens the therapeutic process and makes somatic trauma resolution more effective than regular psychotherapy.

While there are strong similarities between cannabis and other psychedelics, there are also important characteristics that make psychedelic cannabis experiences different from other psychedelic medicines, especially when the medicine is smoked or vaped at the appropriate dose. The psychedelic cannabis experience appears to be more accessible and less overwhelming for a client's ego. Clients are better able to engage and navigate through the experience due to an ongoing sense of agency than with other intense psychedelic experiences, and this increases the potential for postsession integration. Therefore, a primary difference between psychedelic cannabis experiences and other psychedelic experiences is one of agency and continued consent. Clients regularly report a greater capacity to engage their inner experience with skill and intention. Regaining and exploring this sense of agency, contrasted to experiencing the loss of control, is often a key factor in trauma resolution and significant healing in this practice.

Unlike other psychedelics, cannabis gently invites clients into deeper and deeper spaces and generally permits them to go at their own personally chosen pace and chosen direction. It is the primary purpose of the therapist to support this process of gentle, natural unfolding. At any time, a client can even *pause* the experience—for example by shifting positions, removing an eye covering, or taking a break to go to the bathroom—if it becomes overwhelming. Paradoxically, however, psychedelic cannabis journeyers generally choose not to titrate or pause because it feels so safe and within their capacity to navigate. When clients sit up during a DMT experience, they are clearly still fully in it. With cannabis, the same clients, experiencing a journey that is as intense as DMT, could sit up and nearly immediately return their orientation to consensus reality. When they are ready to return to their inner experience, they can do so in just a few minutes at the same level of intensity as before the pause.

These experiences challenge the notion that the typical loss of control associated with psychedelics is a necessary part of the healing process. For someone seeking help in healing a severe trauma, loss of control can at times be detrimental to the process and potentially lead to retraumatization. This is because a lack of agency and consent is often a primary cause of the trauma to begin with. Having a choice in how the healing unfolds is often a corrective experience for our clients when resolving traumatic experiences.

We refer to cannabis as the *somatic psychedelic* because body awareness is uniquely amplified, as well as a specific form of somatic healing. Cannabis addresses physical traumas in the fascia, tendons, muscles, and bones, not just trauma held in the nervous system, memories, emotions, and personality structures. New research indicates that increased cannabinoid receptors in the joints and fascia in a location of injury allow cannabis not only to reduce pain but also to help heal the injury and inflammation itself (O'Brien and McDougall 2018). The role of the therapist during these somatic releases is to trust the process and encourage the client to relax into the releases, to let them happen spontaneously, and not to physically adjust to reduce any discomfort. We invite our clients through probing questions about the physical and energetic symptoms to remain curious about their experience. Usually, if an emotional release also happens through a difficult recollection, we simply encourage our clients to gently stay with the experience until it passes. We then explore the underlying gifts of greater awareness or physical relief that often occur after the discharge.

These somatic releases appear to also be helpful in completing the healing processes that MDMA often initiates. Because current PTSD treatment protocols with MDMA only recommend that MDMA be used a very limited number of times, a protocol could be developed that uses psychedelic cannabis in conjunction with or after an MDMA protocol to deepen and extend the overall healing process.

Dosing and Duration

All doses of cannabis use can be therapeutic, and dosing and duration are interesting concepts with cannabis. How long an experience lasts, as well as its intensity, can be designed with much more flexibility than other psychedelic substances, especially when smoked or vaped. While a lower dose of MDMA or psilocybin would result in a shorter experience, it would also be a much lighter experience. In contrast, cannabis sessions can be designed to create a very strong peak state lasting from about one hour to three hours or more.

Dosing is very subjective, and a higher, psychedelic dose with an appropriately balanced psychedelic cannabis blend is very safe (McQueen 2021). Negative experiences commonly associated with high-dose cannabis use are not typical in this context. Dosing primarily depends on the state the client wishes to achieve, and if the client is a regular user, personal tolerance is taken into account as well. Regular cannabis consumers still have psychedelic cannabis experiences, it may simply require a larger dose than someone new to the medicine. The medicine can be taken in stages and titrated, particularly for new cannabis users, to ensure that they take an amount necessary for the state they wish to achieve but not more than is comfortable for them. Smoking or vaping the medicine achieves a significant altered state in consciousness in just a few minutes, with the peak beginning within ten to fifteen minutes after consumption. Therefore, the optimal dose for a client can be determined very quickly during the session over a few rounds of consumption.

A typical Cannabis-Assisted Psychedelic Therapy session lasts either three or five hours. In the shorter session, a typical psychedelic experience is about two hours in length, with about three to three and a half hours devoted to the psychedelic experience in the five-hour session. The longer session typically has a bathroom break and second dosing in the middle. Psycholytic, cannabis-assisted psychotherapy sessions can be much shorter, one to two hours in length. These are both part of an ongoing protocol that includes regular, nonmedicine psychotherapy sessions for ongoing preparation and integration support.

Intensive psychedelic therapy sessions are either weekly with integration sessions in between or completed in two- or three-day intensives with preparation and integration support happening within the intensive sessions themselves and in pre- and post-nonmedicine preparation and integration appointments. When two or three psychedelic cannabis sessions are completed in a few days' time, the second and third experiences often spontaneously begin where the last one ended. Splitting up the session in shorter sessions allows therapists to more easily care for themselves and for clients to integrate the experience in stages. However, this can sometimes leave the client in the middle of an important therapeutic process that requires tending between sessions, something that could have been completed within a typically longer MDMA or psilocybin psychotherapy session. Again, though, integration appears to be easier due to the interval nature of the sessions. Generally speaking, unlike other psychedelic medicine experiences, sleep is usually not disturbed after cannabis sessions, and most clients report improved sleep patterns afterward.

Difficult Experiences

Unlike any other psychedelic, cannabis provides a natural antidote for difficult psychedelic cannabis experiences. This antidote is literally embedded in the chemical makeup of the plant itself—the cannabinoid cannabidiol, or CBD (McQueen 2021). This antidote is effective for treating difficult psychedelic experiences and the panic, anxiety, increased heart rate, increased breath rate, and even the paranoia that accompanies them (Holland 2010). On the rare occasion that a journey experience is difficult to manage or the client is excessively uncomfortable, ingesting nano-encapsulated tinctures of CBD or vaping pure CBD (without THC) almost immediately drops the experience to a physiologically safe and psychologically manageable level. CBD also increases the empathogenic, MDMA-like nature of the experience and can be used as an adjunct to facilitate the discharge of physical tension (McQueen 2021). This medicine should be in every psychedelic therapist's supply kit as an important tool for psychedelic harm reduction.

In our experience, only a very small fraction of psychedelic cannabis clients have strong negative responses to the medicine, and this number can be reduced significantly with the right preparation, support, and clinical assessment. When difficult experiences do occur, they are often mild to moderate and generally have a psychosomatic component that can be explored with the therapist for greater understanding and healing. This process often reveals the memories and emotions held within the body system. As a client explores a sensation in the body, deeper memory recall, with emotional releases, are activated simultaneously with the somatic discharges and shaking.

Although cannabis is regularly used to treat nausea, psychedelic cannabis experiences may also elicit nausea. This nausea generally corresponds to an emotional release of some sort. Vomiting is rare, unlike ayahuasca, but it occasionally happens. Extreme physical discomfort, indicated by frequent body adjustments, may indicate a need to take the CBD antidote to calm the nervous system. While some anxiety is not uncommon, particularly at the beginning of the session, extreme anxiety is rare. However, extreme anxiety should be immediately addressed and supported by the therapist so that it doesn't spiral into panic and paranoia. Coaching the client to bring awareness to the breath and to breathe slowly and gently into the belly is generally the best antidote for both nausea and anxiety.

If a client reports sometimes getting paranoid on cannabis, it is important to address this before the session begins. We usually ask if there is anything in the room that makes the client feel unsafe, or if there is anything we can shift to increase a sense of safety. We always discuss appropriate boundaries, such as nonsexual, consensual touch and the physical parameters of the experience, before every session begins, and we develop a safety agreement that can support the work if paranoia arises. If it was agreed that the client is safe before the session begins, and paranoia arises during the session, I remind the client of the discussion we had about safety. I then invite the client to look under the experience of fear instead of projecting the fear to an outward source. Usually, paranoia is a projection of an important but sometimes scary process of self-discovery. When a client can stay with the sensation of paranoia, just like any symptom, with acceptance and relaxation, it moves through and out of the client's experience, and beneath it important information is uncovered that is accompanied by a profound sense of relief. In a very real sense, emotional crises in the psychedelic state are incredible opportunities for healing when engaged skillfully.

Therapeutic Interventions

Therapeutic interventions depend on the needs of the client, the therapeutic skill and orientation of the practitioner, and the intention of the journey. Some people require more guidance to stay on track with their intention than others, especially if they are new to medicine experiences or mindfulness practices. Because cannabis provides a sense of agency, sometimes extremely difficult experiences or realizations that benefit the therapeutic process don't automatically activate as with other psychedelic medicine experiences, and instead the client may require support in taking steps toward them. When this happens, therapists can provide resourcing strategies or act as an auxiliary nervous system by staying calm and in contact, while simultaneously supporting clients in turning toward the most noticeable experience in their own bodies.

Clients are encouraged to turn awareness toward body sensations and note what they are most aware of. This is usually a strong somatic or energetic sensation, tension, or pain. When a spot is located, the therapist can guide the client into greater awareness of that sensation by asking certain questions. This is called the *Five Awareness Practice,* and it is part of Cannabis-Assisted Psychedelic Therapy. The practice employs questions that relate to the five ways of sensing and perceiving in psychedelic states: (1) physical sensations, (2) energetic sensations, (3) feelings and emotions, (4) thoughts, memories, and beliefs, and (5) visual, auditory, symbolic, and imaginal content (McQueen 2021).

Generally, simply focusing a relaxed awareness on an area of the body—staying with the experience for many minutes, exploring the many ways of perceiving it—begins to release both the physical tensions held in that location, as well as the psychological structures connected to it. This process supports and helps facilitate a natural holotropic process, toward greater well-being and health, just as a midwife is there to support and help facilitate a natural birthing process.

The therapist offers an awareness of compassionate, accepting curiosity and asks in many different ways: What else is there? What else do you see? The therapist provides probes that support the cultivation of awareness in multiple dimensions of experience and follows the "charge" of the inquiry through staying in contact with the client as sensations that are most present are described. This relaxed awareness, in the presence of a therapist or witness, often leads to further uncovering many layers of therapeutic healing processes. Usually it takes only a few moments of guiding before the journey develops a momentum of its own. At that point, the therapist supports the unfolding or unwinding with encouraging words and presence. If there is shaking or unusual movement in the client's body, the therapist can normalize the experience by simply saying things such as: "This is what healing looks like." "Your body knows exactly what to do." "Trust your body, trust your breath." "Remember, all is well."

FUTURE POSSIBILITIES

I have been openly and legally working as a psychedelic professional for the past seven years with a medicine, *Cannabis sativa,* that is as potent, meaningful, intense, and psychedelic as other classical psychedelic substances. What possibilities could we create together as a psychedelic therapist community if we collectively comprehended the implications of this? What are the societal costs of cannabis being underutilized and misunderstood as a therapeutic tool? Given the state of the world, are we not ethically required to consider it?

15

Iboga

Lessons from the Bwiti Tradition and Therapeutic Use

Svea Nielsen

THE BWITI TRADITION

This chapter introduces the sacred wood iboga and considers its potential in Western therapeutic practices. The name *iboga,* or *eboghe* in Tsogho, originates from the verb *boghaga,* which means "to care for" (Laval-Jeantet 2006). *Tabernanthe iboga* is a shrub from Equatorial Central Africa. The bark of its root contains over a dozen active alkaloids that have been used in traditional medicine and Pygmy initiation ceremonies in Gabon for over two thousand years. Traditionally, the root is ingested by young men as part of a rite of passage toward adulthood, initiating them as full members of the Bwiti. Nowadays, different groups of Bwiti also use the bark with a therapeutic intention, including women. The Bwiti is a philosophy of liberation; it allows men to escape from matter, to leave their shell, to flower.

The Bwiti system is different from other traditional African or South American shamanic systems where a shaman or therapist is designated and has a social function. People are drawn to the Bwiti spiritual practice for different reasons—for physical and emotional healing or simply to learn the music. During the initiation, some initiates reveal themselves as *nganga,* as therapists. They should ideally be inclined toward the healing arts and have knowledge about plants, but they can come from any social group.

Another difference perhaps from other rituals involving teacher plants is that the initiate becomes the protagonist of his therapy, delving into the invisible world to face his issues and treat them. He is also expected to retrieve new information from the invisible world that could be useful for the group that is initiating him. This is one of the reasons why I so appreciate being at this plant's service. The shaman is more of a facilitator who stays behind the scenes, holding the setting where the interaction between the sacred wood and the participant unfolds directly and powerfully.

In central Africa, eating the root is a ritual practice that takes place in a ceremonial setting after much preparation and the help of the entire village. The initiation lasts several days and is carried out in the forest or very close to nature. It is usually done only once in a lifetime, and the integration time is prolonged. Some say you need at least a year to get back on your feet. In Bwiti it is believed that once ingested, the wood works in you for life.

THERAPEUTIC USE OF IBOGA

Howard Lotsof, who had multiple addictions himself at the time, discovered in 1962 that this root was an extraordinarily powerful tool to heal addictions, and he went on to pioneer its use in the Western world (Lotsof and Alexander 2001). Iboga often allows addicts to detox from heroin overnight with few or no withdrawal symptoms, opening a window of opportunity for change. In most cases, little or no craving is felt for several months after the iboga treatment. The root has been found to be useful for working with all kinds of addictions, from physical to emotional withdrawals. The physical detox is so effective that extra precautions are needed when taking any drug after the iboga treatment.

In the beginning, iboga was often administered by groups of ex-addicts who set up underground clinics to treat their peers. The testimonies of drug addicts saved by a night with the wood are numerous, but this is not a miracle cure. It is essential to combine the ritual with several years of therapeutic follow-up. It is often necessary to leave one's living environment for a period of three months to a year. The wood triggers a physical and mental *reset,* and a neutral environment is needed so that the *new person* can fully develop new ways of being in the world.

In the late 1960s, Claudio Naranjo, a Chilean psychiatrist, used iboga with many psychotherapy patients. In his view, this substance has a number of advantages over other psychedelics for therapy. The visions are usually very personal, about the subject herself or her close relatives, and often facilitate a deeper understanding about how the subject's patterns of thoughts and behaviors have evolved through her lifetime and how her self-medicating patterns of addictive behavior have arisen. The clarity of the visions also allows a reexperiencing and processing of traumatic events, so that they untangle and move toward resolution. For example, a young man had been preoccupied for many years with the question of whether his mother had experienced sexual abuse in her childhood. His own intimate couple relationships were often challenging and disrupted. During the ceremony with the wood, he had a vision of his mother as a victim; the wood said very clearly, "This is not your story, go on your way." From that moment, he was able to allow himself relationships with women that were more untroubled and at greater ease from the women in his lineage.

On the other hand, as with other master plants, the healing process often unfolds without understanding it. The visions from the journey are sometimes like a time-lapse cartoon, difficult to follow and with a meaning that eludes us. However, there remains the impression that these mixed visions participate in a great cleansing, as if the root initiates a purifying process. The visions may involve encounters with spirit animals from the lower worlds and are generally better interpreted according to the shamanic tradition.

Naranjo shares the view of Bwiti spiritual chiefs, who believe that iboga can only reveal what the initiates already have inside themselves: "ibogaine cannot open a door by itself, but it is the oil for the hinges" (Naranjo 1969, 224).

How does a ceremony with the wood unfold in a Western context? The practices are varied, with one common denominator: the duration is long, with effects lasting between twenty-four to forty-eight hours. The one to two day session is classically called a "flood dose." The wood does not like being talked about openly, and many elements are very difficult to describe. It is the medicine of the Pygmies, rediscovered by drug addicts in the West and used in marginal circles. It is a precious gift for addicts, people in pain, and those seeking ecstasy, whose healing paths have been complicated by Big Pharma and the War on Drugs. But this teacher plant is one of the few psychedelics that can be lethal, and certain precautions are required, such as an ECG (electrocardiogram) to check for a prolonged QT interval or other cardiac issues. (Prolongation of the QT interval on the ECG is associated with an increased risk of torsades de pointes, an arrhythmia with increased mortality.)

It is said to be the medicine of ancestors and death, a plant that works with our lineage and helps us to reconnect with its resources. It is also a plant that helps us clear the unnecessary burden we may carry from our past and that of our family. During the journey, past events are reexperienced, from our personal past but also from that of our ancestors, sometimes going back hundreds of years and often accompanied by powerful cathartic effects. Sometimes certain visions provide release without requiring understanding. This transgenerational cleansing and rebirth of a *new self* is extremely powerful with iboga. It is not uncommon for initiates to change their life and move closer to the person who performed the ceremony for them. This person is often described as a new father or new mother. The bond linking the initiate and the iboga provider is like a family bond, closer than the bond that one can have with a traditional shaman.

Iboga therapy is mainly known in the Western world as a short-term treatment for addictions. It appeals to the addicted mindset of those who seek a quick and easy solution. In the traditional setting, however, the vibrant heart of the tribe and the omnipresence of nature create a natural container for the integration of profound experiences. How can we achieve this amid our modern lifestyle?

Over the years, I have learned to approximate this experience through iboga microdosing, regular coaching, and brain nutrition. The latter, in the form of a personalized orthomolecular protocol, has the added benefit of extending the time devoted to preparation and integration.

ORTHOMOLECULAR PREPARATION PHASE

At the beginning of my practice in this field, I was trained in the use of specific nutrients to prepare the body and the brain for the iboga ceremony. This method stems from orthomolecular medicine, which was developed in the seventies to treat schizophrenia (Hoffer and Saul 2008). The aim is to repair the nutritional imbalances caused by addiction with high doses of amino-acids, vitamins, and minerals, thereby optimizing the iboga treatment. People without addiction issues can also benefit from a protocol with certain nutrients, for example to treat anxiety or help wean off certain pharmaceutical drugs to prepare for the ceremony. The orthomolecular preparation phase usually starts at least a month before a flood-dose ceremony, or at the same time as a microdosing protocol. Many people report that certain nutrients improve sleep disorders, brain overactivity, anxiety, and depression. We provide education, including the nutrient content of specific foods for each main neurotransmitter. Physical and psychological health requires fresh, organic, and whole foods, which are lacking for many clients, so balancing their nutrient intake with supplements is often necessary. The person who trained me for ceremonies told me: "Often people turn to psychedelics to solve their problems while the solution is in their brains and their food."

MICRODOSING THE WOOD

Microdosing psychedelics has gained popularity in the last few years, often derived from James Fadiman's protocol, consisting of a subthreshold dose every three days. The two-day break between microdoses helps to avoid tolerance buildup. Fadiman encourages the use of a journal as part of the microdosing protocol, which I strongly endorse. The results of his research, with hundreds of people reporting on their microdosing experiences, has shown enhanced overall well-being (Fadiman and Korb 2017).

Compared to other psychedelics, microdosing the sacred wood is less common but produces interesting results. It can be used to prepare a ceremony with the wood, either as a single test dose or as part of a longer preparation phase consisting of several weeks of microdosing. Giving at least one microdose some time before the ceremony is quite common, both as a test and as a first encounter with the spirit of the plant. The effects vary greatly, from feeling energized to feeling sleepy. The latter is more frequent with people who have a tendency toward overstimulation (cocaine addiction, for example).

Microdosing for several weeks is a different matter. It can be done before a ceremony as preparation or after a ceremony to sustain the long-lasting benefits.

Evan's Story:
Microdosing as Preparation for a Ceremony

Evan was a very sweet and sensitive man, hidden behind his armor. He drank liters of wine and beer daily and used crack cocaine on weekends while he also had experiences with LSD and psilocybin. Microdosing and a weekly coaching session helped Evan prepare for the flood-dose ceremony. For Evan, flood-dosing needed to be delayed as abruptly stopping his alcohol consumption could trigger withdrawal symptoms. He began his substance use at thirteen and had become increasingly self-destructive. Over time, he had broken over twenty bones in his body. Despite his addictions, he was working part-time in his father's company and was in a long-term relationship. Evan showed a genuine and strong will to change and had spent a great deal of his money seeking recovery. He had already undergone three detox treatments, one in a hospital and two with a Scientology program (based on a sauna and orthomolecular protocol).

Evan felt that his attraction to drugs was strongly linked to a spiritual quest and that he had become a better person after his numerous psychedelic experiences. When his iboga treatment started with a microdose, he felt instantly connected to the spirit of the plant. He microdosed for seven months before the ceremony, allowing him to slowly taper down his alcohol consumption. He felt that the wood was like a helping spirit, protecting him. He also followed an orthomolecular protocol, with vitamins, minerals, and other GABA precursors. As a result, he felt more peaceful; he slept better than he had for years. He became less hyperactive and less aggressive in his relationships. During his microdosing preparation, he described feeling in-between worlds, which was uncomfortable. He was no longer the old Evan, obediently working in his father's company and enduring the negative energy around him. Yet, he was also not ready to become fully independent. He was eager to change but didn't feel strong enough to initiate these changes. He gradually started to become more independent, getting freelance jobs outside the family company and building up his confidence.

After seven months of microdosing and coaching, his alcohol consumption was low, and he had replaced beer with nonalcoholic beer. He could go for several days without alcohol and rarely used crack. He wanted to do the flood-dose ceremony despite his fears and nightmares about his soul being kidnapped by bad spirits. However, when the time came for the ceremony, he felt ready. The day after the flood-dose, he felt better than ever in his life; radiant and full of hope. The second day, he realized that his life and relationships were not guided from the heart, which saddened him. After a flood-dose, a change of environment is strongly advisable, and he had planned a trip to South America to work as a volunteer and travel. So, a month after the ceremony, Evan was traveling through South America; he was happy with himself, able *to enjoy alcohol without the need to get drunk, and he had no cravings for crack. He felt he had reestablished clear limits within himself but knew he had to become more proactive rather than simply waiting for things to happen. He said the ceremony had matured him and given him the* will to be.

Another application of microdosing with the wood is to extend the effects of a flood-dose ceremony. For people with addictions, it is often useful, combined with ongoing coaching, to use small amounts of the wood to continue detoxifying and deepen the healing process. The wood can also be snorted and if done with respect, it can help to prevent a cocaine relapse for example. In Bwiti, there is a similar practice; some healers propose that the initiate take pinches of grated iboga at intervals in the weeks following the ceremony to sweeten the weaning process and to continue the work that began in the ceremonial initiation.

When Microdosage Is the Treatment in Itself

Microdosing with the sacred wood is a more accessible way to work with the teacher plant for people whose worldview makes them reluctant to participate in a flood-dose ceremony. Elisa, a sixty-year-old woman with a history of bulimia, was one of them. She was struggling with sugar addiction, eating several chocolate bars at night, feeling deeply guilty and unable to stop. She was slightly overweight and did not feel good about herself. She had undergone psychotherapy and nutritional coaching in the past, which helped her understand where her behaviors were coming from and how to lose weight. But this knowledge did not seem sufficient to stop her bulimia. She started microdosing and said it felt like a shield: she was able to go to a friend's party, with delicious cakes on the table, and not overeat. It appears the wood gave Elisa more strength and clarity in the face of everyday temptations.

Iboga microdosage has also been used to help people taper down pharmaceutical drugs like antidepressants. Other promising results are being investigated with conditions such as Parkinson's disease. A dosage much lower than a classical microdose is reported to benefit some

Parkinson's clients to recover their ability with everyday function, but these cases are anecdotal and more research is required.

IBOGA AND INTEGRATION

Nowadays, the need for integration work after ceremonies with psychedelic medicines is increasingly recognized. With iboga, preparing and implementing this integration period is simply a must. Without it, the entire treatment is at risk. There is risk of physical death for ex-addict clients, who, if they use their usual drug dosage, are likely to overdose. There are risks of spiritual and psychological harm if one does not take care of this newly born person. Caring can take many forms. In the iboga providers network of which I am a member, our integration practice for former drug addicts consists of two key elements: first, long-term therapeutic follow-up (one to three years) in person or online, to allow the fruits of the ceremony to be harvested and advance on the healing path; second, a change of environment for at least three months, if possible.

The environment that best supports and welcomes the initiate in the integration phase should, in our experience, have several important characteristics. Most important, it should be a place where nature prevails. Nature calms and refocuses; it is a loving and powerful healing agent. The initiate should be in a community of benevolent humans; experiencing the feeling of belonging to a supportive community helps the initiate to relearn how to build relationships, to communicate needs in a nonviolent way, and to more fully feel and express emotions. A supportive community provides a setting where any spiritual awakening will be welcomed and respected. Eating quality food is also a key element, along with growing vegetables in the garden, cooking them, and enjoying the flavors. Contributing to the household through a few hours of daily work will bring satisfaction to the initiate and may help him or her to develop new habits that hadn't been learned before. Last but not least, the initiate should play: whether playing badminton on the lawn or cards in the house or returning to childhood and playing hide and seek until nightfall. Places with these characteristics, that can accommodate people in psychedelic post-treatment, are still lacking in Europe, and I hope the network of supportive communities will expand in the future.

CONCLUDING OBSERVATIONS

Over the years, some important aspects on the benefits and pitfalls of using the wood have been considered. This may seem obvious, but it is still important to emphasize that respect for the plant is crucial. The therapist should treat and present smaller doses with the same attitude as in a ceremony. The wood itself inspires respect. I remember a client saying: "I can feel the spirit of the wood very strongly, even when the capsules are in my cupboard."

In our Western culture, when something doesn't feel good inside, we tend to cover it up with something external. This tendency begins in infancy, when babies are often given a blanket or soft toy as a transitional or comfort object to, for example, help them fall asleep alone—a practice that is rare in non-Western cultures. Microdosing, together with the nutrient supplements, also act as transitional objects that can help the client stay on track in between coaching sessions. It is important, however, for the client to gradually take responsibility for the treatment, relying increasingly on internal practices like meditation or journaling. This helps avoid dependency on the coach or the medicine and builds resilience. The wood also helps the initiate strengthen awareness of his own body sensations. Exercising and embodied practices are crucial for clearing up the memories that are stored in the body.

When microdosing the sacred wood occurs before a flood-dose, it may impact the protocol of the ceremony. In some Bwiti groups, they don't like it when an initiate has previously ingested iboga. They say they now have to give him "too much wood" for him to travel far enough. Indeed, the client's light habituation to the wood means a higher flood-dose is necessary during the ceremony itself.

On the other hand, the Bwiti do sometimes use a microdosing protocol. It is called *elik,* meaning "solitude," and consists of taking very small quantities of the wood every night for fifteen days followed by talking about one's dreams in the morning with the nganga (Laval-Jeantet 2006). This preparation with microdosing helps to alleviate the fears one can have when facing a flood-dose. As Evan said: "Preparation with the microdoses motivates you to go through the process. You are already changing, and you can feel the call of the ceremony."

The benefits are similar to those of other psychedelic substances, but the wood comes from the deepest part of the forest and acts as a call back to nature, to feel the wonders of the living creation. A client, who had been working for years in a building next to a lake, finally awoke to its beauty and swam in it for the first time. There is a world of difference between looking at the lake through a window every day and feeling the water on your skin!

The effectiveness of the sacred wood, even in small doses, appears to be helpful in the recovery from addictions. We saw it in Evan's story, when he was able to decrease his alcohol consumption from several liters of beer and wine every day to a couple of drinks a day over a few months. Another client told me she microdosed when she went to a party where she knew everyone would drink heavily. It acted as protection, and by the end of the evening, she realized she had only had a couple of drinks but had still enjoyed herself. Microdosing seems to act as a kind of repellent for many addictive substances, including sugar. In my own journey with the wood, I saw sugar as a substance that I needed to be really careful with. Indeed, some consider sugar to be the mother of all addictions.

This medicine, even in microdosing, can help remove layers of *emotional blockage* that have built up over the years. How this actually works is a mystery, but most people who use it report this effect. For example, one client on a microdosing protocol achieved greater connection with her adult son, with whom it had always been difficult to spend time without ending in an argument. Another woman said she felt during her journey in a ceremony that her heart region was full of ice, like a glacier. Then suddenly the ice broke, and there was a white light underneath it. She felt great relief and joy.

The ceremony with the sacred wood usually provides a peace of mind unknown until then. Microdosing can provide a glimpse of this feeling of total peace in the present moment. It can help people be more satisfied with their lives and grateful for the small things. It can support people who have started or are solidifying a meditation practice. The meeting with the sacred wood through microdosing often provides a broader access to spiritual experiences, a finer perception of the connection we have with God or the universe, helping to guide our life on an everyday basis.

Microdosing, together with regular coaching sessions, is a very powerful tool to help the client finally take action and make the changes he has long wanted to make. We work on a long-term basis, building trust in the relationship, which serves as a container for new and positive experiences. Johann Hari's quote has been a guiding principle in my own work: "The opposite of addiction is not sobriety. The opposite of addiction is connection" (2015).

As a final note, it is interesting and beautiful to see in the client how the wood moves slowly but surely inside the psyche, between the unconscious and conscious layers. As Evan once said, "Now I cannot act as if I didn't know."

16

Transformational Coaching, Psychedelic Therapy, and Addiction

Deanne Adamson

NATURE OF ADDICTION

Addiction is an endemic phenomenon that both plagues and enlightens the human race. Addiction, the instant and temporary gratification that comes from the uncontrollable and repeated use of a certain substance or behavior that causes harm, presents itself as a solution to the fear, discomfort, and anxiety that emerges within each individual during dark and disconnected times in his or her life. Addiction follows a journey that progresses through stages: experimentation, social use, habitual use, abuse, continued abuse, loss of control, tolerance, and, lastly, physical dependence.

This journey of addiction starts with many apparent benefits. The instant relief, euphoria, freedom, and assuredness that addictive drugs and behaviors offer is tantalizing and stands in stark contrast to the monotony of pain and suffering. But with this diabolical enchantment comes an unforeseeable and significant cost as the relief, euphoria, and excitement wane, the wounds that lie behind the suffering remain unhealed, and the chemical dependency with all of its unfolding consequences takes hold.

The experience of addiction can feel like a possession, a loss of self-control or being taken over by something else. This something else, whether alter-ego, entity, energy, illness, pain, gene, narrative, or belief, takes precedence over one's own survival and well-being. It is as much a nightmare for the person addicted as it is for the people around him or her.

Addiction lurks in every corner of our world, touching every demographic both in the visible and invisible spaces acting as resistance against our greater awakening. Herein lies the great opportunity for transformation and a reclamation of one's true self, for it is in the absence of oneself that the illusion is finally revealed, paving the way for its opposite to emerge—the true self. Yet to achieve this, one needs to face and transform the root of addiction—the suffering that lies behind it.

What's interesting about the spectrum of suffering is that it is often disguised under layers of social conditioning and material-world distractions, projecting the cause of the pain onto something external to avoid facing the core wound. The desire to avoid suffering, and the belief structures employed to do so, can easily exacerbate the suffering by denying the cause and creating additional problems through dysfunctional behavior. However, when harnessed, suffering and addiction turn one's focus inward, so that the unhealed wound at the center can be healed, so that meaning, passion, and purpose can be found and celebrated. This path of healing and self-actualization is what we've come to call transformational recovery. Although there are many tools and ways to approach a transformational journey of recovery, psychedelic medicines are quickly gaining recognition for their potential to assist with this process.

TRANSFORMATIONAL RECOVERY

Transformational recovery is the process of approaching addiction as an opportunity for growth, healing, and positive change. This holistic approach to recovery takes into account the subjective story of each individual, the roots of his dependence, and the many facets of his life that either contribute to or detract from stepping into his true self and passions.

When someone chooses entheogenic treatment for addiction (or other state of mental suffering), it is important to know that the medicine will not do all the work. Addictions can be interrupted with psychedelic treatment but not cured. What is required to get the most benefit from entheogenic treatment is full participation, excitement about the opportunity, surrender to the process as it unfolds, and commitment to being held accountable and willingness to tolerate discomfort.

One of the greatest assets for people approaching entheogenic addiction treatment is the support of a coach. Since 2010, my online coaching company Being True To You has been refining our transformational recovery coaching model to bring together our highest understandings of both recovery and psychedelic integration to support people undergoing this process. The coaching relationship provides the continuity between pretreatment, preparation, and posttreatment integration, which can help to set the context and to smooth out what could otherwise be an extremely jarring experience that shakes everything up but does not fall back into any recognizable order. Integration of these powerful experiences with the help of an informed supporter is essential, and it begins in the preparation phase.

Preparation for Entheogenic Addiction Treatment

Every entheogenic journey is different, every time, for everyone. While we still don't fully understand how these substances work, cultures that have used them for thousands of years say they carry a sentience or intelligence about them that works with your higher self to produce the exact kind of experience you need in your life at that very moment.

The importance of proper preparation for psychedelic experiences is well known within the psychedelic community, but for those seeking treatment for addiction, preparation assumes an even more critical role. Whereas psychonauts and recreational explorers will often have a fairly strong understanding of psychedelic substances before seeking out a mediated experience with a facilitator, many people in the addiction realm turn to entheogenic treatment out of desperation and without any understanding of or experience with psychedelics. Since psychedelic treatment for addiction is still relatively obscure to the general public, the people who find it are often those who have exhausted every other modality of addiction treatment, such as twelve-steps, detox, rehab, and sober living. They feel despondent, their life is chaotic, and they may be in dire physical condition. They may feel as though the treatment is imposed by their family as a kind of sentence or mandatory prescription. Thus, their preparation needs to be both thorough and approached with a long-term recovery plan in mind.

Transformational recovery coaching begins in the preparation phase when coaches apply their expertise of both entheogens and recovery planning to weave the psychedelic journey into a long-term holistic recovery strategy. This conversation with the coach typically starts even before quitting the addictive behavior, with an appraisal of the individual's current situation, the mapping out of the recovery process, and the creation of a long-term recovery plan.

Our holistic approach to preparation, integration, and recovery looks at six distinct areas of preparation for an entheogenic journey:

- Mental
- Physical
- Spiritual
- Home
- Relationships
- Lifestyle

Mentally, it is important for the individual to clarify his intentions while dropping any expectations, to approach the experience with curiosity and bravery, to be ready for discomfort and challenges, and to try and reduce stress as much as possible before the experience.

Physically, it is critical for the individual to undergo any necessary medical screening, maintain a healthy diet, get enough sleep and exercise, get in tune with her body, and learn how to relax via breathing, stretching, or mindfulness.

Spiritual preparation will be unique to everyone, but the common theme is for the individual to begin contemplating his higher purpose in life, connect with his heart and intuition, start some form of meditation or introspection practice, and open himself to the possibility of a spiritual experience that is perhaps completely new and unexpected.

When it comes to home life, it can be incredibly useful for the individual to begin transforming her living space. Cleaning and organizing the home can have a major impact on stress levels, and removing old triggering items and replacing them with new, inspiring, and tranquil objects can create an ideal landing pad for after the entheogenic experience.

With relationships, it is helpful to move away from toxic or triggering people and inform loved ones about the upcoming treatment so that they can be aware and supporting of this significant stride toward recovery and self-improvement.

In terms of lifestyle, it is great to outline any tasks and responsibilities so they are clear and workable, to cultivate positive daily habits and disciplines, and to build positive momentum for change.

Each person will approach preparation in his own way according to his personality and capability, but we have found that providing this holistic method gives people the best chance to approach their intimidating entheogenic treatment with confidence.

Entheogenic Navigation

As transformational recovery coaches, our role is to remotely help clients prepare for their experience and integrate it afterward: we are not onsite with people while they are undergoing their treatment. While the majority of the treatment experience will be dictated by the set, setting, and facilitator of the clinic or center, we do provide our clients with a set of tools for navigating their journey with an emphasis on openness, surrender, and grounding exercises for when things get too intense. Treatment facilitators and psychedelic psychotherapists will often be the main guides of the experience, but we share the following tools to help clients feel secure and prepared for their inward journey.

Remember to breathe. Awareness of breath is your primary life-line to ground you in both worlds; it will help stabilize you and get you through any challenging moments. The only way out is through, and you can get there through focusing on your breath.

Surrender to the experience. Surrender and let go of the need to control the experience, relax the mind, relinquish the need to know everything, and embrace the infinite love and mystery that is within the psychedelic space.

Go inward. Let go of the outside world, home life, relationships, and all the to-dos. Turn your focus inward, and observe your inner workings and psychological patterns; close your eyes when you can, and truly see yourself.

Observe areas of resistance. Notice when your mind and body get tense, caught up on something, uncomfortable, afraid, in denial, defensive, judgmental, angry, and so on. Consciously release this tension.

Have compassion for yourself. Leave out the self-judgment, criticism, and worry about whether you're doing it right or not. Just be where you are and accept how you and the substance are showing up, whatever that looks like.

Say yes to each moment. Lean into the experiences you encounter, especially very difficult ones. Saying yes opens the gate and allows you to get through to the next level or phase. This is what you are training for and where the rewards come, and this shows your acceptance and appreciation for each opportunity.

Trust you are safe. Have faith that you are where you're supposed to be, doing the work you are intended to do, and having the exact experience you need to get the results you want.

Stay in your process. Continue to introspect, continue your meditative exercises and integration activities after your experience, and don't rush out of your experience and jump into old comforts and patterns.

ADDITIONAL GUIDANCE FOR CLIENTS

Meeting Challenges

Psychedelic experiences can be very intense and produce any number of challenges and difficulties. When these are met with resistance, they can lead to unpleasant and unhelpful "bad trips," but when they are met with courage, acceptance, and proper planning, they can produce the greatest learning and healing opportunities. Being prepared for the unexpected can help you bring yourself to reassurance faster and maintain trust and ease throughout your journey.

There are many things that can challenge you during an entheogenic experience, from the medicine "not working," to not having the experience you were hoping for, to having a very intense experience that feels never-ending. You could feel nausea, pain, physical discomfort, loss of control, or fear of death. You might see terrifying things, face your demons, relive traumas, stir up difficult emotions, or learn truths you don't feel ready for. You might not feel supported in the moment. You might start worrying about things at home or simply be so overwhelmed by the experience that you feel unable to process anything and want to escape.

Psychedelic journeys are known to sometimes bring out your deepest fears and also bestow incredible healing and growth on the other side. To prepare yourself to meet challenges is to prepare yourself to face your fears. You can begin this process of facing fears before you enter your journey by practicing recognizing what those fears are and understanding how to respond to them. Beyond fears, reflect on hardships in your life and ways that you can feel empowered by facing them.

Managing Disappointments

Managing disappointment starts with managing expectations. As soon as you become aware of an expectation during your journey, work to release it and trust that whatever is happening is right for you in this moment. It is important to remain humble and open-minded when working with psychedelics and not impose expectations.

Start by observing your ego's tendencies to compare your experiences to others, to expect a certain kind of psychedelic experience to boast about later, or to be validated in having a life-changing experience. Remind yourself to focus on what the experience is offering in the moment.

If your experience was less than you hoped for, focus on what you noticed, learned, and discovered. Where was your resistance? Where was your disappointment? What moved you, both good or bad? What inspired you, elevated your understanding, or opened you up? Writing down your insights and gifts can help the benefits become more tangible to you.

It's also helpful to talk about these disappointments, to understand them and learn about yourself through your unmet expectations. This is an opportunity for you to see how your reliance on the external is preventing you from connecting with your own power. Remember always to look within and "own" your experience, however it plays out.

The lasting value of any psychedelic experience lies in the integration. There will be many fruits that come to blossom if you stay in your process and don't get hung up on disappointments. Keep in mind that your brain's tendency to ruminate on disappointments stems from the ego and an addictive mind, which is always looking outward, holding you back from experiencing a higher truth and wisdom already within you.

Entheogenic Integration and Recovery

Integration can mean many things:

- Integration of mind, body, and spirit
- Integration of self, other, and Mother Nature

- Integration of inner and outer worlds
- Integration of past, present, and future
- Integration of old self and new self
- Integration of principles and values into real life

When you invite psychedelics into your personal healing and growth process, big energies are unlocked, lifted, and transformed. While the experience itself only lasts for a short period of time, it will continue to unfold for months, years, and potentially a lifetime. Being open to this long journey of unpacking the experience will offer the maximum possible benefit. Psychedelic experiences open the door to transformation, but the lasting benefit comes through integration. Without proper integration, you risk missing most of the benefits of your experience.

Integration works through the conscious application of the insights gained on your psychedelic journey into your daily life. It is where the old aspects of yourself meet and transform into the new you. Often, it takes the shape of unlearning old ingrained habits and beliefs, replacing them with positive ones, exploring new passions and interests, and seeking deeper, more authentic relationships and community connections.

One of the best definitions of addiction by Johann Hari (2018) is that it is "the opposite of connection," and integration can be defined as the process of "making whole again." Thus, we can look at the integration and recovery process as a holistic journey of connection and reconnection to the many aspects of the self and environment. Some examples include:

- Connecting with positive friends and community
- Connecting with passions, hobbies, and interests
- Connecting with your experience through journaling
- Connecting with your goals by outlining and tracking them
- Connecting with breath and inner truth via meditation and breathwork

- Connecting with nature via walking, hiking, or camping
- Connecting with your creative expression through music and visual arts
- Connecting with your body through dance or movement arts
- Connecting with a coach for accountability and support

Everyone will have a unique version of these integrative activities. For some it may be martial arts, twelve-step groups, and journaling, for others it may involve yoga, gardening, and community service. None of these are required, but all of them are viable means to help you integrate and ground yourself in a new, more positive, and healthier version of yourself.

Coaches will generally not make specific recommendations but will encourage you to set healthy habits, patterns, and activities that reflect your own interests and passions. Recovery and integration are not a static process but an evolving process with many phases.

Beyond adopting specific activities, habits, and behaviors, it is also useful to reflect on the entheogenic experience from a holistic conceptual standpoint. Just as we looked at all of these areas in the preparation phase, it is helpful to revisit them after the experience as part of the integration process.

Mentally and emotionally, what did you discover about the relationship between your thoughts, emotions, and behaviors? Where are your strong points and shortcomings in your mental and emotional landscape?

Physically, what did you learn about your physical body and how physical pains or sensations were related to certain ideas or mental patterns? What is your ideal relationship to your mind, body, and emotions, and what needs to change for it to be that way?

Spiritually, what did you learn about your true self, and how would you describe your sense of spirituality now and before? What are the implications of it, and how can you more fully embody these experiences and beliefs?

When you return to your home life, what do you see that you

like and don't like? How does your environment affect your quality of life, and how can you nourish yourself in this way? Looking at your relationships, who do you want to cut out of your life, and who would you like to connect more deeply with? How can you show up better and more fully for those positive people in your life? And in terms of your lifestyle, what did you learn about your daily routines, and what new habits would you like to cultivate to more fully embody your new, recovered self?

While this holistic approach to integration is powerful, it is important that you approach these integrative questions and activities slowly and incrementally. For some people, having a comprehensive map of changes for all aspects of their life can feel empowering; for others, it can be overwhelming. Regardless, changes are made one at a time, and small victories are celebrated. We call this "taking the stairs rather than the elevator," as when the momentum of many small victories adds up, challenges and setbacks are far less devastating. Trying to change everything at once can be counterproductive, and when a setback occurs, it feels like the whole plan is ruined. It is far better to fall down a few stairs and brush yourself off again than reach prematurely for the stars and find yourself in freefall down the elevator shaft.

GUIDING CLIENTS THROUGH LONG-TERM RECOVERY

Just as psychedelic integration can be a long-term process spanning years of uncovering insights, recovery too is a long-term process that happens in phases. At different stages, people need different kinds of support.

Integration and Short-Term Recovery

During the first month after entheogenic treatment, the "honeymoon phase," a person is often still experiencing the afterglow of the treatment, and the substance itself may still be present in their system. If the individual feels a sense of heightened mood and optimism, it may be relatively easy to remain sober and on track with new goals during this time, but it is important to start integrative activities and recovery planning even if the person feels like he or she does not need it. The afterglow will eventually fade, and when it does, recovery and integration will need to be carried onward by the person's own volition and momentum, rather than the reverberations of the medicine.

When the afterglow fades, the "between worlds" phase begins, where the honeymoon phase has ended and a person is at the helm of a somewhat strange new life. This can last for up to six months and can be the most challenging time for people because they are no longer who they were but are not quite who they are becoming. The support of a recovery and integration coach, positive friends and community, and engrossing new, positive tasks will help keep a person on the road to recovery during this time and not fall back into old patterns. This is where the rubber meets the road, and a person's true commitment to integration will make or break recovery efforts.

Beyond the six-month mark, the client enters the long-term recovery and integration phase. If the previous integration phase was navigated successfully with earnest commitment, then staying in recovery and on track in life will become less of a struggle and more about maintenance. During this time, the client must remain consistent in new practices and ground them even deeper. He or she also needs to watch out for any temptations that arise because "you are doing so good" and "you deserve something" or "you can now handle something." Dedication will be tested, but overall, this phase is characterized by the recovery process being smoother, more natural, and less arduous. The more the person commits to new passions and interests and positive communities, the harder it will be for addiction or other chronic states of suffering to creep back in again.

Relapse and Long-Term Recovery

Relapse is sometimes a natural part of the maturation process arising out of addiction and other states of mental suffering. Rather than seeing it as a failure, we have found that a nonjudgmental and curious approach works best. We say to the client: "So, you relapsed—OK! What did you learn? How was it different from before? How do you feel about it now?" People in recovery find this approach very refreshing, and often a final short relapse is the straw that breaks the addiction's back forever. Experiencing their relapse with their new insights is so incongruent with who they are becoming, they realize they never want to do it again. Of course, relapse can be dangerous or even fatal, so maintaining sobriety should be encouraged as much as possible.

Sometimes people will need or want second entheogenic treatments for their addiction. This is not inherently good nor bad, but it is important to emphasize that the medicine is not going to do the work for them. At times people think: "It's fine. I'll have some more fun with my addiction because I can just rely on treatment again." Not only is this dangerous, it also falsely assumes that the substance can do the work for the client and bypass the need for truly looking within and changing what needs to be changed. It is the voice of the addictive mind trying to twist the great opportunity of entheogenic-assisted recovery into a subordinate cycle of ongoing addiction. For some people, their healing process will involve multiple treatments that build on one another and eventually effect true change. Like the psychedelic experience itself, everyone's recovery experience shares larger themes but is entirely unique.

Psychedelic treatment creates a profound window of opportunity, but each person must walk through that portal and dedicate herself to proactive self-cultivation so that the pernicious roots of addiction have no soil to grow in, like weeds that have no room to reemerge in a thriving garden.

At the core of every addictive behavior is a seed of hidden truth that wants to be known and a wound that is calling out to be healed. When we embrace the introspective process of transformational recovery with proper support, guidance, and accountability, the tragedy of addiction is transformed into the journey of self-realization. Once people are securely past their old wounds and old compulsions to use, recovery and integration evolve into an ongoing process of self-discovery and self-reflection that grants resilience, optimism, and fulfilment for the rest of a person's life. This is the great opportunity latent in the crisis of addiction and mental suffering, and the heart of our transformational recovery coaching model.

17

The Deep Dive into *Bufo alvarius* (5-MeO-DMT)

Natasja Pelgrom

My journey to the medicine has been colorful. I have changed from an out-every-night party girl in Amsterdam to a woman who tries to live and heal from a place of gentle awareness. I started clubbing at the age of fourteen, partly because I was fascinated by seeing people in ecstatic states. I have always been interested in self-discovery, and I am no stranger to suppressed shadow; in my youth, I would sometimes take drugs as a way of cutting off my emotions and sensitivities. My first psychedelic experience was with magic mushrooms at the age of fifteen. My intention at the time wasn't self-explorative or even therapeutic, but this journey turned out to be life changing. It opened my eyes to the power of plant medicines, although the real call to fully devote my energies to them came much later.

In my early thirties, I went through a period of feeling lost and stuck in a negative energy cycle that shook my whole world. I knew I needed to change when my relationships started suffering, and when the business I was running—a concept bar with an art, music, fashion platform—felt more like an ego-based endeavor than a real entrepreneurial accomplishment. I was out every night, my inner state was in turmoil, and I felt far removed from my true path and potential.

At this time, I discovered the teachings of esoteric researcher and author Drunvalo Melchizedek and worked with Hira Hosen, a Zen Buddhist nun and teacher of Drumvalo's work. Hira and I organized a number of five-day retreats called Awakening the Illuminated Heart. This was the start of my own spiritual transformation. I discovered through Heartmath that we have a little brain in our heart that has different qualities to the brain in our head. Our heart is not a polarity organ and frees us from the logic loops that our brain can lead us into. Our heart knows us very well; it's been with us a long time, and if we can locate our heart intelligence, it can answer us sometimes before we have even finished the question. My crisis also taught me firsthand that sometimes we have to lose ourselves to find ourselves in a new way.

ENERGY WORK VALUES

Since my teenage years, I have been exposed to many different healers. Through experimental participation I started to understand what the other healers were doing on an energetic level, working intuitively with an inner vision. I learned so much, not just from books but also from observation.

Energy work modalities such as reiki, VortexHealing, ThetaHealing, sound healing, and shamanic healing, to name a few, are useful additional skills to bring to your practice. It's the combination of intuition (feminine or yin) and technique (masculine or yang) that I find works best in healing and shamanic practices. Most people who practice a form of energy work don't necessarily know what they are doing or how they are doing it, but somehow, I am able to see, feel, and understand the energy field they're working in. This has always allowed me to see which techniques are effective and successful and in what context.

Over the years I've spent working with sacred medicines, I've learned to blend my observations, visions, and research with my own special techniques. These are all tried and tested on myself, or by myself, via the spirits that come to work through me. I have come to know that any healer can apply his or her own technique without knowing fully how or why it works. Similarly, a lemon tree knows how to make lemons, but it doesn't know that it knows how to make lemons. It doesn't need to.

THE TOAD MEDICINE

The compound 5-MeO-DMT is consumed by inhaling bufotoxins from the Colorado River toad or Sonoran Desert toad (*Incilius alvarius*). The compound is also known as *Bufo alvarius, Bufo, el sapo* or *el sapito* (which means "the toad" or "the little toad"), and toad. It has become increasingly popular in a variety of underground ceremonial settings in recent years.

One way to consume *Bufo* is by inhaling the smoke produced by burning the substance extracted from the toad's glands. *Bufo* venom contains 5-MeO-DMT and bufotenin, a close chemical analog to DMT. There is no conclusive evidence of bufotenin's psychoactive properties when smoked, although many find that smoking *Bufo* venom produces a stronger experience than taking 5-MeO-DMT alone.

The experience of 5-MeO-DMT lasts anywhere from fifteen to forty minutes. Its effects can kick in after just a few seconds, and the participant generally loses sense of time. *Bufo* can welcome in a vertiginous feeling of eternity and unity with all of existence. During the experience, it is possible to go through moments of catharsis, as well as an oceanic sensation of communion with oneself and with the universe. This dissolution of the ego allows us to perceive the purity of all that exists. One infinite source. The mystical experience is that of the observer merging with the observed and consciousness becoming conscious of itself. In life, we can experience the divine through the human, but with this substance, we experience the human through the divine. The totality of the present moment becomes clear—but no amount of words will ever explain the inexplicable.

I have witnessed about a quarter of participants experience an ineffable sense of divine bliss and love with *Bufo*. Another quarter experience facing and processing their emotional blockages and traumas. The remainder have a range of experiences, often transcending identity and duality but with a more neutral emotional tone. A few people return with no recollection of the journey at all.

Toad Ethics and Synthetics

You might be asking, what about the toads? Well, the pressure on toad populations and those locally subtracting the substance is currently quite severe. Our culture's desire for the toad venom may realistically end up pushing this toad toward an endangered status. Having read the concerns of herpetologists, I've wondered whether synthetics might be the way forward.

From what I've experienced and observed, natural *Bufo* seems to last a little longer, and it seems to take a little longer to come back from the experience. There's something else in the naturally produced *Bufo* that perhaps cannot be re-created in a lab—something natural that works with the heart to support healing. I also believe we bring our limiting beliefs, assumptions, and preferences into these journeys. If you believe organic is "better" than synthetic, who's to say it won't shape your experience? One must also take into consideration the dose or the number of different tryptamines present.

I should note that in the years I have worked collecting the real *Bufo*, the toads were never harmed. They were all returned to their natural habitat by the carriers. However, I cannot say the same is true for all the carriers out there.

HOW THE TOAD FOUND ME

I did not have any ambition to work with *Bufo alvarius*. Rather, it chose me when I met Enrique who has been a facilitator for the medicine since 2012 and has administered *Bufo* to over a thousand people. Born in Mexico, Enrique had a life-changing set of experiences with *Bufo* involving heart healing and addiction recovery. While enjoying a more fulfilling and healthier mental and physical lifestyle, he felt called to work and serve with the medicine, and he's been doing so ever since. Enrique is warm-hearted, genuine, and caring, and he views his role as a humble act of service. He was blessed by the elders of the Seri tribe from the Sonora dessert to share some of the traditions with me. The Seri or Comcaac are an indigenous group of the Mexican Sonora desert.

After my first session with *Bufo alvarius,* with Enrique as facilitator, I felt the medicine had deepened my resilience, strength, and intuition. It saturated me with so much love and expanded my heart in more ways than I had ever anticipated. The same weekend of my first *Bufo* session, Enrique and I facilitated together about twenty-five medicine journeys for others. Within each session, I was able to step into the space with all the gifts I had been crafting over the years, from energy work to shamanic healing tools, neurological programming, and spiritual emergence techniques. Above all, I felt a deeper purpose emerging for the use of my hearing, feeling, and seeing abilities. It became obvious that I had been preparing my whole life for this precise, pivotal moment of remembering. I had come home.

My clients seek out these medicine journeys to treat a number of conditions, such as depression, anxiety, opioid addiction, and fear of death, as well as for personal development purposes. Being forced to let go of the ego is precisely what draws many people to *Bufo alvarius* 5-MeO-DMT. The dissolution experience can impart an understanding and acceptance of mortality that can help us overcome the fear of death. I've witnessed how it can disrupt attachments with past trauma, negative behaviors, and habitual negative thought patterns.

Over the years, I have participated in many different forms of healing with ceremonial graded cacao (not psychoactive), psilocybin, synthetic 5-MeO-DMT, and *Bufo alvarius* 5-MeO-DMT. *Bufo* in particular can shake your soul in ways it has never been shaken. With *Bufo,* you might even find yourself being exposed to the meaning of life.

THE POWER OF OBSERVATION
AND WITNESSING

When I'm aware of an issue relating to an individual's well-being, I'm able to support the healing with song or sound and direct the energies with intuitive communication and/or touch. When I hold small ceremonies, preferably in nature or a teepee, I also ask the group to hold space for the voyager. I've found this to be extremely valuable for everyone involved.

> *Years ago, when I was assisting Enrique in a three-day retreat, several retreat assistants had the idea that the more people were involved in a healing, the better the outcome would be. A woman named Mia came forward with the intention to work on her fear of speaking up and expressing herself. We gathered together as a group of five to work on her, while Enrique lit the pipe. She didn't move much on the teepee's blankets, so it was relatively easy for us to work around her. But when Mia opened her eyes and tried to speak, she complained of a sore throat and said she didn't feel safe.*
>
> *Going into a trance state myself, I was shown that it's better to work one-on-one, with one practitioner. In this case, people were directing energies in different ways, and I realized that even though our intentions might have been good, our varying techniques created confusion rather than peace and relief in her altered state. I could also see that one facilitator was quite ungrounded, and this person may have affected the energy as a whole.*
>
> *Mia slowly got up and went outside, to be by herself. It took some*

persuasion on my part before she came back for a second round. I asked the others to send out love so that I could reach out and harness it and envelope her with it in my own way. When we finished, Mia was smiling and crying. She started singing with a childlike voice, full of wonder and openness. Having witnessed hundreds of similar healings, I can testify they are a magnificent way for people to bond in unconditional love. A sense of transformation, connection, and awe can occur in those witnessing the healing, as well as in the individual experiencing it. From that day on, I made a practice of inviting all my participants to send love to a specific space in the field to support the individual whom they were witnessing for.

HOW TO PREPARE FOR
YOUR SACRED MEDICINE JOURNEY

In my experience, the more you have worked with your unconscious, the more profound the teachings that you will receive from the medicine. In our preceremony session, we may work on healing a person's inner child, banishing limiting beliefs, or use a somatic approach to trauma.

In many sessions I observe that the medicine cleanses the emotional, mental, and physical being before starting to teach what it is the individual needs to learn. It can take several ceremonies before some people receive the profound visions and teachings the medicine has the capacity to provide.

Developing a deeper understanding of yourself as a multidimensional being and having a spiritual practice of meditation will help you navigate the medicine's healing abilities. It will not guarantee an easier expansion, but after the experience, you may be less inclined to return to duality, to a right-wrong, victim-aggressor perspective.

BECOME THE HOLLOW BONE

In the wisdom teachings of the Hopi, which have been shared with me over several years, it is said that our primary spiritual task is to become as a hollow bone. Emptying ourselves of self-limiting beliefs, fears, resentments, unhealed wounds, doubts, and apprehensions can free us and leave us ready to serve others better.

Many other spiritual traditions also speak of the hollow bone (or empty reed) to illustrate the largely misunderstood concept of humility—the most direct path to enlightenment. In my experience, the more shadow work, trauma processing, and self-understanding you have undergone, the clearer you will be as a facilitator. This deep inner work that you do supports your further development as a facilitator and provides a more balanced space for the healing work with your client.

The key to becoming an excellent facilitator lies in holding no expectations for the outcome and knowing it is not you who is actually doing the healing. Becoming a hollow bone means making yourself into a vessel that holds and channels the medicine to others. As is often seen with spiritual concepts, there is more than one level to this teaching. On one level, humility has to do with giving up self-importance to see more clearly. At a higher level, it points to a deceptively simple pathway of self- transformation. A common misconception is that the practice of humility is about humbling yourself. It isn't, really. Nor is it about "knowing your place." It is not something you do, nor is it something that is done to you. The essence of the practice of humility means being completely present and releasing attachment to outcomes. You get out of your own way. Though practicing humility is mentioned in many spiritual teachings, few people actually understand how to accomplish it.

The secret of humility—becoming the hollow bone—involves clearing your resistance to the universal flow of energy in your life, allowing the source of existence to flow through you unobstructed by your conditioning and self-identity. This is analogous to the shamanic practice of nondoing. Nondoing is not the same as inaction; it is about ceasing to micromanage everything by thinking, analyzing, and forcing action, about no longer working your will on life.

THE RULES OF MEDICINE TEACHINGS

All the teachings I have received have held the same core value: you cannot heal another if you haven't healed yourself. As a facilitator you should uphold professional standards of conduct, clarify your professional roles and obligations, accept appropriate responsibility for your behavior, and seek to manage conflicts of interest that could lead to exploitation or harm.

The clients who make their way to you are often reflections of what you might be holding in or working on yourself. I have a personal rule that when I receive three requests in a row with the exact same theme, it's time to understand that I might need to visit this theme myself, even if I think I have healed that part of myself.

I also make it a personal rule never to accept a request if I do not feel aligned with the person and his intentions. When I started implementing this, I began to feel quite liberated and could better recognize wounded healer aspects within myself.

Angela approached me for a one-on-one ceremony. During our exploration call, Angela elaborated that she chose a session with me because I am female. It emerged that her previous experiences with males hadn't healed her. Her feelings were very valid to her, and it became clear to me that during her previous sessions, she had experienced an emotional flashback of her childhood.

After our call, I felt that in her case it would be better to hold a healing session around inner child work before stepping into the 5-MeO-DMT space. This was not what Angela wanted to hear. She argued with me, withdrew from the process, and prematurely ended the sessions. This is where our personal therapy, our own deep inner work, and our intuitions are vital, as our own transferences will usually be unconscious too. We may need help to identify our blind spots. In Angela's case, however, I felt strongly that my decision to do the inner-child work was the right one. She did not return for her sessions, and she ended our connection with an elaborate message disagreeing with my reasoning. I left it at that; we are not meant to step into this space with everybody.

DEATH: THE UNTOUCHED TOPIC

I learn something from every person who comes into my life, and I have met many people over the years who have impacted me in powerful ways. In my very first session assisting Enrique, I saw how one person, Peter, almost died out of awe for the space he was merging into and didn't want to return. This experience created fear for me around death in ceremony: I was determined not to let death take any of my clients. Death was to me something that needed to be avoided, something that cheats us out of living, until another person, Levi, showed me a different viewpoint about the fear of death and the will to live. Through Levi, I learned to invite death into a sacred space, and in doing so, I continue to honor him now that he's passed to the other side.

Levi and his partner, Isis, traveled together from Israel to meet me for a two-day private ceremony. Levi had colon cancer, and before undergoing treatment, he wanted to understand why he'd contracted this disease. He was a kind, talkative, and mentally active person, and every time I tried to explain how the medicine session would work or share the traditions involved with Bufo, *he would interrupt and ask a multitude of questions. His curiosity was based on his need for control and, therefore, the fear of losing it.*

In our first intake conversation, I made it clear that no spiritual energy healing, or substance could be guaranteed to cure him, prevent, or treat his condition, and a sacred medicine facilitator should never make such specific claims. While partaking in Bufo *can be a life-changing* experience of immense significance, ultimately, the journeyer is the one responsible for the way we relate to any challenges we may encounter either during or after the experience.

Levi's first session was extremely challenging for him. Within fifteen minutes of his first intake, he started speaking and sharing. His mind was in resistance mode, and his body was in pain. We took a small break. He seemed to reach the conclusion that he had chosen to be in this space of suffering for a reason, and I invited him to go again. His second session was even more challenging, as he journeyed through the dark night of the soul.

Going through the dark night, the suffering seems unending. There's a deeply profound lack of light and hope. The person feels utterly alone and experiences great difficulty in his session and will face his greatest fears. The dark night of the soul holds a profoundly ominous quality, yet I have seen many people pass through it and find light afterward.

In special cases, I tailor journeys with breathwork and extended coaching sessions. When you slow your breathing, it sends a message to your body that you are safe. Think of it like hitting a switch, only slower. It's an emotional trigger that sends the healing into action.

On day two with Levi, we started with breathwork. The way Levi was breathing was proof of his chronic activated nervous system, and I saw the link to his limiting beliefs (I can't do it, I'm afraid, I'm not worthy, no one will love me, etc.). As I prepared the pipe for his second ceremony, Levi sat in front of me. I closed my eyes and went inward, allowing the emptiness to settle in and the awareness of the hollow bone to come to the surface. I opened my eyes and looked into Levi's kind, yet fearful expression. Something took over me, and I heard myself say: "Levi, it is a good day to die!" In that moment, a part of my identity shot into panic mode. What had I said? But Levi was able to smile and utter, "Yes, it is." He understood that this was the invitation to face death, to invite it to be seen and felt.

His second journey in the teepee was less rocky. While I increased the dose, he still couldn't let go, although his body was calmer than the previous day. I didn't use song or a rattle this time; I felt he needed *the medicine of hearing his own heart. His first words coming into full awareness were directed toward Isis, who was sitting patiently nearby, hoping this would cure his disease. With a tender voice he said, "Isis? . . . I love you. You are the one who needs to hear this." Isis looked up in tears. She grabbed my hand and whispered in my ear that for the past seven years of their relationship, he had never before said, "I love you."*

As I witnessed this unfolding, I understood that living a life without being able to say I love you likely springs from fear. One might fear rejection, feeling shamed, appearing needy, or maybe in Levi's case, hurting Isis by dying. From that day onward, death has not been something I've ever feared. I grieve when appropriate, but I realize now that welcoming death as a friend makes living so much juicier.

The medicine can't prevent anyone from dying, but it can certainly help people prepare for it. I've come to learn that it's not me (or you) against death in a battle of duality. Death isn't the enemy; it is part of it all. We all come to that moment of deep release, where we have to let go of our bodies, but what's important during life is to live as deeply, fully, and fearlessly as possible.

FACILITATOR SELF-CARE: THE ESSENTIAL DECOMPRESSION

Decompression sickness or the bends occurs when a rapid decrease in air pressure releases nitrogen bubbles in the blood causing neurological symptoms, nausea, achy joints, paralysis, and sometimes death. Today, scientists know that the use of a decompression chamber allows for a gradual reduction of pressure, which prevents the nitrogen bubbles from forming. Similarly, even though psychedelic medicine sessions can be uplifting and awe-inspiring, after holding ceremonial space, I always need to schedule in self-care and decompression time. I require an expansive psychic space around me so I can breathe and replenish. Over the years, I've developed a strong hermit side that protects me when I need space. Crowds and loud environments can be exhausting if I don't practice self-care.

As a result of the recent COVID-19 pandemic, we are now collectively stepping out of the modern world, decompressing in our chambers, just as the great spiritual masters did. They embarked on solitary journeys to probe the depths of their being and to find answers in revelatory, transformative experiences. Spiritually, being alone may bring you closer to your inner being. It may allow you to easily and more readily access the creative and intuitive aspects of yourself. Why not allow yourself to embrace it?*

---

*Thanks to Becky Wicks for her editorial assistance.

18

Art Therapy and Psychedelic Integration

Bruce Tobin

No realm of psychedelic experience is more commented on than the perceptual and, in particular, the *visual*. Journeyers describe intensification of colors, visual distortions, synesthesia, and a flow of intricate geometric patterns, shapes, and fantastic architectures. But these perceptual aspects of a psychedelic journey are relatively superficial. On a deeper level, the insights, revealed truths, and transcendent states that can lead to important personal healing and significant positive clinical outcomes are often aided by the medium of visual imagery through visual symbols, metaphors, and pictures—through *visions*. This phenomenon of a journeyer's encounter with spontaneously presented meaning-laden mental images lies at the heart of psychedelic healing.

Art therapy is a psychotherapeutic discipline in which therapists lead clients to use art materials (drawing or painting on paper, making a collage, taking photographs, or sculpting clay) to visually express the personal material relevant to their issues in therapy. It encompasses a set of techniques and activities that can be wedded to a wide range of theoretical bases, from cognitive to Jungian and transpersonal approaches. As an eclectic art therapist, I invite my clients to *show* me with an image rather than just *tell* me. I lead them to draw a picture as an adjunct or alternative to *talking* about their relationships, emotions, or personal issues.

INTEGRATION SESSIONS

Integration sessions serve to weave clients' psychedelic experience into their ongoing lives so that it has an enduring favorable effect. They have two general goals. The first one is *preservation,* where the clinical goal is to assist clients to *consolidate* the gains from their medicine session, to accept their psychedelic experience, to find meaning in it, and appreciate its relevance to their life issues. Healing often stems from profound experiences involving love, redemption, forgiveness, birth, or death and rebirth. Sometimes these experiences are interactive-relational; they involve a healing encounter with another entity, a transcendent being. Perhaps even more clinically significant are so-called mystical-type (or unitive) peak experiences in which the individual self dies and merges with a cosmic self, becoming one with all things. Therapists assist clients to *retain access* to these images and healing experiences and develop ways of keeping them alive. This is akin to inspiring a devotional practice: to tend the sacred fire inside so as to maintain and grow their inner well-being.

The second goal is *closure,* which centers around supporting clients toward emotional cooling, centering, relaxing, regaining composure, confirmation of emotional safety, and readiness to move back into daily life. This may involve clients reviewing and confirming their strengths and resources for handling life's challenges, anticipating those future challenges, and planning for dealing with them effectively.

There are two important aspects of this closure goal. First, some clients may return from their psychedelic journey with certain unresolved encounters with inner material. These clients have a special need for closure. Ideally, we help them process that material to resolution directly following the medicine journey. But sometimes completion is not possible, and we may want to help them close their troubling material down, to temporarily contain it until it can be safely reopened and resolved in later sessions.

Second, we all have to be able to cope when we return home, to stand up to the world with its stresses, responsibilities, and demands. To handle these challenges, we have to find and live from what we might call our inner warrior. As we return from a transcendent world, we need to find our feet on the ground. Warriors must again find their shields and spears and adopt a healthy stance toward the world to defend themselves and advance their interests.

There is a fascinating tension, of course, between these two goals. Clients benefit by staying open to transcendent experience, preserving it, and weaving it into their lives. But they also need to close enough to deal with the vicissitudes and struggles of everyday life. The unitive experience of being the cosmic lotus flower that basks in universal love needs somehow to be balanced with a strong, healthy sense of self. The experience of moving beyond ego will be truly therapeutic only if it leads to a more aware, empowered, stable, and functional sense of self.

So, integration sessions are most deeply about integrating these two aspects of our being: the cosmic self and the warrior, the ego-less unitive experience and a strong self that is capable of a satisfying interactive-relational life in the world. How to honor both? How to integrate the one and the many? How to walk through the world with open-heartedness and still take care of yourself? How to become the warrior-bodhisattva?

INTRODUCING ART MAKING INTO INTEGRATION SESSIONS

Both preservation and closure goals can, of course, be reached through talk therapy alone in which clients use words to create verbal representations of self, relationships, or emotions. But in addition to engaging and supporting clients' verbal voices, we can greatly enrich this process by leading them to develop their visual voices—to encourage image to speak for them.

Not everyone will be open to this art-making process, but many will be—especially if we head off client anxiety by making an important distinction between fine art, found in art schools and art galleries, and rough art, the visual representation made by individuals with no particular art training, talent, or experience. We let clients know that rough art is completely OK; the process we encourage them to enter is about authenticity rather than aesthetics. Every client picture is to be accepted with Rogerian unconditional positive regard; every picture is perfect just as it is.

Most art therapy integration sessions will have two parts: a nonverbal art-making part followed by a therapeutic conversational part in which clients are encouraged to verbally explore the meanings in their work.

Enhancing integration sessions with art making yields many therapeutic dividends:

- Creativity itself is inherently satisfying and an easier, more natural, and intuitive way than words to communicate ideas and emotions.
- Visual expression usually involves greater emotional honesty, less defensive editing of emotional truth; it is likely to be more authentic.
- Through a process of externalization, clients put inner images out there on paper. Client inner experience thus becomes public, sharable with the therapist and available for discussion.
- Images form a permanent record of progress over time, a visual journal of a journey.
- Images can be closed down to enhance emotional safety and opened again later.

But there is an important additional benefit in using image, one specific to psychedelic psychotherapy involving mystical experiences. These transcendent experiences, which are strongly correlated with successful clinical outcomes, are essentially noetic; they involve the subjective sense that deep truths are being revealed. So, naturally, these experiences are perceived as being deeply important to the journeyer. But they are also, by nature, ineffable; verbal description seems futile; we just can't put them into words.

Here, a picture is worth more than a thousand words. The image can show something of what cannot be said. Our language is essentially dualistic, creating a distinction between self and other. So, verbal expression tends to draw us out of unitive experience; it pulls us back into duality, back into our ego selves. There is a time for doing this as part of our closure goal, but there is also a time following a medicine session, especially a well-resolved one, when it is important just to let clients steep in the afterglow of a well-resolved session by staying away from words, encouraging them to stay with nonverbal visual expression. It slows the rate at which the cement sets up and prolongs the time in which emotion and cognition are still malleable and open to further therapeutic movement.

TEN ART ACTIVITIES
FOR INTEGRATION SESSIONS

I offer ten art activities that can be helpful in reaching our two goals of preservation and closure. Each activity plays a role in enhancing the integration process. The first four activities have preservation themes, and the six that follow are for closure. In a well-resolved session, while clients are still open from their psychedelic experience, we usually begin with the preservation themes and move toward closure themes as they prepare to reengage with their day-to-day worlds. However, when a medicine session has not been well resolved, we may choose to lead with closure themes. The following activities can be used flexibly and be adapted to the client's pace and process.

Artwork for Preservation

1. My Encounter with Transcendence

This activity is particularly valuable following a well-resolved session, leading clients to consolidate their healing experiences. Our invitation

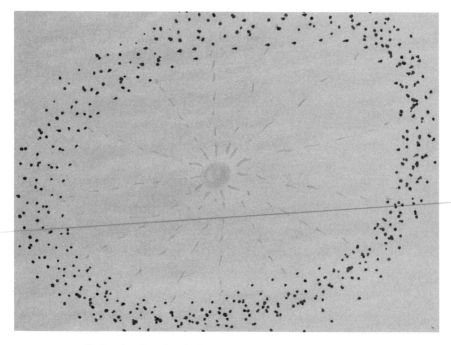

Patient artwork: *My Encounter with Transcendence.*
See plate 1 of the color insert.

is: "Create a visual image that represents your experience. It can be abstract, just using colors, lines, and shapes. Let your picture show whatever treasures, truths, wisdom, or healing you have gained from your journey." We encourage clients to invest themselves in this picture, to steep themselves in it, and give them at least half an hour to work on this. We invite them to move beyond thinking and allow whatever wants to emerge out onto the paper. When completed, we may encourage clients to sit silently with their image, as an object of meditation, breathing its goodness in as they inhale. Later, we gently invite clients to verbalize the picture's content: "What is this picture showing us about your healing experience?" At session's end, I may encourage clients to take their icon home, letting it serve as a subliminal reminder of those healing energies they experienced. The picture thus becomes a touchstone to help maintain access to that healing experience.

Arthur, a thirty-one-year-old man, suffered from chronic anxiety and depression. His image making is a great example of how effective this modality can be even with patients who have no prior experience with art.

Arthur: "I came to this oneness, an infinite space, absolute emptiness, but it contained everything. And at the center of everything was this . . . golden light, this infinite love that radiated right through me. I felt a profound gratitude for having been allowed to see and feel this. I cried and cried, but I was beyond joy or grief. For the first time in my life, I felt fundamentally loved and felt a profound healing, not just with my emotions but right down to my soul."

2. Tending the Fire

For this picture, we encourage clients to focus on preserving and nourishing the parts of their psychedelic experience that they find

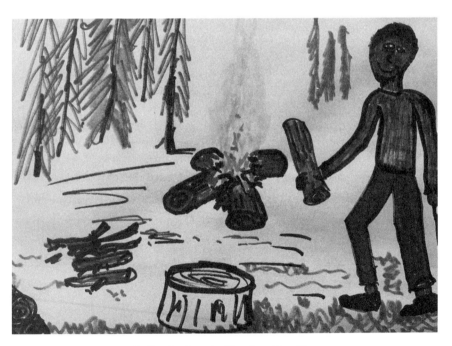

Patient artwork: *Tending the Fire*.
See plate 2 of the color insert.

most valuable. Our invitation is: "Choose a metaphor that represents the precious new life you have discovered inside. Create a picture that shows you taking care of it, helping it flourish." Clients might draw themselves tending a fire, keeping it alive with fresh wood, but they could also choose another metaphor, such as watering a beautiful plant or cultivating a garden. In the conversational part of our session, we invite clients to talk about their picture, asking, for example, "How are you nurturing the fire in your picture? What's it like to nurture that fire? And how will you nurture what's important to you from your psychedelic session? What practical steps can you take to keep your inner light and warmth alive?"

> Arthur expressed misgivings about drawing this picture: "I'm the world's worst artist. I can't draw people at all!" But he was an avid camper, and he knew a lot about getting and keeping a fire going. This picture became a wonderful conversation starter: What counts as fuel to sustain your inner fire? How will you know when your fire needs more nourishment? Where will you get it from? How will you feel as you're able to maintain your inner fire? Arthur pointed out the importance of the size of the fire: not too big, not too small. He also commented on how much he began to enjoy the art materials once he let go of worrying about how his picture looked.

3. Obstacles along My Way

This picture leads clients to focus closely on the threats that pose the biggest challenges to their process. We encourage them to: "Show in a picture the people, places, or situations that are the most likely obstacles to keeping your inner light alive." Then we engage them in a discussion about how they can effectively deal with those obstacles and what success might be like. We may invite clients, in subsequent pictures, to show themselves dealing effectively with those obstacles. This becomes a way of road-testing a new plan and rehearsing new behavior in fantasy.

Artwork for Closure

4. Closing Mandala

This Jungian-informed activity promotes emotional closure and containment by using a process of visual closure. A mandala is a design built around a center. Here, we invite clients to create a mandala that expresses how they are right now. We advise clients to begin their design on the outside perimeter and work in toward the center.

5. My Strengths and Resources

Clients are asked to make an image that shows their strengths: "Create something—it can be realistic or abstract, using colors, lines, shapes, or symbols—that shows the strong part of you, the survivor who can successfully overcome your challenges." Later, we look at it together and ask: "What is this image showing us about your strengths? Where did they come from? How will you use them? How will they help you in specific situations?" This focus encourages positive self-regard, readies clients for what's ahead in their lives, and orients them to the resources they'll need to meet those challenges.

> Arthur: "I came out of this experience feeling that I could finally love myself. Here's me, feeling cleansed and strong and resourceful. When I feel this good inside, I want to share it around! My greatest strength and resource is that I feel connected to myself and my world; I feel access to a well of love in the center of my being, and I find joy in letting that out into the world." (See the image on page 238.)

6. Me as the Lotus Flower and Me as the Warrior

This activity, essentially a set of three self-portraits, is particularly relevant for those who have had a significant mystical experience. It invites clients to visually represent the two sides of their being and to integrate the two. My invitation to clients is: "Create two pictures. The first abstract one will show your cosmic self, at one with everything. The other, using more realism, will show you, the warrior, with your sword and shield, strong and ready to deal with the challenges in your life."

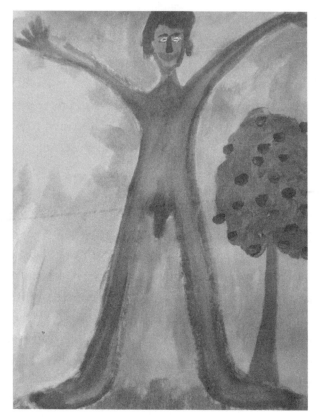

Patient artwork: *My Strengths and Resources.*
See plate 3 of the color insert.

Moving from the abstract to the realistic depiction of a human body has a grounding and embodying effect. We then ask clients to create a third picture that combines the first two. We ask: "How can these two aspects of you work together in an integrated way? What does each contribute to the whole? What would balance between these two sides of your being look like in your life?"

7. My Problem Image
Sometimes, clients emerge from a psychedelic session with unresolved issues relating to a person or situation, and we will make the decision to lead them to explicitly confront that unfinished business. An

invitation to create a relevant visual image can be very helpful: "Draw your problem image, person, memory. Bring this image out of the shadows right onto the page." When drawn, we invite clients to stay with the image, to dance with it, to let the image move them. We may encourage them to verbally dialogue with the image as a way of closure. We may supplement this problem image with an invitation to "draw something that shows how you feel right now about this person or situation."

> *This image terrorized Arthur through much of his medicine session: "A monster that just wouldn't stop chasing me. He's trying to destroy me; he's relentless!" Arthur acknowledged in his first integration session that this image had "stalked me through my whole life." He came to see this figure as representing his "rage-aholic" father who emotionally abused him, but the figure also represented his own rage. After much cathartic expression of anger using large brushes and copious amounts of red and black paint, Arthur looked at this image with new eyes: "He looks so young, so defenseless, and in so much fear and pain." Arthur cried as he realized this image is himself as a child and how frightened he was for so many years. (See the image on page 240.)*

In cases where emotional agitation persists and resolution appears unlikely within the current session, we can choose colors and media that enhances client safety and closure. Options here include:

- Directing clients to use cool colors, such as blue and green, can help them cool emotionally.
- Moving clients toward media in which they have more manual control can enhance their sense of emotional control; for example, move from painting with large brushes to using felt pens or even pencils.
- Suggesting clients use smaller pieces of paper to attenuate the volume of expression.

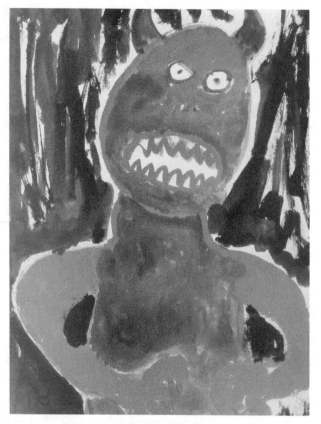

Patient artwork: *My Problem Image.*
See plate 4 of the color insert.

- Inviting clients to use containment techniques, such as drawing or painting a border around their pictures, when there is a need for emotional containment. For example, "John, you have done some really good work today. Your picture really shows how upset you are about X. How about if you take a color from the crayon box that for you is really strong. Try putting a border around your picture that will be strong enough to contain all these feelings so that they don't bother you too much through this coming week until we meet again. Make your border as thick and as strong as you need it to be."

• Inviting clients to use metaphorical acts of closure. We may suggest that clients fold the paper with the troubling image: "Is it time to close this image down for now? How about folding your paper?" When done, we continue: "How about folding it again—and again. How does it feel to do that?" If clients report a calming effect, we might continue: "OK, and now how about wrapping this string (or elastic band) around this folded paper? And how about we put this little package in the back of this filing cabinet, and no one is going to open this cabinet until you decide to." We can enhance this containment process by actually giving the drawer key to clients and inviting them to put their work into the drawer and locking it.

8. Relaxxx

This activity uses a combination of drawing and body movement to facilitate reduction of emotional or physical agitation: "Choose colors

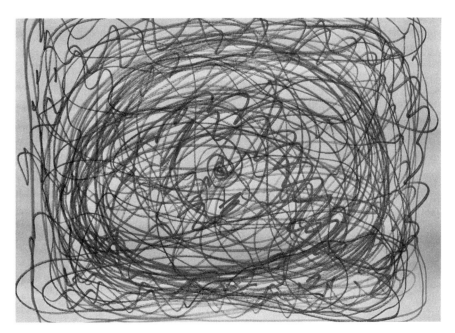

Patient artwork: *Relaxxx*.
See plate 5 of the color insert.

from your box of felt pens that most represent your troubling emotion or body tension. I'm going to invite you, on this large paper, to imagine that you can drain all that tension out onto the page. As you let your crayon scribble all over this page, let your tension empty out of your body, through your arm, your hand, and your crayon onto the page. Let your crayon move as quickly or slowly as you'd like. Let your felt pen move for as long as it wants to."

> Arthur: "Yes, I needed to let that stuff out—the after-birth! I seemed to want to start with the warm colors and then I wanted to continue with the cooler colors. I could feel my breath relax as I widened those loops. At first, I thought 'Yuck, look at this tension still inside of me.' I didn't like to see it on the page. But then, as I kept going, I started to like what I saw on the page: 'Hey! This is me; this is my energy!' And it felt pretty good! It also felt good to end right in the center; I feel a sense of balance."

9. My Safe Place

We invite clients to draw a safe place: "Draw a picture that shows you in your safe place, a place—real or imaginary—where you can rest and heal without fear. Make it as safe as you need it to be." Visiting their safe place following an encounter with difficult inner material promotes emotional closure for clients, especially when the session has not been resolved.

As clients in medicine work relax their defenses against looking at the painful parts of their lives, they will inevitably experience anxiety and vulnerability. In the closure process we want to enhance clients' sense of control. We want to help them to experience a sense of efficacy in relation to their therapy process. As Arthur noted, "I can open up; I can also close down. I am in charge of my process. And I have a safe place inside myself where I can return to after I have gone out into the difficult places."

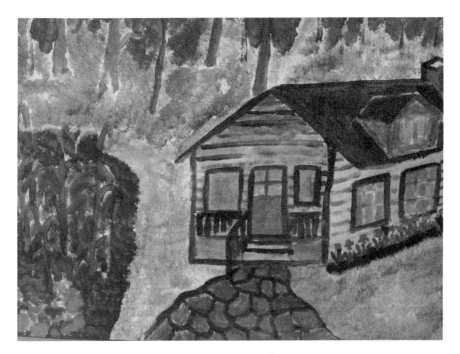

Patient artwork: *My Safe Place.*
See plate 6 of the color insert.

Arthur: "I've made this cabin for myself—in the woods. It's warm and cozy inside. I've got vegetables growing in the garden, and I can sustain myself here until I decide to venture back into the world. There's a paved path for when I want to seek company, but right now, I like it that it's quiet here and no one will bother me. I can rest and heal here. This is my space, my ground, a place where it's very easy for me to just be me. I feel peace when I look at this picture. I feel warm inside, just like my little cabin looks warm inside."

10. Good-bye

At the end of integration work, interpersonal closure is also important; it's a time to for the therapist and client, who have by now established a relationship of warmth and intimacy, to say good-bye. Here, an exchange of an art memento or a symbolic transitional object between

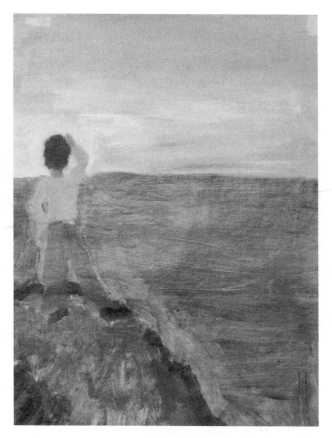

Patient artwork: *Good-bye.*
See plate 7 of the color insert.

client and therapist can be a great way to mark the importance of the established relationship.

> Arthur: "We've come so far together in this process. Now, in this last meeting we'll be having together, I feel I'm at the end of one journey and about to begin a whole new one. As I look at my picture, I realize I feel alone as I look out across the open water and sky that represents my future. But you have been close by as I have made it to this point, and I feel that I will carry you in my heart as I find the boat that will carry me across these waters to a new land."

THERAPEUTIC CONVERSATIONS
ABOUT CLIENT ART

Our discussion of the foregoing activities offers some general guidelines to how therapists might lead clients to discuss their created images for therapeutic benefit. Assume a stance of enlightened ignorance. Our role will be to ask the questions. Real progress occurs when clients do the work of interpreting their images, not us. Let them be the authority on the meanings of their work. Our therapeutic questions fall into three groups:

- **About process.** Before attending to the image itself, we begin by asking about the clients' experience of creating the image: "What was it like to work on this picture? What went on inside as you created this image? What did you notice in your body as you worked on it?" Responses to these give us clues as to how to proceed.
- **About content.** These questions seek to identify what the image presents. We usually begin with general questions that clarify the big picture: "What is this picture showing us?" We then move toward more detail: "Who is this? What is that?"
- **About meaning.** These questions help clients focus on the semantic content of their picture and help them digest it: "What is this picture showing us? What message does it express? How does this picture relate to your current life situation? Does this (color or symbol) have a meaning for you here? What does this face, mouth, stance, hand, eye say? What is X feeling about self, other, situation? What is X saying, thinking, wanting, looking at?"

SUMMARY

Integration is the process by which therapeutic psychedelic experience translates into enduring life changes. Outward expression of inner personal imagery with art materials can enhance integration by both honoring the experience that cannot be described and showing more clearly what can be spoken about. Therapeutic conversations about client images lead to greater clarity for clients about self, the meaning of their journey experience, and how that meaning may be sustained in practical ways as the future unfolds.

19

Integration Using Mandalas

A Personal Perspective

John Ablett

F or centuries, stylized circular images known as mandalas, from the
Sanskrit word for circle, have been used as a focus for spiritual contemplation. In some traditions, they take the form of cosmological representations of celestial realms or maps of inner territory (see pages 248
and 249). The modern Western interest in their therapeutic potential
derives from the psychiatrist Carl Jung, who noticed that when he began
making circular images daily during a time of personal crisis, it helped
him organize his thoughts, as well as providing a visual record of his psychological process. Intrigued by the spontaneous appearance of mandala
symbols in the dreams of his patients during similar periods of profound
inner transformation, he also made cross-cultural comparisons between
mandala images in diverse traditions worldwide.

The therapeutic use of mandalas in psychedelic research was pioneered by Joan Kellogg, an art therapist on Stanislav Grof's team at
the Maryland Psychiatric Research Center in the 1970s. She encouraged test subjects to create mandalas before and after their psychedelic
experiences as a way of documenting and comparing the outcome of

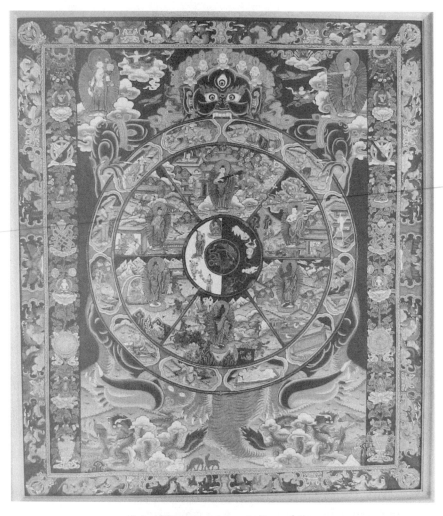

A traditional representation of the
bhāvacakra (wheel of becoming) of Tibetan Buddhism.
See plate 8 of the color insert.

sessions. Stanislav Grof subsequently incorporated mandala drawing as an integration process when he developed Holotropic Breathwork. In this context, mandalas are used to help make a nonintellectual connection with the content of a Breathwork session as well as provide a visual aid when describing the experience in a sharing group during the integration phase of the work.

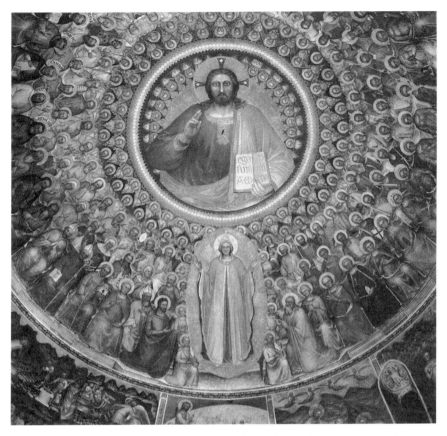

Paradise, a fresco at the Baptistery of the Padua Duomo painted by Giusto de' Menabuoi. See plate 9 of the color insert.

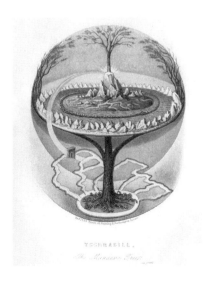

Yggdrasil of Norse mythology. This image is from the 1847 English translation of the *Prose Edda*, translated by Oluf Olufsen Bagge. See plate 10 of the color insert.

IMAGE AS SYMBOL

Staring at a blank circle on a sheet of paper after an intense experience, it can often be difficult to work out where to begin. An integration mandala for a session in an expanded state of awareness doesn't have to be complicated or even necessarily depict the experience in a literal way. It only needs to connect imaginatively and emotionally with something that feels important, or that might otherwise be difficult to verbalize.

The image at the top of the next page, for example, is a simple yellow circle. It recalls my earliest memory of recognizing and using transcendent imagery to change my state of consciousness when, as a child, I used to rub my closed eyes before bedtime to stimulate the optic nerves and then watch the phosphene rings fade as I went to sleep (figure on next page). The same image has connections to a family secret and my mother's death, in a single symbol that demonstrates for me the enduring nature of love and grief. Imagine, if you will, that we're sitting together in a sharing group at the end of a long day's inner journeying, and I'll tell you the story.

I'm a scared teenager, sitting with my mum. She is dying of cancer and has started hallucinating under the influence of her morphine medication. She is sitting up in bed with a pudding dish of pineapple rings when she suddenly asks me to bring her some tissues, whispering conspiratorially that she wants to "make it nice" for my father. I watch in horror as she spoons the pineapple rings carefully onto the tissues and wraps each one individually, telling me to keep them as a present for my dad when he returns home from work. As the tissue turns transparent with wet juice, my memory of this event becomes one of symbolic grief, marking the moment when I can no longer recognize or relate to my mother's experience meaningfully.

Thirty-some years later, at a Holotropic Breathwork workshop in Spain, I "dream" in my session that I am back at my mum's bedside as she folds the corners of the tissue around the pineapple ring like a nappy.

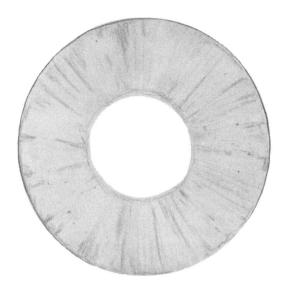

A simple yellow circle that evokes a childhood memory of the author's mother eating pineapple. Image by John Ablett.
See plate 11 of the color insert.

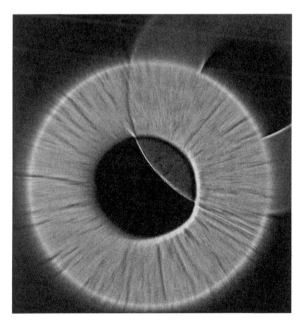

Phosphene rings. The same symbol of the circle represents a gateway to deeper unconscious material. Image by John Ablett.
See plate 12 of the color insert.

Like a master puppeteer, she looks meaningfully from me to the fruit and back again, as if telling a wordless story, and it suddenly seems to me that the subject of the tale she is telling is me, as a baby.

Although alike in every other way, the second parcel that she wraps is just a wet sticky mess. It feels like a tiny corpse in a white shroud, a second, dead, baby. My mother wants to keep it a secret. She wants to wrap us both up in her love in order to "make it nice" for my father. In this moment, my teenage experience of sitting with her in shame and terror, not knowing what to do, appears to exactly reflect her own experience of having a stillborn child.

In real life, although I had intuited that I had a twin who died in the womb, I had never known or been able to talk to my mother about it while she was alive. It was overwhelming to think that, all along, she had already told me everything I needed to know in this miniature symbolic drama. Finally experiencing the full circle of our collective emotions, it seemed to me that our respective love and grief dissolved into the same sea of tears.

The first time that I recounted this experience, using my mandala as a visual aid, I was sitting on the rocks outside the holotropic workshop venue, which was a hotel overlooking the sea. In an almost unbelievable moment of synchronicity, a freak wave rose up and completely drenched the painting in salt water, just as I finished telling the story. Using tissues to soak up the tide, I saw the yellow halo of my mother's love shining, as if through the veil of memory itself, exactly as I had done thirty years earlier.

Integration is a process, not an event, so the "meaning" of an image like this will never be found neatly defined in a dictionary of symbols. This pineapple ring is woven inextricably into my life, through events in different times and states of consciousness. Its meaning evolves fluidly from the act of remembering how those experiences felt, retelling them in narrative form and reframing them to see how they speak anew to different stages of my life.

IMAGE AS TRANSLATION

It sometimes surprises people who look at my mandalas to know that they are not actually records of visionary experiences. In fact, I very rarely "see" anything in my holotropic sessions at all. Although picture books excited me tremendously as a child, when I remember what it was like to have them read to me, I realize I would more often imagine what they felt like in my body than actually picture them in my mind's eye. Like a storyteller, I would assume the postures of the characters in the picture book and imagine what it would feel like to make their voices inside my own throat.

In the same way, I experience work in different states of consciousness as profoundly body based, so that integration becomes an act of translation, a process first of attaching a narrative to what I feel in the holotropic dream space and then subsequently finding a way to portray it visually. In the mandala on page 254, it was my own hands that spun quickly in a circular motion as if turning a wheel, my hands that stirred an imaginary pot of bones and excrement as I cackled on the workshop mat, and my hands that caressed my torso as if smearing myself with blood.

The identification of these dark and strange symbolic instincts with the three crones seen in this image was an association of ideas. Earlier in the session, I had experienced a lot of traumatic choking, which reminded me of the poisoned apple that Snow White eats in the classic folktale. A piece of the apple becomes lodged in her throat so that she can't swallow it, causing her to remain in a strangely dissociated state in a glass coffin, cut off from the rest of the world. When, as a five-year-old, my parents took me to see the animated Disney version of the story, they told me not be scared because the witch wouldn't come onstage to capture me, and the very idea of this scenario terrified me more than any film ever could. In this mandala, the specters of my fears are onstage, and I am walking down the aisle of a cinema in flames, thrusting myself through the screen to experience the filmlike narrative alongside them.

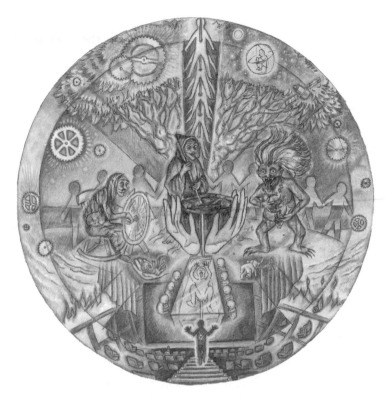

The Cauldron of Transformation by John Ablett.
Turn to plate 13 in the color insert.

At the time of this particular session, I was working as a trainee social worker in a child protection team, a field where the external stresses and risks are often obvious, but the real dangers lie in losing awareness of the dark places in one's own psyche. In this role, I was reading medical case notes on a regular basis, which described horrific acts of sexual abuse, alongside somewhat distant daily conversations with the children and adults who held disembodied versions of these experiences inside themselves. My holotropic experience seemed to be a way of reconciling the things I had intuited in my body but hadn't fully come to terms with, about the reality of sexual abuse and the way it can distort sense of self and body image.

Along both axes of the circle, I drew a linked chain of figures, some skewered as if on a long pole, others multiplied like paper cut-out figures. This is a direct translation of the feeling in the session that my own body was somehow amplified, as if in a hall of mirrors, by collective experiences of trauma. Too much for any one person to contain, these experiences extended into the roots of my biological family tree through hormonal information encoded in the blood of my own ancestors.

What has never been fully brought into awareness can neither be truly remembered nor forgotten, so the act of translating such an experience into words or images is a process of making connections between different parts of oneself: between inside and outside, between body and mind, and between memory and experience. In the case of trauma, toxic material is often dismembered, experienced as symptoms in cut-off parts of the body, unidentified remains that are boiled up to make integration soup in the cauldron of the psyche.

Following this particular session, I struggled with composing a mandala for many weeks. It wouldn't assemble itself properly until I finally put that pot of bones and excrement where it belonged—right there in the center. In doing so, I was able to honor the idea that the three figures whose hands I had felt inside my own were both personifications of childhood fears and ancient archetypes of the deep psyche.

But every image that roots itself in something transcendent has an element that ultimately goes beyond language. It's one thing to recognize intellectually that frightening images can contribute to the work of healing by personifying important symbolic processes and quite another to truly feel comfortable with those processes inside one's own body. In this mandala, the final set of hands, the flame-like ones that safely contain the cauldron, belong to one of the workshop facilitators. She held my head at the end of the session as I let out a series of screams—again, and again, and again—to an empty workshop space where everyone else had long since finished their sessions and gone to lunch. If I listen carefully, I can still almost hear the inhuman noise that came from my own throat that day.

COMPOSITION AS INTEGRATION

Like dreams, events in nonordinary states of consciousness can often contain complex details whose relationship to the experience as a whole is not obvious. As part of my integration process, I have trained myself to make a numbered list of every individual element I can remember from a session. This can sometimes take several weeks because the memories often continue to be triggered days after the experience. They also often occur in clusters, which can give clues as to their relationship with one another.

I regularly go back through notes from old sessions to see what elements remain unintegrated, and the mandala on the next page is a composite drawn from approximately ten years' worth of experiences. To give a sense of scale, the pineapple ring symbol is shown here hanging from the branches of a tree (top center) where it acquires additional layers of meaning simply by being depicted in a new contextual relationship with other symbols.

The mandala took nearly three years to complete, and it contains too many stories to be able to tell them all in a single setting. I want to highlight the peacock's tail of hands around the top outer edge of the circle, each representing a different bodily sensation from a holotropic session. Depicted here are times when my fingers felt cramped, as if they were rigid like animal claws, tree roots, or ossified bone. In between were extraordinary occasions when my hands reached out to touch another person, or something invisible seemed to reach out to touch me.

The central image of the figure dragging the boat originates from a dream I had in my adolescence in which I stood watching a procession of spectral figures parading through a narrow Renaissance-style Venetian street, accompanied by a powerful wind. That dream was one of several that heralded a period of profound psychospiritual crisis in my early twenties, culminating in a six-month episode in which I believed that I was enlightened and played the role of a guru (Ablett 2020). It took many years of holotropic reintegration before I was able to finally approach the heart of that experience again, and when I

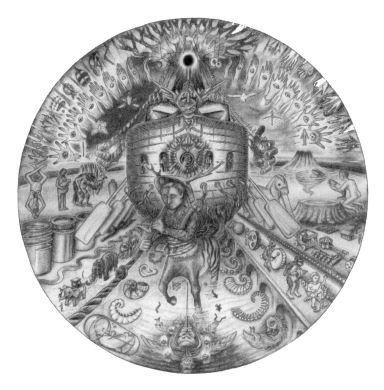

The Harbor of the Psyche by John Ablett.
Turn to plate 14 of the color insert.

finally did, I "dreamed" in my session that the person hauling the boat was me.

> On this occasion, it is the solar boat of the sun god, the sacred vessel of the archetypes, and when I try to move it, like a strong man towing a juggernaut single-handedly with a noose between his teeth, it moves less than a fraction of a millimeter. I feel deeply ashamed of how little I have been able to contribute to the collective experience of the world—until I become aware of a whole army of invisible helpers who are actually doing the hard work of pulling the ship behind me. "This is the speed that it moves at," they tell me, "and we all move it between us. It was never your responsibility to carry, but it touches us that you even tried."

Lasting personal and cultural change moves at a glacial pace. While it can be common to have spiritual experiences that feel so important and profound that everyone needs to know about them *immediately*, it is equally important to have experiences that shrink our sense of self-importance right down to size. In one tiny section of this mandala, my hands that once turned the spinning wheel of fate become the smaller hands of myself as a child, moving the pedals on an upturned tricycle as I play at being a train driver in the family garden. Neither image is more correct than the other, rather they are both different perspectives on the same reality. In one version, profound truths are shown to be essentially playful; in the other, deep profundity is shown to be present in the heart of play.

The completion of this mandala coincided with the end of my training in Holotropic Breathwork theory and facilitation, and I celebrated by floating in the sea with fellow trainees. I'm not a confident swimmer, so I chose a sheltered cove where the tide was not too strong and there was a rope to hold onto in the deeper waters. Using that rope to pull myself back to the shore, I realized that I had missed something important about having depicted myself as the heroic central figure of my mandala. It wasn't just that I wasn't really pulling the boat; I wasn't even fully aware of what I had actually been doing instead. I realized I was hanging on, with all my strength, trying to haul myself out of the deep waters of the psyche in an attempt to avoid being dragged back into them. I was half-human, half-animal, paddling in early traumas that had receded in intensity, and when I realized I had reached land, I suddenly felt enormously privileged to have been a part of such a celebratory parade of experiences. The mandala's title, *The Harbor of the Psyche,* reflects the relationship between an experience and the process of visual translation. For me, drawing a mandala is a way to ground an experience in something that can be shared and spoken about, even if not fully understood. The alternative is to be faced with the prospect of experiences without boundaries or horizons, nor even any maps with which to navigate them safely.

SHARING AS INTEGRATION

There comes a time when the accumulation of extraordinary experiences in nonordinary states of consciousness no longer works as an end in itself. While the possibilities for personal insight and development are undoubtedly endless, I sometimes found myself on lonely and expansive shores where the basic human need to connect was the only thing that anchored me to sanity. In these circumstances, the telling of my story wasn't just a wide-eyed sharing of remarkable travels, nor even a therapeutic process to aid positive integration, it was a real movement of the heart. I had something that I knew I needed to find a way to share with others or else a part of me would forever die internally.

> In my session, I "dream" that I am a pharaoh entombed alive in my own pyramid (see the mandala on the next page). I have been cursed for a terrible act of family treachery with what amounts to an increasingly dull and inconvenient immortality. My most trusted servants, also buried alive with me, have all died slow and painful deaths. Here, in the quiet darkness, I reflect on all my royal treasures, all those items of gold and jewel-encrusted furniture piled high in the antechambers, and I consider what a waste it has been to hoard such an obscene collection of riches for the kind of afterlife I am now experiencing. In my despair, I even find myself longing for the tomb robbers to break in and discover me because the indignity of having that ritual space desecrated would not be worse than the knowledge that its contents might never see the light of day.

There can be a peculiar narcissism involved in assuming that the "purpose" of therapeutic work in nonordinary states of consciousness is to heal one's own trauma or to advance one's own personal development. In reality though, the dilemmas and traumas that we face are often human traumas that many people struggle collectively to integrate and make sense of. In such a context, there can logically be no such thing as a deep archetypal meaning that only speaks to me and

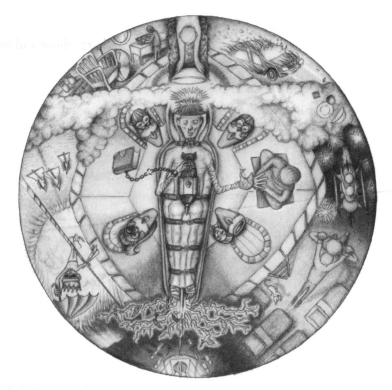

The Greatest of All Illusions by John Ablett.
Turn to plate 15 in the color insert.

my concerns. Sharing with other people, therefore, is about learning the generosity of allowing the material to integrate itself collectively, in other minds and hearts.

But how can we hold such head-turning experiences lightly without either self-aggrandizing or diluting the narrative? It is all too easy for personal stories to be misused to influence other people, to stockpile personal power, or to attract judgments, both positive and negative. For me, being aware of that risk and accepting it is part of the unspoken contract involved in being able to have this incredibly privileged access to deep realms of the psyche. We do this work knowing that many others who would benefit from it are not able to, and I believe that conveys a duty to return and share whatever we can.

Sharing also encourages us to let go of our own interpretations.

Watching someone else find a personal meaning in your story or mandala is much like watching one's child make friends at school and begin to forge his or her own way in the world. It's bittersweet, anticipating a future time when the things you gave birth to, or that you have shaped or created from your life, may actually be all that other people know and remember of you.

Later in the session, I find myself talking to my own body, much as one might imagine a conversation between an out-of-body soul and its host. My body asks, like an earnest child, what it will be like to die and who will be there to take care of it. I say, tenderly, that I know that its parents won't be there to hold it and that I, as a consciousness or sense of self, probably won't be there by that stage either. I say that I think it might be a lot like not breathing any more, and we both hold our breath for about ten seconds to see what that might feel like. I speculate that there might even be another person that neither of us currently knows, perhaps a nurse or a complete stranger, to hold my body's hand while it stops breathing, and we agree that that would be nice, probably enough to make it feel OK.

When we do work in expanded states of consciousness, through meditation, Breathwork, or psychedelics, unfamiliar thoughts flash through our brains and unfamiliar energies move our hands and bodies. There are any number of explanations for what is happening at these times, but as an artist, I tend toward the poetic. For me, it is the ancient gods and archetypes who, for the briefest of timeless moments, live again in us. When those bright experiences fade and the colorful cast of mythical characters, deities, and ancestors solemnly process back into the places from which they came, they leave us knowing that it might be almost a whole generation before their stories are heard or told.

It's true that after each new experience I may well weep for sheer beauty in the emptiness of my own tomb for a while, like a monk keeping vigil after the death of a saint. As the years roll on, however, I trust that there will always be ways to convert what I have felt, seen, and heard into new images, proud hieroglyphs and stick figures, to decorate the ritual spaces and hymn the stories to new generations. It's an act of service, honoring the family and friends that traveled with me and all those others whose ancient labors built the collective structures on which my life depends.

Ultimately, it also foreshadows the death of the body in which I have my experiences, both those which are transcendent and those that are gloriously ordinary. This work suggests to me that in our own way, whether we know it or not, every single one of us deserves to have a royal burial in keeping with the dignity of our collective ancestry. Even while we construct our own mausoleums of the deep psyche, we owe it to one another to keep the doors of those internal sacred places open, to keep them as places of welcome and contemplation, and to decorate their walls as comprehensively as we know how, with images from all the stories that have been entrusted to us.

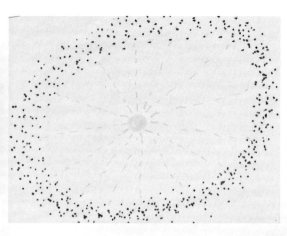

Plate 1. Patient artwork:
My Encounter with Transcendence

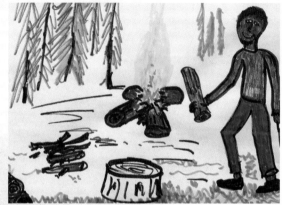

Plate 2. Patient artwork:
Tending the Fire

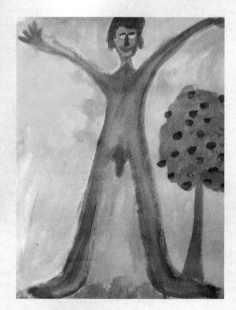

Plate 3. Patient artwork:
My Strengths and Resources

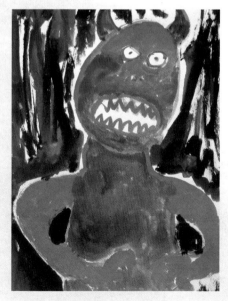

Plate 4. Patient artwork:
My Problem Image

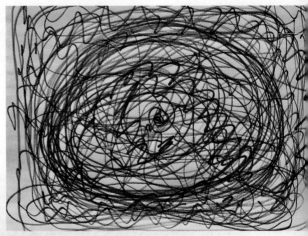

Plate 5. Patient artwork: *Relaxxx*

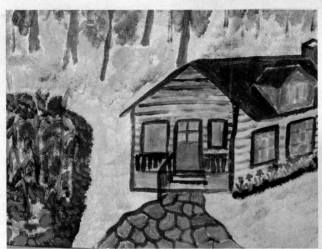

Plate 6. Patient artwork: *My Safe Place*

Plate 7. Patient artwork: *Goodbye*

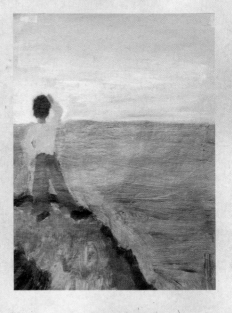

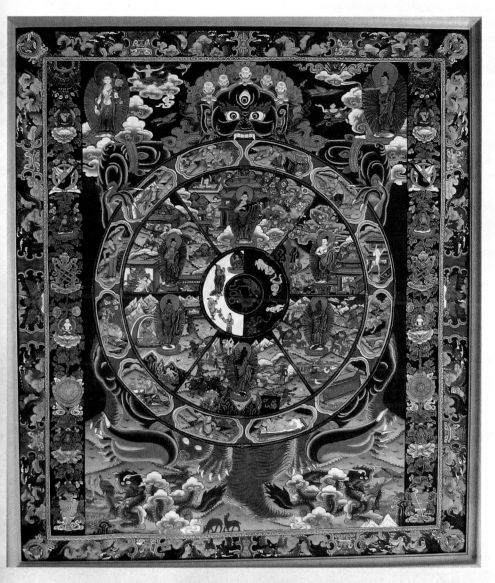

Plate 8. A traditional representation of the bhāvacakra (wheel of becoming) of Tibetan Buddhism.

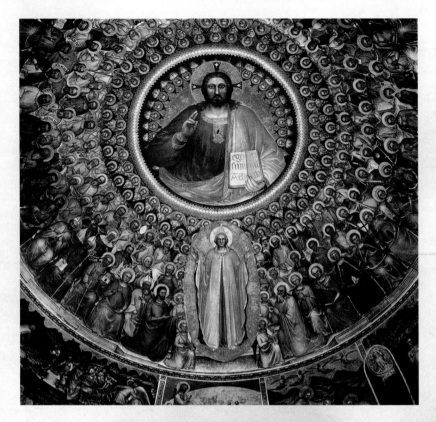

Plate 9. *Paradise*, a fresco at the Bapistery of the Padua Duomo painted by Giusto de' Menabuoi.

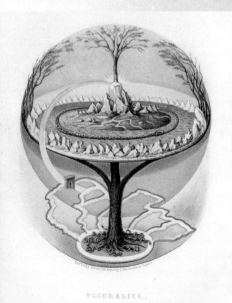

Plate 10. Yggdrasil of Norse mythology. This image is from the 1847 English translation of the Prose Edda, translated by Oluf Olufsen Bagge.

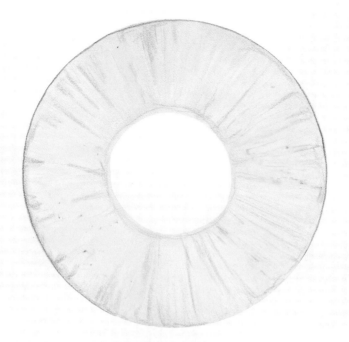

Plate 11. A simple yellow circle that evokes a childhood memory of the author's mother eating pineapple. Image by John Ablett.

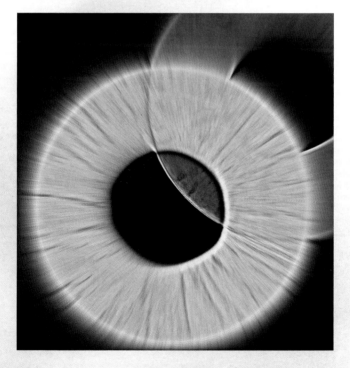

Plate 12. Phosphene rings. The same symbol of the circle represents a gateway to deeper unconscious material. Image by John Ablett.

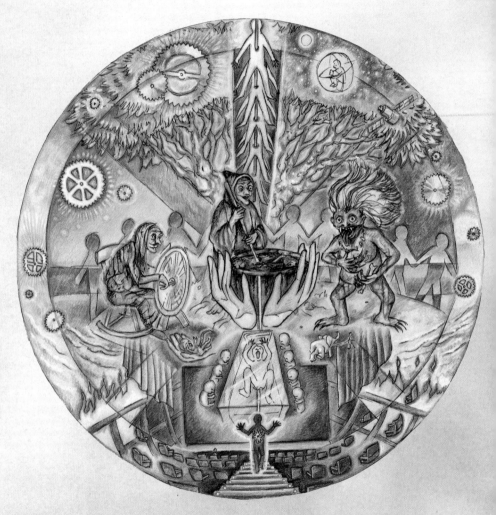

Plate 13. *The Cauldron of Transformation* by John Ablett

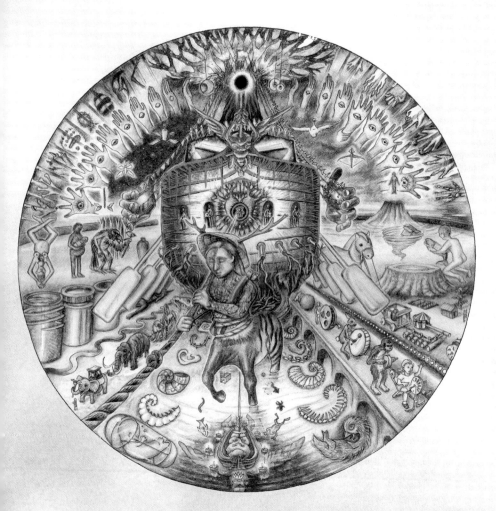

Plate 14. *The Harbor of the Psyche* by John Ablett

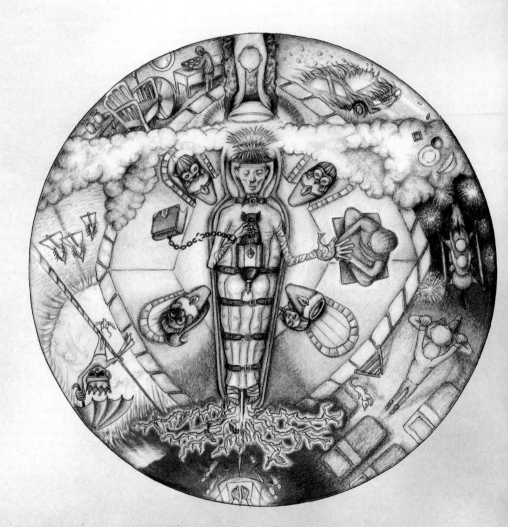

Plate 15. *The Greatest of All Illusions* by John Ablett

20

Harm Reduction, Peer Support, and the First Steps of Integration

Nir Tadmor

Psychedelic harm reduction was born during the iconic days of the 1960s when Western society was confronted for the first time with the chaotic yet transformative powers of psychedelic use outside the clinical context. Psychedelic concerts and festivals were a new playground where some had transcendent experiences of unity and unconditional love, some experienced profound inner transformations that propelled them toward a new way of being in the world, some were confronted with terrifying mental, emotional, and spiritual phenomena, and some were experiencing a severe mental and emotional breakdown.

The roots of psychedelic harm reduction can be traced back to organizations like the Parking Lot Medics, which served the sometimes lost crowd at Grateful Dead concerts, and the Hog Farm, the longest running commune in the United States, founded by peace activist and clown Wavy Gravy, which through its "please force" served the needs of the massive crowd at Woodstock in 1969. These groups inspired many more people to take responsibility and support those who were having challenging psychedelic experiences and thus paved the way toward a more compassionate approach to supporting psychedelic crises. Inspired by this approach, psychedelic harm reduction teams like the Zendo Project, who offer harm reduction and peer support services to Burning Man and other events, and Kosmicare, who support Boom Festival and other events, together with many other contributors, wrote the principles, guidelines, and manuals of the field that is commonly referred to today as psychedelic harm reduction and peer support.

Inspired by this work myself, I cofounded a psychedelic harm reduction and peer support project in Israel called Safe Shore. During the last six years, we have attended thirty-eight events, supported nine hundred people in expanded states of consciousness, and trained more than five hundred psychedelic harm reduction sitters. Many of the people we supported just needed a safe place to rest, some needed someone to quietly listen to their experience, and others were having unexpected intense mystical experiences. Many were reliving a traumatic experience from their past or were suffering the consequences of consuming the wrong combination of drugs. Only five out of nine hundred people were dangerous to themselves or others and needed sedation by a medic. *All* of these people, sooner or later, returned to their ordinary state of consciousness.

Some remembered very well what unfolded; others had little or no memory. While most of them were eager to get as much information from us as possible about what had happened, a few preferred not to talk about it even in the follow-up call days after. With some, we could spend hours of peaceful conversations to help them integrate; with others, we had limited time to talk before another person needed our immediate attention. The psychedelic harm reduction setting is less than ideal for integration, but as this is what we have, we try to make the best out of it.

The psychedelic state often serves as a gate through which previously unconscious traumatic material can arise to conscious awareness. Although such encounters with one's shadow can allow an opportunity for profound healing when supported professionally in a therapeutic setting, in cases where such an experience takes place in a nonsupportive environment, severe anxiety, retraumatization, or even a psychotic reaction may unfold. Since a psychedelic experience in a festival or at a party can sometimes be the first visceral encounter people have with these deep hidden wounds of their psyche, it is crucial that a safe setting and compassionate support are provided so that people can encounter, process, and begin to integrate what emerges.

This chapter is an attempt to share some of the insights and lessons we have experienced in our team while supporting people during these events on their transit from an expanded to an ordinary state of consciousness.

Jacob's Military Trauma

During a four-day festival we received a call about someone having a crisis by the lake. When our sitters* got there, they found a young man punching the ground, his hands bleeding, repeating: "I just want to go to swim, I just want to go to swim." He responded to their initial attempts to engage him, and although he insisted on wanting to swim, the sitters observed that he was not attempting to do so. It took two hours of talking to him by the shore of the lake before he was able to discuss his experiences as a soldier. Four months earlier he had gone with two friends from his unit to a place they were strictly forbidden from entering; they were discovered by hostile forces and shot at. His two friends died in front of him, and he was wounded in his shoulder.

The sitters listened and held him physically in his distress. They offered the privacy of our harm reduction space, a geodesic dome, where he could drink, eat, and rest. As he talked, he shared his will to swim as far as he could into the lake until he ran out of energy to swim back, as a way of ridding himself from the torrent of traumatic memories

---

*The terms *sitter* or *trip-sitter* describe a person that soberly accompanies people on their psychedelic experiences. The term is used as an alternative to *guide,* as one of the cornerstones of trip-sitting is to refrain from actively guiding another person's experience.

that had erupted with such unbearable force under the influence of the LSD-MDMA combination he had taken. He asked us to find his trusted friend, and when we found him, we had to make sure that he was in a state of ordinary consciousness himself before taking him into the dome. We stayed present, with his permission, and supported him as he was sharing his experience with his friend, revealing for the first time the guilt, the shame, and the pain that had filled his life during these months. He had seen an army psychiatrist immediately after the event, who told him he was "OK" but who did not give him the opportunity to unpack his experience and did not follow up with him. He did not receive any therapy.

After a short rest, he felt ready to return to the party, and we suggested he keep a slow pace and refrain from drinking or tripping during the event. He accepted it with a nod and some disappointment but thanked us deeply. He returned the day after to tell us we had saved his life and that he felt motivated to offer other people the help that he had received himself. The sitter that was leading the intervention had a follow-up with him where they both shared their experience of what had happened and agreed to have a further follow-up after the event. On the first working day after the festival, the sitter visited Jacob in his workplace, and they discussed grounding and self-care practices like the importance of eating and sleeping well and various physical exercises to release pent-up energy. Advice was offered about integration tools and methods so that the wounds that had been exposed could move toward healing rather than remain open. The advice included keeping a journal to help integrate intense experiences, sharing of feelings and challenges with at least one other person, and the usefulness of psychotherapy as a space to process this experience further.

INTEGRATION IN A
NONTHERAPEUTIC CONTEXT

In psychedelic-assisted psychotherapy, the integration process will naturally look very different. Psychedelic psychotherapy, like any other psychotherapy, is based on a trusting relationship between the therapist and the patient, who has come to therapy sober and with the intention to explore his or her inner experiences. In a psychedelic harm reduction context, there is no previously established relationship, no appropriate setting for therapy, and, most importantly, no sober consent—and thus no *real* consent to embark on a therapeutic process. Although our lead sitters are experienced with trauma work, we are all well aware that the festival is not the time or place to open these wounds beyond what is naturally occurring, nor is it the time to process the traumatic contents from all the aforementioned reasons. That being said, we help our guests connect to their feelings and encourage them to keep a curious mindset, as we believe expanded states hold a profound healing potential and are an opportunity for psychospiritual growth.

What does it mean to support the first steps of integration in a non-therapeutic context? First, it means establishing trust and improving the setting as much as possible to increase the guests' sense of safety. This will enable the guests to share their experience, or if they prefer to let the experience sink in before they share it, it will allow them a quiet space that will support their rest and contemplation. Once they have returned to ordinary consciousness, we will support them in forming a coherent narrative of their experience. This process usually begins with an invitation to share or ask anything they would like, and only when the guests have finished sharing their experience, we ask if they are interested to hear more about it from our perspective. If the answer is affirmative, we share with them the way the events unfolded from our perspective, while concentrating on the meaningful moments and on assimilating the specific experiences that were remembered by the guests. We also encourage our guests, especially those who don't want to share the details of their journey with us, to write down their experiences and add new information as it comes up later, thus facilitating the development, in due course, of their own coherent narrative.

Since often a verbal expression is either challenging or perceived as a narrowing of the vastness and abstract nature of the experience, we bring with us to festivals and parties a painting kit that allows guests to express their inner dynamics in an artistic way. The process of translating inner dynamics into an external form is important for the psychedelic integration process, allowing a greater agency over these forces and also an opportunity to connect with one's inner experience from a different angle through symbolic and archetypal expressions.

We also strongly encourage our guests to notice their somatic experience and to take care of their body after (and, if possible, during) the experience, whether through breathing, short walks, basic yoga asanas, or healthy nutrition. Reactions like restlessness, shaking, insomnia, or aggressiveness are usually signs of pent-up energy stored in the body and can be greatly supported by attuning to the body's needs and discharging it using simple practices like running, screaming into a pillow, dancing, gardening, or any other safe physical expression one finds beneficial.

Another important aspect for our consideration of their integration process is the setting to which the person returns to after the party. In some cases, we will have to talk to our guests' partners, parents, or roommates to prepare the ground for their safe landing. Since we keep all details of our guests and their experiences fully confidential, we do not share anything with anyone without our guests' permission. The only exception is if a person requires the involvement of the medical team when we share anything that can help him or her better understand the situation. In some cases, guests give us their consent to contact their family or friends so that we can help them return home, but they ask us not to share any details regarding the substances they used or the events that took place. In these cases, we try to convey to those that will receive them the importance of a soft, nonjudgmental approach toward the person who just had a very intense experience, and if we are asked to provide further information, we explain our commitment to confidentiality. We emphasize in these conversations with both our guests and their loved ones the importance of grounding, sleeping and eating well, and drinking plenty of water. Some of our guests return from their expanded states determined to make abrupt changes in their personal or social life, and we urge them to take a few weeks or at least days, before taking any crucial decisions that might have a major impact on their life. Often, the insights one has during a psychedelic experience can seem very different later from a more grounded state of mind.

The integration process is not only a psychological and metaphorical one but also a biological one. The research by Carhart-Harris et al. (2014) has shown that the psychedelic state is characterized by unconstrained cognition and high-entropy neurodynamics, and that when the person shifts back to an ordinary state of consciousness, his or her brain goes through a process of reorganization (entropy-suppression). This is why the set and setting of the hours and days of transition between one state of consciousness to another are sometimes critical for the shaping of new beliefs and behaviors. The intense somatic, cognitive, emotional, and often spiritual processes that are taking place at the same time may leave the body and mind deeply exhausted after the many hours of the experience, which is why the importance of sleep and nourishment cannot be overemphasized.

THE UNINTENDED MYSTICAL EXPERIENCE

Psychedelic experiences have been known for thousands of years to awaken powerful mystical experiences, but modern recreational users often embark on their psychedelic journeys with the intention of having fun, bypassing their social and sexual boundaries, and staying awake and energetic through the night. This mindset tends to leave people completely unprepared not only for a confrontation with the shadow side of their psyche, where untreated wounds from the past are contained, but also with the spiritual dimension of their lives and the extraordinary powers it holds.

David's Explosive Mystical Experience

David was escorted to our space by security and two of his friends, who were very concerned about him. At first, he appeared potentially violent, furiously throwing his arms in the air while shouting and mumbling broken sentences. I spent a few moments with him in the secluded outdoor area of our safe space, observing and trying to make some sense of his seemingly wild behavior. After a while I discerned that the content of his mumbled speech concerned unity, the messiah, and Mount Sinai. It was clear that he did not intend to hurt anyone, and even though he appeared to be angry, he seemed to be dealing with the often-frightening somatic energies that can be awakened during a mystical experience. After a moment, he lay down on the grass and started twitching and shaking; four of our sitters immediately sat around him, laying their hands gently below his head, on his heart, and on his feet. The immediate task was to keep him physically safe, and they were prepared to hold him more firmly if necessary, to "ground" him energetically, and also to give him a nonverbal confirmation that he was not alone in his experience.

While my colleagues were busy containing him, I was talking to his friends, gathering as many details as possible about what he had taken and the sequence of events; I also enquired about any preexisting medical conditions. They had all taken MDMA, but since his reactions didn't look like a typical MDMA experience, I also needed to consider the possibility of any preexisting mental health issues. His friends told me he had stopped his SSRI antidepressant a few days before the festival in order to prepare for his psychedelic experience. They did not know his diagnosis. We assured them that he was safe and suggested they go to the dance floor to release the energy that was still building up from the MDMA and dance off some of the stress from the experience. One of our sitters joined them so that we could contact them in case of need. Meanwhile, our guest was still shouting and mumbling while his whole body was contracting and releasing with immense force. We were concerned enough to ask the medics to assess his vital signs while he was moving in and out of an intense-looking mystical experience. His state fluctuated; there were periods when he had his eyes closed while he shook, moaned, and incoherently mumbled different religious terminologies and verses. At other times he opened his eyes, looked frightened, and asked us for reassurance: "Is this OK? Will I be fine?" We responded that he was safe, that we were with him, and that he could fully surrender to his experience. When he was frightened by the tremendous amounts of energy that rushed through his body, we reassured (while gently holding him) that this was OK and that he could allow his body to shake and move in any way that it needed to.

Three and a half hours later, he slowly stood up, still with eyes closed. We all stood with him, curious to see what would unfold. He asked us to sing a Jewish prayer song with him. He started singing, and we all hugged as we joined him. When the song was finished, he crouched, and as I crouched in front of him, he raised his gaze, looked straight into my eyes, and said: "Where can I get more MDMA?" I couldn't help myself from laughing as I hugged him and welcomed him back.

One of our lead sitters, who is a somatic psychotherapist and an experienced bodyworker, spent the next few hours supporting his transition back to everyday consciousness. The separation from unity and his direct contact with the divine was painful and confusing. He was shocked and exhausted but remembered many profound moments and visions and was deeply grateful for the compassionate support of the team. He ate and drank after hours of very little hydration (the sitters managed to get him to sip some water whenever possible). The intense pulses of energy had left his body feeling stiff, tense, and exhausted. Our lead sitter helped him release the tension he felt, mainly in the shoulders and neck, using various massaging techniques.

He rested for a while before trying to share his experiences with the sitter. They acknowledged the ineffability of the experience and talked about God and the sacred, his day-to-day life, and the religious background of his family, while making room for the different emotions, body sensations, and mental images that came up. This experience prompted him to begin psychotherapy to continue the integrative journey over the longer term.

DIFFICULT IS NOT THE SAME AS BAD

Time and time again, we find that with adequate holding, even the most challenging experiences can become a fruitful ground for our mental, emotional, interpersonal, and spiritual growth. Sometimes, especially where traumatic content has emerged, processing the experience with an experienced psychotherapist may eventually be necessary. In other cases, peer support will be enough to allow the person to engage with the psychedelic integration process, where the knowledge and insights could be translated into actions through different practices and changes in perspective to support the person's psychospiritual development and self-actualizing process. One way or another, it is of crucial importance to acknowledge these experiences as meaningful and potentially transformative rather than simply a bad trip. The term *bad trip* conveys a judgmental outlook on a potentially transformative experience and may prevent us from properly opening to the experience with a compassionate and curious attitude. It may also ingrain a notion that challenging experiences are not a healthy part of our healing journey and thus prevent us from taking responsibility for our personal and transpersonal issues.

Another significant aspect of the harm reduction perspective is to respect the person's increased suggestibility by avoiding the imposition of interpretations, opinions, or dogmas on the consolidating psyche of the guest. For example, we do not use spiritual terminologies like chakras to explain physical phenomena, we do not use religious frameworks, we do not give guests mantras to reduce anxiety, and we do not offer explanatory models for the phenomena that our guests experience, even if we feel that we "understand" what is unfolding. We keep our input to a minimum and do our best to allow our guests to meet themselves rather than us. We have observed that some people who were supported on their journey by religious officials end up becoming religious themselves; others may become obsessively attached to ideas and concepts that they were introduced to by the supporting figure.

Providing compassionate support for expanded states of consciousness in festivals and parties is delicate work that requires weeks of preparation for a single event. A team of trained sitters—half female, half male—needs to be recruited (the size of the team depends on the size and duration of the event), including a few professional therapists who supervise each shift and lead the support of any cases that are particularly challenging. The sitters need to be well acquainted with psychedelic harm reduction ethics and guidelines (Zendo Project 2017), the effects and risks involved with each substance, and active listening practices. They also need to be willing to work voluntarily in shifts around the clock during the whole event, to sleep well (not always an easy task in a festival), and, of course, to stay sober. Holding space for challenging psychedelic experiences is a practice that involves encountering the total spectrum of mental and emotional states and thus requires practitioners who are willing to be in service for the mystical and the ecstatic as much as for the painful and perplexing.

These extreme states can also trigger strong emotional reactions for the sitters, who naturally share many of the traumas and wounds of our guests. To take care of their own needs and prevent secondary trauma, the sitters are encouraged during the opening circle to notice their inner dynamics carefully and the way these change with each guest, as some guests might trigger a strong emotional reaction for some sitters and thus prevent them from providing support. The shift leader's role is to stay tuned to the different sitters and notice if they become uncomfortable, tired, or triggered. If so, the shift leader needs to choose the right sitter to replace the tired or triggered sitter, a process that might take a while, once trust has been established between a guest and a sitter. Sitters are also encouraged to look out for one another and to share their experiences and feelings within the team as the event unfolds. Each event ends with an integration circle where we discuss each guest, while focusing on the challenging moments and the lessons that were learned during the process with that person. After multiple-day events, we do a short closing ceremony and meet for a long integration circle a few days after.

During the time we spend together, a deeply intimate connection is formed not only between the sitters and the guests but also among the team members, who have shared humbling moments of vulnerability, catharsis, and gratitude. The comfortable space we build, the bond among the team members and their awareness moment by moment of their own inner experience, are all core aspects of the safe container we invite our guests to. This open and accepting atmosphere enables a safe and nonjudgmental transition into an ordinary state of consciousness and allows the guests to be fully focused on their inner experience, as the sitters are there to make sure all other needs are met.

A healthy unfolding of the first hours of integration is crucial for our psychospiritual well-being, but to create long-lasting changes in our everyday life and our way of being in the world, a conscious engagement with our unfolding psychic process during the weeks and months after the experience is required. Practices that support this process include psychotherapy, intimate conversations with loved ones, journaling, painting, singing, dancing, yoga, spending time in nature, engagement with symbolism, and any other way one finds beneficial in facilitating a space for contemplation, expression, and development.

At every event we attend, people approach us with anxiety and distress that are not related to psychedelics at all but associated with pre-existing mental health conditions, social dynamics, or personal issues. Thus, another important aspect of psychedelic harm reduction is that it gives many people who are on the margins of society (and many who are not) an opportunity to receive compassionate support outside an official therapeutic context and thus take the first steps toward a deeper healing process.

Looking ahead, I am hopeful that safe spaces in festivals and parties will become a mandatory service worldwide and that more mental health professionals, whether interested in the therapeutic applications of psychedelics or not, will get to join a psychedelic harm reduction team, integrate lessons from the field into their professional practice, and experience the profound transformations that occur when extreme states of consciousness are met with loving presence.

21

Psychedelic Peace Building

Relational Processes in Ayahuasca Rituals of Palestinians and Israelis

Leor Roseman

The current dominant model of psychedelic-assisted therapy is that of the *inner healer*. While this model supports personal growth, it might also divert us from relational elements of the psychedelic journey by emphasizing the experience *within* us and neglecting the experience *between* us. Revealing and reminding relational elements of psychedelic use is important for the expansion of the model and prevention of certain problems that can occur through overemphasis of the inner model (Ferrer 2002).

These problems are related to disengagement from sociopolitical realities that can be counterproductive both to the healing of the individual and to society at large. More anxiety can be created within the individual when he does not recognize that some elements of his suffering are contextual and not just psychospiritual. Furthermore, when relational elements are ignored, it is harder to integrate spiritual events back to day-to-day relational life. Trauma and alienation, which are common relational wounds, should also be addressed in relational ways. Healing these wounds should decrease the risk of similar traumas being perpetuated in the future. While many critiques of psychiatry and psychology have addressed social causes of mental health concerns, psychedelic therapy is not immune from this critique. As we come to recognize that many of our world problems are social, ecological, and systemic, momentary spiritual union remains just a patch—perhaps a more effective patch than psychiatric pills but still just a patch.

Yet, psychedelic use is not just inner oriented, and spirituality is not just within. Those who are engaged in other psychedelic practices are well aware of the relational elements of psychedelics, whether it is in rituals, festivals, or simply full-moon tripping with friends in the desert. My research up until recently was centered on neuroscience and therapy, and I have decided to reorient my research to the direction of the relational. To discuss the relational potential of psychedelics, I needed a relational problem—a conflict. So I chose to investigate the one in my homeland: the Israeli-Palestinian conflict, the holy grail of conflicts. I teamed up with Natalie Ginsberg from MAPS and Antwan Saca, a Palestinian activist, and we started enquiring into psychedelic-assisted peace building. This enquiry has revealed some fascinating processes and opened up some challenging questions, some of which are reported in other papers and will be briefly summarized here (Roseman et al. 2021). However, as this book is aimed for people who are interested in psychedelic therapy, I would like to emphasize here how relational and participatory processes and approaches, which were raised in the interviews, are relevant for therapy as well. These are (1) human connection and the therapeutic alliance; (2) recognition and acceptance; (3) participatory spirituality; (4) becoming part of the psychedelic community; and (5) liberation and prophetic-messianic consciousness.

SET AND SETTING

We interviewed Jewish-Israelis and Arab-Palestinians who drank aya-huasca together (for a full description of the groups, see Roseman et al. 2021). Our intention was to understand how this unique setting influenced participants' processes, during and after the rituals. None of these ceremonies were conducted with peace building in mind; they were all Western neoshamanic ceremonies in which different tradi-tions were fused and in which psychospiritual personal growth was the main intention. Furthermore, the groups were asymmetrical: in most of these ceremonies, there was a minority of Arab-Palestinians and most of the facilitators were Jewish-Israelis. While the setting was apolitical, there were many times in which political reality leaked into the ceremony. This happened by the presence of both sides in the same space, or through other elements outside the ceremony serving as reminders of political reality, such as the calling to the prayer of the muezzin, hearing military training, the location of the ceremony, which has historical significance concerning the conflict, or simply the land itself, which plays an important role in people's experiences, both through her sacredness and through her history of bloodshed. Furthermore, most participants had been exposed to conflict-related trauma or grief to some extent, which was active in them when they met the other, especially in initial encounters. Most ceremonies were done at night, with a focus on the participant's inner processes. However, usually in the second half of the ceremony, participants had an opportunity to sing or play their own music and share it with the rest of the group. The participatory nature of these ceremonies was conducive for intercultural and interfaith themes to emerge and for intimate human connection to occur.

THE RELATIONAL IN RITUAL AND THERAPY

Below are elements that emerged from the interviews. I will try to show how these elements are important for therapy. Each section will begin with a relational theme that was observed in the investigated groups and will continue with its relationship to therapy. As many therapists are already inclined toward relational approaches, these elements might be intuitive to some. I believe that these elements are of value for psychedelic therapy. Being aware of them can increase not just the therapeutic efficacy but also the potential for broader change. The social dimension of our existence, which is so often omitted when we think of our difficulties, can bring a wider lens and understanding of the systemic nature of trauma. While many holistic approaches take into account mind-body-spirit, they can move into greater wholeness by incorporating *society*. Rather than focusing on coping with symptoms that arise from an alienating lifestyle, we must turn toward deeper causes that are closer to the source of the wound, and the wound in many cases is contextual. While alienation can be temporarily reduced by a momentary spiritual connection to some higher force within or without, it is by learning the spirituality of *the in between* of day-to-day human relations and connection to nature that can foster a more stable sense of belonging for the longer term (Buber [1923] 1970)

HUMAN CONNECTION AND
THE THERAPEUTIC ALLIANCE

Participants in the rituals experienced *unity-based universal connection*. This was described as connection beyond identities, in which a sense of oneness is experienced by group members that transcends national identity. This connection beyond identity is the social counterpart of psychedelic-induced ego dissolution and mystical-type experiences. This can be seen as a group peak experience and is similar to the Turners' description of *communitas*, which originates in anthropological research of the ritual process (Turner [1969] 2017; Turner 2012). Communitas is a temporary group state of collective joy and antistructure in which interpersonal connection is based on shared humanity and not on regular social structure and power dynamics. Communitas has already been observed in a large sample of participants in psychedelic ceremonies and was found to be a mediator of long-term psychosocial changes (Kettner et al. 2021). Though many of our interviewees reported that they use ayahuasca for personal spiritual growth, they also expressed that they return to the ceremonies because of the community and for human connection.

As all therapists know, human connection is essential in therapy. Like any form of psychotherapy, the therapeutic alliance plays a crucial role in psychedelic therapy as well and maybe even more important as patients are in a highly open and suggestible state. The importance of the therapeutic alliance is dual: (1) the trust the patient has in the therapist will increase the trust in letting go and enhance the therapeutic process; and (2) the therapeutic alliance can reignite a sense of human connection and belonging, especially to those who have suffered from some sort of alienation and/or trauma. The psychedelic-induced communitas mentioned above, in which participants felt oneness and connection beyond social hierarchies and ego relations, is sometimes the hidden reason why participants continue to return to ceremonies. Edith and Victor Turner theorized that these moments of collective joy do not just create a bond within the group; group members also want to celebrate this connection with humanity at large (Turner [1969] 2017; Turner 2012). Martin Buber also suggests that I-Thou relationships can incite a person to continue to appreciate human connection and reduce alienation (Buber [1923] 1970). I believe that the intimacy that is shared through the therapeutic alliance serves a similar function: it can nurture in the patient further appreciation for human connection and a desire to seek it beyond the therapeutic alliance.

RECOGNITION AND ACCEPTANCE

The counterpart of moments of *universal* connection is *diversity-based connections*. These are connections based on nonuniversal local identities in which an expression of cultural and religious diversity, usually through music, leads to intense emotional and spiritual experiences.

Interviewees reported that in these moments "something powerful is happening in the space," and people experience a sense of togetherness due to a unique shared moment. In these moments, people report an expansion in which all of the group is in silent attention: hearts are open, and peace is felt in the air. It was reported that each language has its own vibration and that listening to the others' language in the ceremony created a shift in how the other culture is perceived.

> *Jewish-Israeli woman: "When someone is saying Allahu akbar in a ceremony, one can feel how the room is flooded with love and how people burst the limits of their normal consciousness and connect to something beyond . . . It is a moment of great expansion." (Allahu akbar means "God is the greatest" in Arabic. It is a common Islamic expression, but it is also related with fear by Jewish-Israelis, as it is associated with an Islamist terror battle cry.)*

> *Arab-Palestinian Muslim woman from Israel: "I feel in the language of my present origin, I am an Arab now; Arabic is my mother tongue. I sing from the source, so it really reaches everyone. I can feel that I sing from a full connection. I feel everyone rises; I open another gate."*

Participation through expression of different parts of one's identity can empower an individual. *Being true to oneself* was reported in our interviews as the most essential personal change that ayahuasca practice can facilitate. Almost all interviewees reported that in the past they have felt as outsiders, and their ayahuasca experiences has taught them to be "comfortable with who they are." Some of the most pivotal moments for individuals were moments in which they expressed and revealed themselves to the group, allowing themselves to be seen and witnessed. When acceptance is nurtured among group members, then individuals have the space to express themselves in ways that they never did before, revealing elements of their identity that might have been suppressed or oppressed in the past. When an Arab woman finds the courage to sing to the rest of the group, which is mainly Jewish, she is not the only one who is empowered. The rest of the group is also empowered and becomes more complete by including a previously excluded part. One of the Jewish participants described the atmosphere of the space in these moments as a "larger whole," hinting at the holotropic nature of these moments.

In psychedelic therapy, *being seen* by the therapist can be a corrective event. In a nonjudgmental space, patients expose themselves in ways they might not even express to their loved ones. By fostering this safe relational space, the therapeutic relationship can provide a blueprint for other relationships in everyday life that can eventually increase their well-being, as well as the well-being of others around them. The reciprocity between acceptance and self-acceptance is crucial here. While many argue that self-acceptance leads to acceptance, the opposite is also true. As many conflicts arise from a perceived lack of recognition, finding or creating social structures in which people are easily seen can support social change and prevent future wounds due to judgment and lack of recognition. Therapy, rituals, and festivals sometimes nurture that field of acceptance, participation, and recognition, that can leak into day to day life through integration.

PARTICIPATORY SPIRITUALITY

Ferrer (2002) suggested that Western spirituality has gone through a participatory turn. This was evident in the ayahuasca groups we interviewed in which more experienced participants were encouraged to participate in the ceremony by singing their own songs, and the ceremonies were led not only by the facilitators but sometimes also by the participants. Some facilitators suggested that one of the goals is to "move from I to we." The rituals provided space for cocreation, and this increased the "tribal" connection between participants while retaining each participant's individuality.

Can the therapeutic setting be participatory? I believe so. Encouraging participation and expression in the right moments can be highly beneficial and empowering. This can easily happen in a group setting during the interactive periods. Music, singing, and dancing are the most obvious ways for this to happen, but also verbal expression between participants has its place as long as it is feels authentic in the moment.

Participation in this context is a relational act that can lead to recognition by the therapists and reduce the feeling of alienation. While the predominant therapeutic paradigm places the focus on the individual inner work, being able to expand this framework to include the other would potentially enrich the work and the healing process. Yet, regardless of the participation of the participants, the participation of the therapists is also needed for the relational act. This does not always necessarily mean an active participation but can mean nurturing a mindset in which the therapist enters the relation to learn something herself and to grow from the intimacy, an I-Thou relationship with the patient (Buber [1923] 1970). Sitters and therapists are aware that they can get a contact high in the session, and I suspect that this contact high is a clue to a healthy I-Thou relationship. Cultivating *presence* is critical for this to happen. The politics of holding space, which is usually framed in a way that the facilitator is just allowing the patient or participant to enter his own process within (Gearin 2015), can be expanded to include the facilitator herself, acknowledging that growth might come to her as well.

BECOMING PART OF THE PSYCHEDELIC COMMUNITY

Many of our participants reported some form of "tribal" relations among group members, even when they came from both sides of the conflict. One's own identity becomes more fused with the new tribal identity of the group and also goes through a process of extended fusion (Swann et al. 2012) to the larger global ayahuasca family and psychedelic culture. The same can happen in psychedelic therapy. The experience itself and the relationship with the therapists is also an unofficial initiation process to psychedelic culture. Often after therapy, the patient finds a new sense of meaning and wants to contribute to the broader movement. In my opinion, this is an important element of the therapy, to be taken seriously. When patients want to find ways to contribute to the broader community, the therapist can support their way of doing so. Cultivating this kind of reciprocity provides a way in which the patient can see himself as an active agent in a wider movement and renew a sense of meaning in his life.

LIBERATION AND MESSIANIC CONSCIOUSNESS

Ferrer (2002) argues that liberation is common for many mystical traditions, but that transcendent states are not an achievement of liberation but tools on the way toward this achievement. Psychedelics offer the potential to liberate oneself from ego boundaries or from wider social structures, yet this temporary liberation should be used for the reformation of psychological and social structures to maintain that freedom. One of the Palestinian interviewees from the West Bank said: "How can you heal trauma if the trauma is ongoing" and "I cannot go to checkpoint and say 'I am a human being let me go through, I'm a spiritual light being,' you know." While trauma healing is becoming popular for both spiritual practices and peace building, there is a need to emphasize that it is not just PTSD that affects people's well-being and narratives but CTSD (continuous traumatic stress disorder)—a long-term exposure to stress, whether from repeated domestic abuse or living in a hostile political environment.

While most ayahuasca process were apolitical and related to the participants' own personal life, we noted some processes that were related to the political reality as well (after all, for many in the land, political is very personal). Many participants described conflict-related revelations that occurred during ceremonies. These revelations were mainly visionary, experienced as visual scenes; though sometimes they were cognitive or emotional insights. In the visions, the participants experienced traumatic events related to the conflict. Sometimes these were from their own autobiographical history, from the collective history, or from the potential future (e.g., future war on Temple Mount). Some examples include visions from the army service, the Holocaust, the Nakba (the deportation of many Palestinians from their homes in 1948), and the bleeding land, and visions in which participants saw themselves on the other side of the conflict. These revelations were in most cases triggered by members from the outgroup or by other intentional or nonintentional elements in the ritual that related to the conflict. In a few occasions, these painful revelations drove the participant to share "the message" from her revelations to other group members, usually through music and in what seems like a prophetic process of channeling truth.

> *Arab-Palestinian Muslim woman from Israel:* "It was on Yom Kippur *[Day of Atonement, holiest day in Judaism],* and out of me came the opening paragraph of the Quran . . . and another frequency opened up, and I understood how much pain is in Pachamama, Mother Earth, how it hurts her, all the red in this country, the blood, how much pain, how much anger, and when I sang it, I was fully present, no right or left. It came from my center, in a voice of—I can't say in the voice of God—but in the voice of a messenger: Listen and awaken, there is a battle here between light and dark. The dark is growing more than the light, so understand where we are now . . . In that session they were vomiting, and when I was done, [other participants] said, we have to talk to you in the morning, and they said how their understanding grew. I felt each one, each and every one, where he was, with his fears and his doubt and his ego, where he is, the net each person places himself in . . . I will not forget this session . . . It was a very strong vision, very painful, and after that I couldn't stop crying."

Besides having these personal-political visions, there is another relational element associated with the aftermath of these revelations. Some of our interviewees mentioned that after having conflict-related revelations, they had an urge to transmit a message to the rest of the group. They had a sense of becoming a prophet; they might be ignited by anger toward the political structure but usually it was a message of love. Many interviewees were hesitant to share these experiences as they were worried about being ridiculed as messianic. Failing to recognize this broader vision and experience might inhibit an important opportunity for a collective and individual process of resolution.

Not all transcendent experiences are of the same quality. Different scholars have compared the mystical and the prophetic-messianic experiences (e.g., Thorner 1965). Mystical consciousness is considered the archetypal inward-facing spiritual process while prophetic-messianic consciousness is the archetypical outward-facing process. Mystical consciousness is associated with self-orientation, unitive experience, acceptance, lack of moral judgment, being apolitical, general compassion to all, and passivity. Prophetic consciousness is other oriented and outer oriented as it is directed toward sociopolitical structures. It is associated with conflict coupled with tension relief, resistance, affecting the public sphere, moral judgment and even anger, and being active for change. Mystical consciousness is sometimes associated with elitism, as acceptance is easier for those with healthy life conditions and therefore considered as conservative and serving the status quo, while prophetic consciousness is associated with mass movements and related to the search for change. In some ways, prophetic consciousness is a form of spiritual politics.

From the interviewees, we learned that psychedelics can potentiate both of these spiritual processes and that while both have their obvious self-aggrandizing risks they can be channeled to positive outcomes. While mystical consciousness is well acknowledged as one of the primary mediators of successful therapy (Roseman et al. 2017), the prophetic-messianic consciousness is considered a shadow that is not widely discussed. If someone finds *a calling* during a therapy session filled with a sense of mission, the therapist could learn together with him how to channel this to a positive direction for both the person and the larger society. This requires a delicate dance between containing impulsivity while also appreciating the wisdom of the impulsive insight before day-to-day tensions reintroduce doubt. Furthermore, as mystical consciousness holds the risk of leading to detachment by retreating inward, prophetic consciousness holds the risk of externalization without the appropriate inner work. Both can be spiritual bypasses, and what is bypassed can be both psychological and societal. For a better future through psychedelic therapy, the balance between the two is required, integrating acceptance with resistance.

RECLAIMING A RELATIONAL LANGUAGE

Psychedelic use is also relational, even when not presented as such. The relational acts presented here are of human connection, intimacy, recognition, belonging, love, and mission in life. All of these are potential remedies for what might be the main cause of the rise of mental health concerns—alienation and disconnection. Reclaiming a relational language alongside the dominant inner language will expand the intention, the experience, and the interpretive framework for the psychedelic experience. For those therapists who are concerned about the state of the world and believe that psychedelics can offer solutions, they should be mindful of developing a practice that is engaged with actively addressing social concerns. Integration can be broadened to include engagement with the lived realities of the patient's relational wounds—be it alienation or trauma—and empower the patient to modify the set and setting she is embedded in, which may also support others around her to do the same.

The online version of *Merriam-Webster's Collegiate Dictionary* suggests that reconciliation is the antonym of both alienation and conflict. To become less alienated is to reconcile. This suggests that alienation also means living in a state of conflict. Buber calls this the "It-world," the world in which human relations are used, like one uses an object; while the "You-world" is for the relationship itself (both the It and You worlds exist together). Conflict is not just between nations; all who feel alienated are embedded in conflict. We are embedded in the It-world of having things and using of people. Encouraging participation and relation in life and therapy are required for actualizing the You-world. To enter the world of relation, we all need to cultivate presence, which provides the space for authentic participation. Participation allows us to recognize one another, and that recognition is required for reconciliation—whether we reconcile from conflict or from a state of alienation. Reconciliation is the return to the You-world.

> The I that steps out of the event of the relation into detachment and the self-consciousness accompanying that, does not lose its actuality. Participation remains in it as a living potentiality. To use words that originally refer to the highest relation but may also be applied to all others: the seed remains in him (Buber [1923] 1970, 113).

22
Celestial Integration

Psychedelics and Archetypal Astrology

Becca Tarnas

The air was thick and heavy with rain; the waters came pouring out of the steel-gray sky in punishing streaks, turning the ruined ground into slick mud. Sky and ground had no horizon to differentiate them. All was muddy gray, an infinite field of bloodied and torn corpses, stretching beyond sight, beyond comprehension. This feels like the Battle of the Somme, *I thought. I could feel the depth of suffering, the tremendous lack of meaning permeating this moment, saturating my very being with a sense of hopeless nihilism. Every feeling of despair, depression, and abyssal anxiety felt concentrated into this moment, as the scene from the Great War dissolved into an existential grief without discernible images. And in feeling that grief, in letting the waves of pain pass through me, something was released with those salty tears—something intangible yet meaningful, something that offered some clarity of consciousness in the darkness. How to make sense of such a moment? Why was the distraught battlefield the vision that came, and universal suffering and grief the emotional experience to be digested?*

∙ ∙ ∙

The range of experiences a participant can have using psychedelic medicines is as complex as the human psyche and as vast and diverse as the starry infinity of the cosmos. Every encounter is multifaceted and multilayered and can be somatic, emotional, psychological, perinatal, relational, historical, philosophical, prophetic, or spiritual. Understanding how to integrate such a complex, nuanced, and at times overwhelming array of experiences is essential for transforming what might otherwise be a curious, fun, or terrifying yet potentially inconsequential incident into a powerful modality for healing. Integration takes a moment of insight and transmutes it into a changed life. Awakenings become new practices and habits; unexpected breakthroughs become new world views.

There are many different tools for integration, complementary approaches to digesting the rich plethora of material that psychedelics open up within us. There is one such tool that offers a cornucopia of support not only for psychedelic integration but also for preparation, timing, and a certain level of prediction regarding the nature of one's experience; however, this tool is, in the words of Stanislav Grof, "more controversial than the psychedelics themselves" (2009, 66). The tool is *astrology,* a practice and discipline that has long been rejected by the modern academic and scientific paradigm.

ASTROLOGY AND TRANSPERSONAL RESEARCH

The story behind astrology's unexpected alliance with psychedelic psychotherapy and transpersonal research began in the mid-1970s at Esalen Institute, on California's epic Big Sur coastline (Tarnas 2019). While at Esalen, Stanislav Grof and Richard Tarnas turned their attention to the problem of the unpredictable experiential variability of psychedelic sessions. During one of Grof's workshops, a seminarian named Arne Trettevik suggested that they look into transit astrology as a means to predict and interpret the nature of patients' psychedelic sessions (Tarnas 2019). Transit astrology tracks the movements of the planets through the solar system, taking note of significant angles that the planets make to one another, and then interprets these placements based on the meanings astrologers have come to recognize are correlated with the planetary bodies. After learning the basics for calculating astrological birth charts and planetary transits from Trettevik, Tarnas and Grof compared the detailed notes from their own and others' psychedelic sessions with the corresponding transits and were amazed to find that the symbolic meanings astrologers associate with the planets accurately reflected the nature of their sessions (Tarnas 2019).

Richard Tarnas went on to conduct an in-depth study of the natal charts and transits of the members of the wider Esalen community, before turning the same astrological lens upon significant cultural figures and events in various epochs of history. Tarnas uncovered a vast body of evidence substantiating the claim that the movements of the planets and the archetypal meanings associated with the planetary bodies correlate with the unfolding of human history, culture, the arts, and biography (for a comprehensive study demonstrating the correlations between the movements of the planets and the unfolding of human history, see Tarnas 2006). Astrologers have come to recognize that each planet in our solar system, as well as the Sun and the Moon, correspond with a particular complex archetype or set of metaphorically interrelated meanings. Whether one studies the birth chart of a person or the transits for a historical event, one can recognize the combinations of archetypes expressed through that concrete manifestation and how they mirror the alignment of the planets at the time of the birth or event.

Tarnas and Grof came to recognize that the planetary correlations they were seeing were not materially caused by the *physical* planets; astrology operates through a different kind of causality, one that is archetypal. To use a metaphor articulated by Grof, when a clock states that it is 12:30 p.m., the clock is not physically *causing* the time to be half past noon (2009, 72). Rather, the clock is simply indicating what time it is. The same can be understood of the solar system: the planets are not causing the symbolically relevant events to unfold on Earth through physical means but rather are indicating the *quality* of the time, the archetypal zeitgeist of that moment. Astrology is a demonstration of what the depth psychologist C. G. Jung called *synchronicity,* a meaningful coincidence of an inner psychological experience with an outer event that shares the same archetypal or symbolic core (Tarnas 2006). Thus, astrology can be understood, as Tarnas often writes, to be "not concretely predictive, but, rather, *archetypally* predictive" (2006, 67). In relation to psychedelic experiences, astrology can tell us the archetypal quality of the session, offering the spectrum of meanings associated with the planetary combinations activated at the time, but it will not predict the concrete nature of the experiences. Such archetypal prediction can help orient both the participant and the guide toward what symbolic themes will be present, without narrowly determining the specific material that will unfold.

ASTROLOGY'S THREE FORMS
OF CORRESPONDENCE

The archetypal astrology that Tarnas developed out of this psychological, biographical, and historical research has three essential "forms of correspondence": the natal chart, world transits, and personal transits (2006, 103).

The natal chart depicts the positions of the planets relative to one another in relation to the native's position on Earth. One can recognize in the birth chart the archetypal dynamics of the individual's life as can be seen in her or his psychology and emotional development, childhood experiences and familial constellations, relationships and sexuality, mental and intellectual capacities, spiritual orientation, instinctual patterns, and so forth. The birth chart is like a seed, and the plant that grows and develops from that seed will continue to change and evolve over a lifetime while still reflecting the core archetypal potential. To paraphrase from the astrologer Jan Spiller, at the moment of our birth we are each given a unique slice of time that we then have the opportunity to perfect over the course of our lifetime (1997, 4).

The world transits, which is the second form of correspondence, are the positions of the planets at any given moment in time and correlate with the collective experience unfolding on Earth. These events will be diverse and reflective of several different overlapping astrological factors, and yet there is clear evidence of consistent patterns of correlations throughout history when the same planetary configurations come into alignment. The centuries are punctuated by these overlapping cycles, whether it is the revolutionary cultural upheavals that correlate with Uranus-Pluto alignments, the geopolitical conflicts and crises that align with Saturn-Pluto aspects, the periods of spiritual awakening and visionary innovation associated with Uranus-Neptune periods, or the rise and fall of great civilizations and paradigms correlated with Neptune-Pluto (for more on these astrological cycles in history, see Tarnas 2006). While all of the planetary archetypes can be recognized in significant correlations, it is especially the aspects between the slower-moving outer planets—Jupiter, Saturn, Uranus, Neptune, and Pluto—that define particular historical epochs and cultural movements.

The third form of correspondence is the personal transits, which shows how the world transits align with any given natal chart. Although the birth chart captures the planetary image of a fixed moment in time, the planets continue moving through the heavens and thus continue to make new geometrical relationships or what are called astrological *aspects* to the natal planetary positions. Outer planet transits last for several months to years, depending on the transiting planet, and thus will define the archetypal quality of that period of time in someone's life. The inner planets, which move faster, have much shorter transiting periods and yet are still highly significant and can affect the outer planetary transits in dynamic and catalytic ways. When considering astrology in the context of a psychedelic session, one would look to all three forms of correspondence, first to see what the inherent natal conditions are, then at the larger collective dynamics through the world transits, and finally studying the interaction of the two to see how the individual will be personally affected by the collective situation.

BASIC PERINATAL MATRICES

During the first few decades of Stanislav Grof's research on psychedelics and holotropic states of consciousness, he observed in the sessions an unfolding pattern of patients returning to their births and reliving the perinatal process. Often the subsequent life events of each patient would symbolically reflect the birth process in certain meaningful and significant ways, whether re-creating certain traumatic episodes or mirroring how the patient would approach a challenging task or problem. Grof referred to these symbolically interconnected chains of experience that are rooted in the birth narrative as *systems of condensed experience,* or COEX systems (2009, 78–79).

Grof also observed four distinct stages to the birth process that he came to call the *basic perinatal matrices* (BPMs) (2019, 147–69). Each matrix has a particular character and set of qualities associated with it that would manifest in the psychedelic session in multivalent ways, bringing forth images, emotions, and somatic sensations that all reflected the symbolic nature of the particular perinatal matrix. (Recall chapter 6 of this book.)

Significantly, it is at the moment of birth, when the baby separates from the mother's body after the long journey of gestation (BPM I), labor contractions (BPM II), propulsion through the birth canal (BPM III), and sudden emergence into the external world (BPM IV), that the astrological birth chart is set—usually at the exact time of the first breath, if it is possible to record. The first breath signifies the baby's first moment as an air-breathing, terrestrial being physically separated from the mother's aquatic womb. Thus, the pivotal experience of birth not only deeply shapes an individual's psychology, it also is the moment when the planetary positions are recorded to cast the natal chart. This significant connection between birth and astrology can clearly be seen in an extraordinary parallel: when Richard Tarnas compared the basic perinatal matrices independently observed and delineated by Grof in psychedelic sessions, he was amazed to realize that the qualities of the four BPMs exactly mirror the archetypes that astrologers associate with the four outer planets—Neptune, Saturn, Pluto, and Uranus (Tarnas 2019).

THE TRANSPERSONAL PLANETARY ARCHETYPES

The archetype of Neptune is related to the transcendent, the spiritual, the numinous, the mystical, and the divine. Water is symbolic of Neptune, and thus the archetype is flowing, dissolving, permeating, saturating, and unifying. The experience of oneness and of merging or uniting with divinity, God, or the sacred dimensions of the cosmos are all qualities associated with the archetypal Neptune. The image, imagination, fantasy, enchantment, magic, mirage, illusion, delusion, symbols, and archetypes—these are all Neptune's realm. And yet, these archetypal qualities also exactly correlate with the reported psychedelic experiences that constitute BPM I, when the baby is in the womb, surrounded by amniotic fluid, and still merged with the mother's body.

Saturn's archetypal qualities are heavy, contracting, negating, difficult, challenging, disciplined, structured, punitive, and hard. Time, tradition, the past, finitude, endings, mortality, death, and dying are all Saturn's domain. Yet the archetype of Saturn is also expressed in maturity, responsibility, solidity, commitment, gravitas, and the wisdom of experience. BPM II, which corresponds to the onset of labor and the contractions of the womb before the cervix has dilated, greatly resembles Saturn's archetypal principles, especially in their more challenging and negative forms. However, once the birth process is seen in its full context, one can also recognize how the difficulty and pain of the birth contractions are necessary to bring the baby forth. Indeed, from the mother's perspective, the Saturnian qualities of BPM II can be perceived as the solid container of the womb, contracting with the force of labor, coming through in the tremendous strength of the mother, and providing the Saturnian initiation for both mother and child.

The archetype associated with the planet Pluto relates to the death-rebirth mystery, to transformation and transmutation, to the biological processes of birth, sex, and death, and to the libidinal and instinctual drive. The Plutonic archetype intensifies and pushes all things to extremes, propelling with a powerful force of will. Evolution, destruction and creation, and catharsis are all expressions of Pluto. The underworld—mythically, religiously, politically, criminally—are realms of the Plutonic archetype. The experiential imagery of BPM III, the stage of birth when the baby is being pushed through the birth canal, is diverse and complex—ranging from the sense of a life-and-death struggle, confrontation with biological matter such as blood, urine, and feces, images of fiery hells, devils, wild animals, volcanic magma, and pyrocatharsis. But these qualities also all align with the equally complex archetype of Pluto.

Finally, the planet Uranus is archetypally associated with liberation, freedom, rebellion, awakening, and breakthrough. Uranus is the inventive, insightful, brilliant genius, and it brings innovative change like a revolutionary or disruption like a trickster. Alive with electrical impulses, the Uranian archetype is oriented toward what is new, different, quirky, unusual, unexpected, and sudden. The final stage of the birth process, BPM IV, carries all of these symbolic qualities as the newborn bursts forth and awakens to a radically new reality and world, and the struggle for life through the birth canal is joyfully, suddenly, unexpectedly successful and filled with awe, joy, and wonder.

In seeing these remarkable parallels among the four basic perinatal matrices and the astrological meanings of the four outer planets, Tarnas and Grof came to realize that significant transits from these outer planets correlated with the activation of these particular BPMs during psychedelic sessions. By looking at the patient's natal chart, personal transits, and the world transits, a complex picture emerges of the kind of archetypal experience that would be activated during the session, and thus one could understand why such great variability existed not only among different individuals taking psychedelics but also among different sessions for the same patient. As Stanislav Grof said, they had found the "Rosetta stone" for research into consciousness and the human psyche (2009, 61).

SYNCHRONICITY, SATURN-NEPTUNE, AND THE BATTLE OF THE SOMME

When I found myself immersed in the psychedelic rainstorm of a century-old French battlefield during the Great War, I knew at some level I was having a transpersonal experience: I had transcended my own individual life and entered into a moment in history. During this medium-dose psychedelic session, I not only felt like one soldier dying in no-man's land, I also felt like every soldier whose life had ever drained away into the mud. The rain, soot, and sludge were one with the tears on my face. I felt hollow grief and existential doubt, and a sense of dissolving into timeless suffering.

The experience I was undergoing felt like the Saturn-Neptune archetypal complex, bringing together the qualities associated with Saturn and BPM II, and Neptune and BPM I. The archetype of Saturn was present in the death, dying, suffering, loss, and grief, while Neptune could be perceived in the water and the rain, and in the pervasive, saturating, encompassing, and eternal essence of the experience. The heaviness of Saturn combined with the water of Neptune to make mud and darkened storm clouds, expressing all that dying in the mud can symbolize.

As a practicing astrologer working within the lineage of archetypal astrology, I had in the back of my mind the world transits and my personal transits at the time of this session. The archetypal complex of Saturn-Neptune as I felt it in the experience was the first to crystallize, but as I contemplated these planetary archetypes I recalled that at that moment in the sky there was actually an alignment of these two planets: Saturn was making a 90 degree angle, or what astrologers call a *square,* to Neptune. The world transits at that moment correlated precisely with the psychedelic experience I was having. Furthermore, the

Saturn-Neptune square in the sky was aligned closely on my natal Sun placement. The archetype associated with the Sun signifies the individual, the self, the identity, our autonomous individuality and our shining will to be and to exist. The personal transit of the Saturn-Neptune square crossing my natal Sun correlated with the strong sense of being personally present at the Battle of the Somme and suffering as one of the soldiers who perished there.

Another layer of recognition was revealed to me later, as I researched the Battle of the Somme further. The Somme was an offensive during World War I organized by the British generals that began on July 1, 1916. The long and tragic battle has been condemned for its *lack of imagination:* the British generals could not conceive of a different kind of warfare, one that took into account the development of new technologies such as the machine gun and the tank, and thus sent row upon row of young men to charge headlong into a rain of bullets as though they were still just charging against swords, bayonets, and cavalry (Fussell 2013, 13–14). On the first day of the Somme alone, one hundred thousand men bravely entered no-man's land, and a full fifth were cut down by machine gun fire, while twice as many more were wounded. This battle continued its long defeat for five agonizing months. Throughout this time, the planets Saturn and Neptune were in a conjunction, appearing next to each other in the sky from an earthly perspective and corresponding with the same archetypal conditions I had encountered in my psychedelic session. To reiterate: the experiential qualities of my session reflected the archetypal complex associated with Saturn and Neptune when they are combined; when I had the psychedelic experience of the Battle of the Somme, Saturn and Neptune were in alignment with each other in the sky; Saturn and Neptune were also concurrently aligned with the position of my natal Sun; and finally, when the historical Battle of the Somme took place in 1916, Saturn and Neptune were also in aspect at that time.

The sense of meaninglessness, nihilism, grief, suffering, existential loss, disconnection, depression, doubt, and uncertainty about the existence of the divine are all characteristic of the Saturn-Neptune complex and were part of what I experienced during my Somme session. However, upon the recognition of the multiple layers of the world transits, my personal transits, and the transits in 1916 when the battle took place, I realized that even in the most archetypally meaningless place I could find tremendously significant meaning. Indeed, it was a meaning that paradoxically reflected the meaninglessness I felt. In that paradox, I felt the presence of the sacred and an interconnection between my personal psyche, the records of history, and the largest movements of our solar system. Meaning and wonder were restored not in spite of the suffering I was feeling but *because of it*. Seeing that this suffering was connected to something beyond me allowed me to feel personally held by the cosmos through a deeply painful and vulnerable moment of eternity.

INTEGRATING PSYCHEDELICS
WITH ASTROLOGY

Astrology can be used not only to predict archetypally the kinds of psychedelic experiences one might have in a session but can also be engaged to interpret and integrate those experiences afterward. One can look forward to an upcoming session through an astrological lens, or alternatively, one can look backward to a session that has already passed to understand better what has unfolded. There is value in both approaches, although they can yield different results. When using astrology in an archetypally predictive manner, one can receive a glimpse of the astrological "weather" forecast. If the time of the psychedelic session is already set and scheduled, then one can study the transits for that day and prepare psychospiritually for the territory ahead.

One also can use astrology to *choose* the time of an upcoming session, which can be especially helpful when planning an initial session for a psychedelic novice. A time favorable for an initiatory experience could be chosen, selecting for factors that might be supportive for a breakthrough or positive outcome. However, one must be careful of this approach, since having an astrological prediction available can lead one to want to find the perfect archetypal conditions and to eliminate all possibly negative experiences. This attempt to use astrology to overly control an experience may backfire, since an astrologer cannot perceive every possible detail in the transits or natal chart. Furthermore, it is often the more challenging psychedelic experiences that ultimately lead to greater psychospiritual growth, and thus one might not want to avoid more archetypally difficult conditions because they could provide exactly the pressures needed to lead to the kind of growth and transformation one seeks from a psychedelic experience. Astrology should not be used to control, but rather to gain knowledge and cultivate informed preparation for what lies ahead.

As a retrospective tool used for integration, astrology provides a symbolic language that can help organize and disentangle the complex and multilayered experiences that emerge in psychedelic sessions. The astrological language of archetypes can provide metaphorical connections between seemingly disparate parts of the session, demonstrating how certain biographical, perinatal, and transpersonal elements may all be archetypally interconnected and reflective of one's personal transits, natal chart, or the world transits—and likely all three in dynamic interaction. An astrologer can also help to differentiate the layers of the various forms of correspondence, revealing which parts of a session might be most expressive of the birth chart, and thus inherent to the client's ongoing psychedelic experiences, and which parts might be reflective of the personal and world transits, and thus will change within a set period of time. Since archetypes are *multivalent,* and thus have a wide range of possible expressions while still remaining consistent with the archetypal core of meaning, an astrologer can also direct the client toward other more life-enhancing expressions of the archetypal complexes present in both the natal chart and transits.

If the client is new to astrology, the revelation that there are correlations between one's innermost psychedelic experiences and the movements of the planets through the solar system can have a profoundly transformative effect on one's world view. Astrology undermines the materialistic scientific paradigm because it demonstrates that there are other forms of causality beyond material and efficient mechanisms. When paired with astrological correlations, psychedelics have the potential to shatter all belief that we live in a random, meaningless, indifferent cosmos in which conscious human beings are a strange and lonely anomaly. Rather, they provide tangible and experiential evidence that we are in a universe saturated with meaning, numinosity, and divinity and that through all of our experiences—even those of deep existential despair and suffering—we are being witnessed and mirrored by the great archetypal movements of the cosmos.

23

The Challenges of Integrating an Extreme Psychedelic Journey

Christopher Bache

My book *LSD and the Mind of the Universe* describes an intense psychedelic practice I undertook between 1979 and 1999: seventy-three fully internalized, therapeutically focused, high-dose LSD sessions following protocols set out by Stanislav Grof in *LSD Psychotherapy* (1980). I worked at 500 to 600 mcg. Knowing what I know today, I don't recommend such an extreme regimen. If I were doing it over again, I would take a gentler approach. And yet, I am also deeply grateful to have taken this journey and consider these seventy-three days to be the most important of my life.

This extreme journey generated many challenges around integration. The dilemma I have describing these challenges is that there is not space here to describe the journey itself or the states of consciousness that opened on it. This creates an impossible situation, for information vital to the discussion is missing. What follows, therefore, is not a complete account but a series of compressed observations, which I hope will serve as an invitation to the larger study.

The psychedelic agents we have access to today are so powerful that they mark a new frontier in human experience. We can shatter the shell of our earthbound mind so consistently, grind our physical existence to dust so completely that it becomes hard to describe the depths of cosmic communion that follow. By taking our life to its limits and repeatedly shattering those limits, we dissolve for hours at a time into flows of life that transcend all measures. By entering these states with focus and clear intent, by submitting to the harsh demands of death and rebirth, we surrender all we have been to become something utterly new. A being who can do things "we" could never do, know things "we" could never know. A being who breathes time, who dances in the stratosphere of planetary consciousness, who dissolves into the One that cradles all. As we enter larger and older levels of existence, the universe receives us and tutors us. It rewards our tenacity and perhaps foolhardy courage with exquisite intimacies, drawing us into almost unspeakable ecstasies of discovery.

Just as dreams build on one another if we attend to them carefully, psychedelic sessions build on one another if we engage them conscientiously, at least they did in my case. Over the years, a systematic deepening of my visionary journey took place. I think that the standardization of the procedures I used in my sessions—same set and setting, same medicine and dose, same sitter, same location, and same recording process—contributed to the stability and continuity of my visionary conversation. Being taken into great depth one step at a time allows our cognitive faculties to stabilize at each level before we are ushered into the next; otherwise we would be swallowed whole by the enormity of the encounter, and what would be accomplished but a transient ecstasy that built little?

As I have experienced it, consciousness is an ocean of infinite experiential possibilities. When we take these amplifying medicines, the mind we drop into this ocean acts as a seed crystal that catalyzes a certain set of experiences from its infinite potential. As we are gradually healed, purified, and transformed by these encounters, the seed crystal of our mind is changed. In subsequent sessions, it catalyzes still deeper experiences from this ocean. If we repeat this process many times, a sequence of initiations into successively deeper levels of consciousness takes place and a deepening visionary communion unfolds. Each segment of this communion tends to pick up where the previous segment stopped. Sometimes there is a very tight continuity between the sessions, sometimes it is broader, but it's always there woven into the fabric of engagement. In Jorge Ferrer's language, psychedelic experience, like all spiritual experience, is *participatory*: "The participatory approach presents an enactive understanding of the sacred that conceives spiritual phenomena, experiences, and insights as *cocreated events*" (Ferrer 2011, 2; see also Ferrer 2002; Ferrer and Sherman 2008).

I entered this psychedelic arena as a philosopher of religion, not a clinician. Working at these dosage levels, my journey became less a therapeutic enterprise and more a journey of cosmic exploration. My sessions were not focused on healing the personal self, though healing always flowed from them. Accordingly, the demands of integration were not primarily the therapeutic demands of integrating my personal shadow or even our collective shadow into my conscious awareness, as important as this work is. The deeper challenge was integrating experiences that were breaking all the rules as they ushered me into levels of reality that operated by completely different laws than space-time.

The four challenges I will address in this chapter are: the challenge of retaining the radically new, the challenge of assimilating experiences of transcendence into one's physical body, the challenge of managing the impact that one's "private" sessions can have on others, and the challenge of navigating the loneliness of return.

THE CHALLENGE OF RECALL

Integration begins with accurate recall, and the farther a session throws you into novel and unfamiliar territory, the more challenging recall can become. On those precious days when I would break through to a new level of consciousness, holding on to my experiences could be difficult.

My write-up would have gaps. Sometimes I could recall only fragments of a particularly deep set of experiences, the rest disappearing into the shadows. When I first moved beyond linear time, for example, and entered what I came to call Deep Time, the experiences were so unlike anything I had ever known that I simply lost them. My mind had no points of reference to anchor them. I found, however, that with repetition, my recall and comprehension improved. When I returned to the same level of consciousness in subsequent sessions, I was able to retain the experiences more completely. My system was acclimating to the new territory, and I was able to remember things I had previously forgotten. The pieces began to fit together into more complete gestalts, meanings became clearer. As a result, my session narratives became more complete.

This is an important epistemological point. *With persistence and practice, cognition can be trained to operate in these extreme conditions.* Profound experiences are not simply given to you; you have to train yourself to receive them and hold on to them. I cannot emphasize this too strongly.

Preserving an accurate memory of our psychedelic experience completes the circle of learning and lays a strong foundation for our next session. Part of my protocol, therefore, included writing a phenomenologically complete account of each session within twenty-four hours. This often required writing at the very limits of my understanding as I struggled to describe experiences that were deeply mysterious to me at the time. To help with this, I developed a strategy.

When I would write up a session, I would listen to the music used in the session in the same order it had been played inside the session. I played each piece over and over until I felt I had captured the essence of the experience I had had with this music; then I moved on to the next segment. The day after a session, you are still porous around the edges. I found that by listening to the music in this porous state with my verbal functions restored, I was able to reenter the edges of my psychedelic experience and get it down on paper more effectively. I called it "standing at the edge of the well." Once I have written up a session, I do not change or edit it. I have learned that attempting to make improvements in the account may distort something contained in the original raw language, so I leave it alone.

THE CHALLENGE OF PHYSICAL INTEGRATION

While psychedelic experiences are usually spoken of as states of consciousness, they are profound states of body as well, as every journeyer learns. Mind-opening states are body-opening states that deeply impact our physical and subtle energy systems, requiring careful preparation before a session and careful processing afterward.

In my experience, each step deeper into our multidimensional universe is a step into a more intense field of energy. *Deeper* states of consciousness are *higher* states of energy. This is an unmistakable sensation and a widely recognized principle in spiritual traditions. One may have glancing contact with deep levels of reality without this becoming apparent, but to have *stable experience* of a given level of reality, one must acclimate to its energy; otherwise, our experiences there will be fragmented and chaotic. Just as when climbing a mountain, we must acclimate to the atmospheric conditions of higher elevations, here we must acclimate to the energetic conditions of deeper levels of reality. By stable experience I mean that we have entered a certain level of consciousness often enough that we have acclimated to the territory and learned the terrain. Our psychophysical system has undergone the necessary purifications and adaptations for us to maintain coherent awareness and good recall at this particular level.

Entering deeper states of consciousness triggers a spontaneous purging of impurities from our body and mind. This pattern of breakthrough followed by detoxification repeated itself like clockwork in my sessions. I found that after each major breakthrough to a deeper level of consciousness, there was often a turgid "carrying out the garbage" quality to the sessions that followed, so much so that I came to dread the sessions that immediately followed a breakthrough. An analogy from mining comes to mind. After an explosion opens a new vein of ore in the mountain, you still have to carry away the rocks to get complete access to its riches.

This pattern continued even late into my practice. During the last five years of my journey when I was being taken into that supremely clear reality that I called the Diamond Luminosity and Buddhism calls the *dharmakaya* (the Clear Light of Absolute Reality), the Diamond Light began to crunch itself into my physical being. It felt like the Light was actually restructuring me at a physiological level, remaking my biology and subtle energy system. This triggered new cycles of purification as my system worked to absorb these ultrapure states of being

The cycle of purification is the combustion cycle of sustained psychedelic practice. The essence of the cycle is this. Being propelled into a deeper level of reality shifts one into a higher energetic state, and this higher energy "shakes loose" impurities from one's mental, emotional, and physical being. In subsequent sessions, one's system works to empty itself of these toxins as it continues to absorb the purity and intensity of this new energy. By sweeping out the old to make way for the new, eventually a clearer and stronger energetic platform is established on which future sessions will build.

In deep psychedelic sessions, you open yourself to enormous tidal waves of energy. They carry you into vast landscapes that are fascinating to experience, but after the session ends, it can leave your subtle energy system feeling stretched and achy. This short-term effect usually fades within a few days, but the deeper your work takes you, the more you must actively manage the energetic consequences of entering these powerful states.

My experience has been that once I make solid contact with a given level of transpersonal reality in a session, I continue to have a living connection with that reality even after the session ends. It is as though when a stable window into the universe opens, after it closes a small filament continues to connect me to this level and a trickle of its energy flows into me through this filament. Just a trickle, but trickles add up.

As my practice deepened through the years and I made stable contact with more levels of spiritual reality, multiple strands of energy were formed connecting me permanently to all these levels. Through these strands, different shades of energy flowed into my body and mind every day. This energy nourished me, but it also became something of a problem. My sessions were so far-reaching that eventually my system was having difficulty managing all this "extra" energy. What do you do with all the energy that is continuously flowing into you between your sessions? Now that you are no longer in the visionary state and your system has shrunk back to its "normal" shape and size, how do you integrate the new energetic being you are slowly becoming?

I found that doing Vajrayana Buddhist practices helped me manage this energy by giving it a place to run. (For me it was Vajrayana, but I think practices from other spiritual traditions would produce similar results.) For years, the pattern had been that this energy would build up inside my body making me periodically very uncomfortable. When I started doing Chöd and other Tibetan practices, these symptoms of energy overload began to subside. These ancient rituals connected me to the universe in a way that allowed this energy to run more freely. They allowed my system to ventilate between sessions. Singing these prayers tuned my "body, speech, and mind" to the universe in a way that allowed the energy flowing inside me to merge with a greater surround. It was as if these practices gave me a way of communing with the universe that was midway between my earthly reality and my session reality. When I danced with the *dakinis,* I felt relaxed, cleansed, and exercised. My energy began to run cooler, and I was able to breathe more comfortably in my skin.

THE CHALLENGE OF SOCIAL INTEGRATION

For obvious legal reasons, I never spoke to my students at the university about my psychedelic practice. For my own protection, I built a firewall between my professional life and my personal life in this regard. And yet despite this tight compartmentalization, nature did not honor the boundaries I had so carefully drawn. The effects of my psychedelic practice began to spill over and touch the lives of some of my students.

It was as though by entering into conscious communion with the deeper fabric of life, the threads of that fabric were being activated in the physical world around me.

About five years into my teaching and four years into my psychedelic work, students began to come up to me after class and tell me that an example I had used in my lecture that day was exactly what had happened to them recently. In my experience, I was simply pulling these examples out of thin air to illustrate some point I was making, but in their experience, I was describing their life in precise detail. This pattern grew stronger through the years. As I entered progressively deeper levels of consciousness in my psychedelic work, these synchronicities became more frequent. They also began touching increasingly sensitive areas in my students' lives. It was as though a radar had been activated that was zeroing in on some part of their life that was hurting or constricted. Sometimes it lanced a private pain that had been festering inside them for years or triggered an insight that they desperately needed to grow.

Students taking my courses during these years often found themselves undergoing life-changing transformations without any encouragement from me to do so, as though the very act of our coming together in class was giving them added leverage in their lives. Some chose to end bad marriages or to heal wounded ones. Others left careers they had outgrown, while still others began to confront their addictions. While the activation these students experienced was sometimes quite powerful, there were no casualties and many positive breakthroughs. On the rare occasion that a student's self-transformation became particularly turbulent, I referred them to a gifted therapist in the area with whom they could process what was emerging in a safe setting.

Some of my students also started having unusually deep experiences of the concepts I was presenting in class. As I was simply going about my work describing the perennial truths of the world's religions, students began to have powerful spiritual openings around these concepts—such as impermanence, interdependence, oneness, no-self, and the divine within. Insights long dormant in their unconscious suddenly sprang to life. They felt their energy shifting to higher centers of awareness, though they often did not have the vocabulary to describe it this way. It was as though they were being activated by more than just the verbal presentation of ideas, as though they were being touched by the actual *experience* of these realities that now lived in me to some degree because of my psychedelic practice.

Those who don't know me may suspect that these things were happening because I had crossed the line between education and persuasion, but I assure you that this is not the case, and my department chair will back me up on this. It was not a misplaced missionary zeal that was triggering these events but something much more subtle and difficult to comprehend. What was triggering these effects was not what I was *doing* but what I had *become* through my psychedelic practice. A field of energy moving through me or around me was growing stronger, causing spontaneous *energetic resonances* to spring up underneath the exchange of ideas. (There are other layers of this story I can't address here, including the emergence of *group fields* surrounding courses I taught for many years.)

These synchronicities and activations became such a prominent part of my classroom experience that I was forced to pay them close attention. I began to track what was happening in my classes and watch for signs of student activation. In time I came to understand that the experiences my students were having were demonstrating a simple truth about consciousness, namely, that consciousness is an open field and within this field, states of consciousness are contagious. My personal efforts to realize deeper states of awareness had changed something in me that caused my person to begin functioning as a kind of lightning rod, triggering sparks of a similar awakening among those around me who were receptive to this influence. This was due not to any calculated effort on my part but simply to the seamless nature of consciousness itself. Like ripples spreading across water, this is an utterly natural effect. Our spiritual ecology simply does not permit private awakening. *The ecology of consciousness is an inherently collective ecology.*

To teach in a world where minds are separate at one level and entangled at another calls for a new pedagogy, a truly integral pedagogy that places new demands on the instructor and opens new possibilities for accelerated learning. After experimenting and developing this new pedagogy for a number of years, I wrote *The Living Classroom* (2008). It's important to emphasize that what I describe there has nothing inherently to do with psychedelics. *The Living Classroom* does not even mention psychedelics. My psychedelic practice was simply the trigger that exposed and activated these natural dynamics of consciousness in my particular setting.

That said, the experiences my students were having demonstrate that it is not just we who are touched by our psychedelic practice but potentially anyone in our social network. And the deeper our practice, the more pronounced these effects may become. Integration, therefore, is not just psychological, it's also social. *To fully integrate our psychedelic experience, we must support those around us who are being activated by our work.* I don't think we need to be afraid of the rings of influence that spread out around us from this work. We need to be careful, of course, and to act responsibly and compassionately at all times, but I think we can trust that we are where we are supposed to be, doing what we are supposed to be doing, and so are they.

THE CHALLENGE OF RETURN

Over all, I think I did a good job of integrating my sessions as I went along. I recorded them faithfully, spent many hours pondering their meaning, followed the personal guidance they gave me, and tried to incorporate their teachings into my life. Because of this, I thought that stopping my sessions would be a fairly straightforward process. I thought that I could simply step away and be nourished by the many blessings I had received on this journey, blessings I have not tried to describe here. What I found, however, was that integrating an entire journey is different than integrating individual sessions. Because I had pressed my journey as long and as far as I did, coming off the psychedelic mountain turned out to be a challenging journey in its own right.

In the years after stopping my sessions, I found myself entering a deep existential sadness. There was joy in my life, but my enthusiasm for life itself was fading. Once you have known the ecstasy and freedom of becoming Light, of dissolving completely into the crystalline body of the Divine, life on Earth can begin to feel dried up. I began to feel marooned, separated from my Beloved by the very conditions of my earthly existence. Eventually, I reached a point where I realized I was just waiting to die. I was doing my work, taking care of my family, and giving my lectures, but in my heart of hearts, I was waiting to die so that I could return to my Beloved. I was suffering from the loss of communion with the Divine. (Though I sometimes speak of the Creative Intelligence of the universe as the Divine and use personal language for it, I am not, in fact, a theist. In my hands, "Divine" does not reduce to the God of our monotheistic traditions. My metaphysical commitments run in the direction of monism and panpsychism. My God is the Cosmos. I see all reality, both physical and spiritual reality, as the manifestation of a single intelligence, power, and mystery that may be beyond our capacity to fully fathom but is not beyond our capacity to experience.)

If I had touched the Divine only once or twice, perhaps it would have been different. Perhaps then the joy of embrace would have carried everything along, and the memory would have been sufficient. But my Beloved had taken me into her so deeply so many times that the wound of absence was particularly deep. I knew that the universe was my Beloved's body, that it was impossible to ever really step away from her. I knew that I was every moment immersed in her, that she was the root and flower of my existence. But this knowledge did not spare me the pain of being separated from the full intensity of her presence.

Living one's life waiting to die is not a good way to live, and I knew it was not the way this work was supposed to end. Everything about my life was screaming "failure to integrate," but because I had taken so much care to integrate each session, it was not clear to me where my failure lay. As I turned to get to the root of my dilemma, I came to realize that despite my best efforts to stay grounded on my journey, despite all the spiritual practice I had done, all the reflection and writing, somewhere along the way I had lost a critical balance between transcendence and immanence, between going beyond the physical universe and living in it. I had become so enraptured with the world beyond space-time that I lost my footing inside space-time. I had pushed so deeply into the Great Expanse that I was suffering not from too much God, because all is God, but from too much transcendence.

What a delicate balancing act. A little transcendence is a good thing. It is healing, reassuring, and illuminating. It can remind us who and what we are. It can teach us what we are doing here and what "here" is. But if we drink too deeply from the bliss of transcendence, it can undermine our sense of belonging to Earth, and this is an equally important truth. All of this came crashing into me after I stopped my sessions. As long as I was returning periodically to this deeper reality, the depth of my imbalance had not fully registered. I had been protected from it, buffered from it by the steady rhythm of my return. It was only after I stopped my sessions that the full brunt of my imbalance hit me. It was only then that I realized how transcendentally overextended I had become despite my best intentions.

It took me about ten years to get fully grounded in life again. I did so by grabbing my life firmly, partly by action and partly by sheer commitment. I tempered my memories of transcendence by embracing the immanent Divine more deeply. I made a conscious choice to live where I was, as I was. I renewed my daily meditation practice not to change what will happen to me when I die, for that victory is won, nor to try to reach these distant shores again in this present lifetime. I practice to sing to my Beloved, to become a better vessel of her creation in my remaining years on this Earth.

Along the way I realized that there was a second factor contributing to my sadness, and this was the burden of living in the silence imposed on me by our psychedelic-phobic culture. When I began my unsanctioned experiment in 1979, I knew that the price of this undertaking would be my silence, and I paid this price willingly because it was the only way I could do this work. But I did not foresee the harm I would be doing myself by splitting myself in half in this way. When you divide yourself to live in your culture, when you can say this to one but not to another, you make compromises on the outside of your life that begin to work their way into your insides. Chronic holding back creates cracks with uncertain consequences. In the end, the secrecy that made it possible for me to do this work also made it impossible for me to fully integrate it into my life.

Because of our culture's restrictive laws around psychedelics, I could not bring my visionary experiences back into my world. I integrated my sessions as best I could, but my integration, like the work itself, was private and surreptitious. Though I kept myself whole in my personal life, I was not allowed to be whole in my public life, and if you are not whole in your public life, can you ever be truly whole? How can a teacher who loves sharing knowledge be at peace with himself while hiding his deepest knowledge? How can transcendence and immanence find their proper balance in such compromised circumstances?

The opportunity to share with others what I had learned in my sessions was a missing piece in my integration process. My deep sadness was caused not just by the loss of communion but also by having no community with whom to share my experiences and receive their experiences in return. In his beautiful book on near-death experiences, *Consciousness Beyond Life,* Pim van Lommel writes: "The process of integration cannot get under way properly until the experience can be shared" (2010, 51). What is true for near-death experiences is also true for deep psychedelic experience. In my case, there was a level of integration that took place during my years of silence and a deeper level that opened only when I began to share the full story of my journey.

As I was writing *LSD and the Mind of the Universe,* my absorption of my psychedelic experiences deepened in unexpected ways. They began to live in me differently than before. It was as though all my memories congealed to form a greater living whole. There is a saying from the Navajo: "When you put a thing in order, and give it a name, and you are all in accord, it becomes" (Waters 1970). By telling my story, by giving it a name and owning my experience, something new was set in motion. A new peace settled over me. At first this peace just eased my existential loneliness and made the loss of communion more bearable, but then it deepened further. As I was finishing the book and beginning to speak about it publicly, a new spiritual transparency began to open in my life. It sometimes feels as though the Beloved is not waiting for me to die but is coming for me here. Where this will lead, I don't know. It is still unfolding, taking me to new places, but surely this is the work of integration: to own, internalize, and manifest our experiences as deeply as we can; to let them flow through us and shape our full presence on this Earth.

But I continue to have deep questions about integration. I think we are still in the early stages of understanding how entering these extreme states of consciousness is affecting us. What does it do to a person to hold the kind of memories that I am holding? As long as our sessions stay close to the shoreline of the known world, uncovering the pains of our past, we have therapeutic models for how to work with them. When we travel a bit farther out to experience the intelligence running through all things and the continuity of life after death, we have spiritual models for absorbing these insights. But when our journeys take us great distances from the known world, when we enter the truly deep waters of the universe, how are these adventures being integrated by us then? What does "integration" even mean in this context?

How does a finite being, exquisitely tuned to the conditions of space-time, digest our forays into the Infinite? How does a time-bound being absorb excursions into Deep Time? What is the residual impact of merging with all of existence after we have returned to being just one among many? How does our day-to-day self manage such extreme fluctuations of the membrane of consciousness, not once or twice, but forty, fifty, sixty times?

I am asking more questions than I have answers for. My life has become a living experiment in these matters with the outcome still being determined.

24

Training Psychedelic Therapists

Renee Harvey

*Before you embark on any path ask the question: Does this
path have a heart? If the answer is no, you will know it,
and then you must choose another path. . . . A path without
a heart is never enjoyable. You have to work hard even to
take it. On the other hand, a path with heart is easy; it
does not make you work at liking it."*

CARLOS CASTANEDA, 1990

Setting up training for people who want to become psychedelic therapists starts with some fundamental questions: Who is asking for
this training? Why do they want to do it? What do they want to do
with it? Who are the appropriate teachers, trainers, or mentors to
deliver this training?

A dilemma arises around eligibility for training as a psychedelic
therapist. On one hand, there may be people who are psychedelic
aware but who have no formal qualifications in the psychological or
clinical field. On the other hand, there may be academically qualified

professional people, like psychiatrists, who have little or no real experience in conducting psychological therapy and may not have spent time working on their own issues in personal therapy, or those who are trained and skilled as therapists but who are naive and inexperienced with psychedelics.

Two programs have been at the founding forefront of developing training for psychedelic therapy, one from the Multidisciplinary Association for Psychedelic Science (MAPS) and the other from the California Institute of Integral Studies (CIIS). In recent times we see a great flourishing of new training programs, and an even greater number of shorter courses from sources available across the world, often online. Some are significant new contributions to the field, some are of questionable quality, and some maybe have extremely low standards when compared to better-established programs. There is a risk of people taking such courses and proclaiming themselves trained to provide psychedelic therapy, without having been subject to any scrutiny of their clinical work by a qualified mentor, or without having worked through their wounding, as would be expected in professional therapy trainings. To be properly trained requires direct observation and feedback of practice with ongoing supervision to avoid the pitfalls of unintentional mistakes, which may cause real harm to people. It also requires sustained inner enquiry and process. The focus here will be on standards set by these established programs to form the basis for understanding what constitutes a comprehensive and high-quality professional development approach for psychedelic therapists.

MAPS was established in 1986 by Rick Doblin, a psychologist who initiated research on MDMA for PTSD (Emerson et al. 2014). The MAPS MDMA Therapy Training Program focuses strongly on developing clinicians' skills for working in a research setting. The CIIS Certificate in Psychedelic-Assisted Therapies and Research was developed in 2014 by Janis Phelps, with advice and support from many leading researchers and organizations in the field of psychedelic medicine, including MAPS, Usona, and the Heffter Institute. Leading figures at Johns Hopkins University, such as Roland Griffiths and Elizabeth

Nielsen, provided input into the CIIS training. The aim of the program was to train people to work in research settings, with an additional focus on training therapists to help people negotiate the mystical or spiritual experiences they may encounter (Phelps 2017). This may be regarded as controversial by more conservative scientists, but the key role of the mystical experience was identified by Griffiths et al. (2018) as an essential component in facilitating lasting change.

The training of psychedelic therapists rests on a willingness to be open to new paradigms, especially when therapists come from a conventional training and are naive about psychedelics. There is an overemphasis on accepting only evidence from randomized controlled trials as the gold standard for determining outcomes for therapy. This risks ignoring or devaluing the validity of evidence from other approaches to research, or risks rendering the complexity of elements that together contribute toward positive therapeutic outcomes harder to isolate and identify as being significant facilitators of change. But "absence of evidence is not evidence of absence," as Phil Alderson has stated (2004, 476). The paradigm changes inherent in psychedelic training require a wider perspective and an increased openness to a range of models, ranging from neuroscience to psychospiritual perspectives. A balance is required: an attitude of denigrating science or devaluing the work done by professionally trained clinicians runs the risk of falling prey to unknowing ignorance—not knowing what you don't know—and the potential harms this can cause (O'Carroll 2015).

A comprehensive training program needs to integrate a broad spectrum of theoretical and practical approaches so that trainees are equipped to respond therapeutically in the most helpful way. A science-based approach includes understanding the physiological effects of various substances and being up to date on clinical research, while a mind-based approach includes knowledge of models of change, psychological processes, and risk management. Alongside these approaches, the trainee needs to cultivate skills to work with the embodied mystical, spiritual, or transpersonal aspects of the psychedelic experience, which are encountered so frequently, while being engaged with their own inner work.

Skepticism and a critical attitude toward different approaches from across this spectrum need to be put aside so that the psychedelic therapist can respond flexibly to whatever arises within the session. The therapist may have personal views regarding the relevance of science, for example, or the validity and even acceptability of spiritual or mystical elements, but these disparate views need to be reconciled or at least held in abeyance. The psychedelic experience heightens sensitivity, and any expression of insincerity, patronization, or incongruence could be easily picked up by the experiencer and compromise the trust required for a safely held process.

INTEGRATING ASPECTS OF FUNCTIONING IN PSYCHEDELIC-ASSISTED THERAPY

The aspects of functioning described in this section constitute components that need to be integrated within the therapist into a harmonious, smoothly functioning entity, helping to foster to the maximum extent the opportunity for healing and growth for the person having a therapeutically-held psychedelic experience. Training of therapists will need to cover all of these aspects: they not only need to acquire intellectually based knowledge, they also need to gain the knowledge and tools for managing set and setting and for applying their skills as therapists in the heat of the healing space. Live training with feedback is an essential component of this learning process.

> **The therapist's own insight and experience.** For therapists who understand psychedelic therapy in depth, this path will have followed their own experiences with these medicines. There is a degree of consensus that if you've experienced taking a psychedelic substance yourself, you are more likely to be better at helping others with it (Nielson 2018). They will be able to relate to spiritual and mystical content in an accepting way, acknowledg-

ing its validity for the experiencer and holding a flexible framework within which the person can extract meaning out of these experiences.

In the MAPS training, there has been an opportunity for trainees to have an experience with MDMA as part of their course. At the time of this writing, in both the MAPS and CIIS courses, this is not possible, so a weekend practicum with Holotropic Breathwork has been incorporated, instead, for people to experience expanded states of consciousness, both as a journeyer and as a sitter. This training model provides the dual experience of being taken care of while in an expanded state and of caring for another going through a similar experience. These deeply meaningful experiences have allowed the trainees to navigate the very same territories they would need to be acquainted with for supporting a psychedelic experience, and work with the complexities these may hold.

Knowledge and understanding. The psychedelic therapist needs to understand the actions and effects of different substances, the current status of clinical research, various models of therapy, and the rationale for the various therapeutic techniques that underpin this work. There needs to be a good grasp of interpersonal processes such as transference and projection.

Deep inner work. Conventional training for psychological therapists focuses on the importance of empathy, insight, or compassion, which are mostly experientially acquired capacities. These traits or abilities are more likely to be developed and fostered through the trainees' experiences in their own personal therapy. They may build to some extent on a natural ability, or be hard-won insights stemming from personal suffering. It is generally acknowledged that the best therapists are those who have experienced challenges in their own lives, lived through their suffering, and worked through therapy or other ways to heal their own trauma. In Jungian terms, they have confronted and worked with the shadow aspects in themselves—the parts they would rather not face, often deeply buried and hard to access. Bringing such personal capacities and qualities into the encounter with the person in psychedelic therapy helps them to meet the fear and pain that may arise in the experiencer's sessions with greater compassion.

Somatic aspects. The therapist needs to know and understand the kinds of physical reactions that may arise during the psychedelic experience. He or she must carefully observe and monitor bodily reactions in the experiencer, as well as be prepared to work with these therapeutically. This can include the application of somatic therapy techniques that may, for example, encourage movement or enhance the tension in a muscle to unlock meaning and support the experiencer's process in greater fullness and depth.

Knowing what actions to take in the setting. The therapist needs to be attentive to the physical needs of the experiencer during a dosing session, such as assisting when the person is nauseous, needs to go to the toilet, or needs food or drink. This includes developing skills and techniques for supporting the experiencer should he or she becomes agitated, or managing situations of potential risk, for example where the experiencer attempts to leave the clinical space before the experience has been concluded.

IMPORTANT ELEMENTS FOR THE EXPERIENCER

Preparation before and during a Session

The preparation process shapes the set leading up to the dosing session. The therapists provide preparation sessions so that the experiencer can enter the session with an attitude of trust, confident that their therapists are capable practitioners who will fully accept anything that may arise and who will not reject, abandon, or let the experiencer down. The experiencer also needs to trust that there will be support afterward, and the therapist needs to discuss how this might be structured.

The physical setting will be part of what helps foster a safe and positive mindset in the psychedelic session. A psychedelic therapist needs to understand the importance of the space that is created as the container for the work, both as a physical space as well as an emotional and potentially transpersonal space. The setting itself needs to be contained in an environment where it is protected from anything that could impinge from the outside. Therefore, if a need arises to move the session outside the space for reasons of safety (if, for example, medical intervention is needed, or a fire alarm goes off), the therapist must be able to negotiate this by having already considered the wider setting.

Integration of the Experience after the Session

Mystical experiences may be welcomed or cause great fear. They may inspire awe, or they might occasion experiences of ego death and give rise to terror. The containing power of a well-managed integration group where the person can share what happened with others who can relate in an accepting and understanding manner is invaluable and can harness such experiences to powerful and life-lasting positive changes. A skillful, insightful, and compassionate therapist to work with an experiencer on a one-to-one basis may be also be needed for a continued period after the experience.

Personal insights, memories of trauma, or other emotionally charged events of the past or present may require integration. Often people describe an experience with psychedelics as years of psychotherapy condensed into a few hours. This takes patience and careful processing to help the person rebalance and make sense of the experiences. Encouraging the experiencer to engage with inner work in an ongoing manner by following practices like meditation, journaling, or creative expressions will support the unfolding and embedding of discoveries.

One of the biggest opportunities for making lasting change arises when the person is able to work with old attitudes, behaviors, and ways of being in a way that translates into real change. Often, it's about returning to a life that is much the same but with a new attitude or set of behaviors. It can be challenging for a person to integrate these new experiences, while carrying on with life as before, and to resist sinking back into old patterns and old ways of thinking or the urge to leave everything behind and retreat to a forest or a mountaintop. The paradox here is achieving a balance between the perception that "everything is different" and "nothing is different." As the Zen proverb goes: "Before enlightenment, chop wood, carry water. After enlightenment, chop wood, carry water." Holding and eventually resolving the tension between the transcended realms and everyday life is part of the integration process.

But while the external world and the demands of everyday life may still be the same, the person has an opportunity for deep change in personal meaning-making; in how he or she makes sense of life with all its associated structures, a shift that potentially brings about change at a fundamental, personal level of functioning. If this shift can be carried over to the person's external relationships with the world, profound changes can be initiated. Family work is an invaluable element of this transformative process.

All of the above considerations need to be incorporated into psychedelic therapy training to equip therapists with the necessary skills and synergistic balance that will help them navigate the territory for themselves and for those they will accompany through this path.

ASSESSING CANDIDATES

One of the major challenges of current trainings is the widespread interest they receive, and one of their primary tasks is to discern and assess who would be a suitable candidate for what the course offers. The queries will often come from people with many different backgrounds, varied trainings, and personal degrees of experience with psychedelics, including some with years of working as underground psychedelic therapists. Some will have been trained in the medical field; some will have had no formal training at all but will report they've been actively working in this field for twenty years or more. Others will have undergone an alternative training, such as in various shamanic traditions.

Acknowledging that psychedelic therapist trainings cannot practically aim to re-create all the basic levels of knowledge in the field of medical and psychological treatment approaches, while respecting the fact that there are many diverse backgrounds, it is often necessary to start by recognizing the foundational value of some previous professional trainings. Future course developments may aim to cater to additional roles for diversely qualified people who could still have a useful part in working in teams with more formally qualified colleagues, but often the starting point is to develop a training where previously trained professionals acquire additional skills or modify skills already learned. In addition, qualifying in these professions requires adherence to codes of practice, forming an invaluable foundation of values and ethics upon which psychedelic therapy can build.

Psychedelic-assisted therapy courses that strive to ensure a solid clinical baseline will often rely on three requirements as a clear basis for admission. The first two are relatively clear-cut: First, as a minimum, candidates need to have at least a graduate level qualification in a field related to mental health. This should ensure that time does not need to be spent repeating basic knowledge, such as the definition of PTSD. Second, candidates need to have worked for a few years in delivering some form of psychological therapy or counselling requiring supervised clinical work. This ensures that candidates have acquired at least the basic skills in conducting themselves in a therapeutic environment with a patient or client and know how to follow legal, practical, and ethical principles.

The third requirement is more challenging and involves assessing the qualitative aspects and motives of candidates wanting to be trained. The aim is to establish to what extent candidates are able to convey empathy, compassion, and depth of understanding without an impulse to direct the process the experiencer is going through. The right candidates for psychedelic training need to be able to balance a high level of ethical and moral standards while being open to whatever arises during psychedelic sessions as well as to be able to tolerate uncertainty and ambiguity and willingly accept challenges to any preconceived belief systems. Candidates are required to have engaged in considerable self-examination and deep inner work to resolve their own potential issues of narcissism so that they can approach the work without heroic grandiosity, of seeing the work as a way to compensate for their own personal difficulties and shortcomings. Suitable candidates would have worked on their own issues and are clearly aware of their own starting points and motivations for engaging in this work. Once again, a basic platform is needed here for the training to have a foothold on which to build.

Skillset Requirements

Janis Phelps, director of CIIS, developed five core competencies for the institute's training, mapping out the necessary and essential skills for the development of safe and competent psychedelic practitioners.

1. **Empathic abiding presence.** Described as "a universally agreed-upon quality of a properly trained psychedelic therapist" (2017, 11). It incorporates "composure, evenly suspended attention, mindfulness, empathic listening, 'doing by not doing,' responding to distress with calmness, and equanimity" (2017, 12).

2. **Trust enhancement.** Phelps highlights three aspects of this skill. The therapist needs to enhance the participant's view of the therapist as a trustworthy guide and the participant's ability to trust his or her own inner healing capacity, as well as "the ability to reliably normalize for the participant that paradoxical transformations and radically unexpected moments in sessions are to be expected and thus trusted as part of the process" (2017, 14).

3. **Spiritual intelligence.** The capacity to work with spiritual and mystical aspects as well as having had some personal experiences to support their understanding of such encounters.

4. **Knowledge of the physical and psychological effects of psychedelics.**

5. **Therapist self-awareness and ethical integrity.** The therapist needs to be self-aware, know what his or her motives are for doing the work, know about boundary issues and the therapeutic alliance, and understand relationship dynamics such as transference and countertransference. The role of clinical supervision is emphasized as crucial to doing work with insight and integrity

and is a strong justification for selecting therapist trainees with this background understanding and requirements in their training and experience.

6. **Proficiency in Complementary Techniques.** Therapists ideally should have knowledge and proficiency in other techniques, such as somatic-oriented work, meditation, and family systems work.

Janis Phelps (2017) describes twelve domains of training as foundational for any course in psychedelic therapy. These are aimed at enhancing the development of the core competencies described above. She writes that future benchmarks of success in training could be evaluated based on the coherent linking of the competencies with the overall aims and objectives of the training and its intended scope.

To meet the highest standards of training, it is important for programs to have well thought-out integrative theoretical underpinnings. Neuroscience and research needs to be supported by psychotherapeutic theory and practice with the addition of somatic therapeutics and transpersonal approaches. Theory needs to be supported by experiential components, which in some trainings is psychedelic-assisted therapeutic experiences in legal frameworks and in other trainings are viable alternatives, such as Holotropic Breathwork. Trainees should be encouraged to develop awareness of set and setting and learn to work collaboratively with other professions, referrals, and treatment pathways. Clinicians should also be challenged to examine their own practice, identify and focus on their own developmental needs, and expand and integrate their skills. As trainees incorporate new facts, weave together theory and practice in how to work with people, and simultaneously open themselves to the inevitable personal growth and learning inherent in this work, they develop a solid foundation for helping others.

After the training program ends, the mentoring and supervised practice should continue as part of an ongoing commitment and engagement in deepening one's learning and clinical capacity. For trainees in Australia there are currently programs in their early stages of development that can offer trainees access to research programs with opportunities for supervised practice.

While this book is being edited, we are witnessing a proliferation of courses being offered across the world in psychedelic-assisted therapy, many with promising potential for supporting the wider dialogue around working with expanded states and integration to open in novel and exciting ways. The Psychedelic Therapy Training offered by ONCA strengthens the dialogue between indigenous and Western cosmological frameworks and offers a training that can cater to those who might not have an initial qualification in psychotherapy. The Depth Relational Process training offered by the Institute of Psychedelic Therapy brings in a focus on personal process alongside an integrative framework that brings together animistic, depth, transpersonal, and systemic approaches. These two examples point to the fact that we are moving toward greater theoretical diversity that will support and take this work forward, and that the future field of psychedelic therapy will reflect the diversity of orientation that we see in the field of psychotherapy.

The current expectations are that these medicines might become available as legal prescriptions through medical professionals, following the paradigm that has already been set in the United States with the medicinal use of cannabis. In building these trainings, we look forward to a future where there are legal clinical settings offering psychedelic-assisted treatment by providing the medicine alongside integrative psychotherapy of sufficient quality and duration to support the fullest expression and unfolding of this process.

25

Psychedelic Psychotherapy Supervision

Shared Learning and Reflective Practice

*Tim Read, Michelle Baker-Jones, Sven Kimenai,
Jonny Martell, Roberta Murphy,
Ashleigh Murphy-Beiner, Rosalind Watts*

Supervision is an integral part of psychotherapy practice. It offers a safe, reflective space where the complexity of the work can be unpacked and processed so that people can continue their professional development and build on their previous training. Ideally, therapists under supervision should have core competencies in psychological treatment and, in this context, some knowledge of expanded states. However, some people attending supervision may be experienced psychotherapists but quite new to work with psychedelics while others may be comfortable in the psychedelic space but less familiar with concepts such as transference, projection, and boundaries.

A well-held supervision group is a shared journey of learning and an adventure in consciousness that celebrates the diversity of training and experience of those who attend. The psychedelic experience has layers of complexity that simply do not occur in conventional treatment with the amplification of intensity and the archetypal nature of some of the material, as well as the duration and intimacy of the therapeutic encounter. But the relational aspects must not be ignored: we are relational beings with our unique histories, psychodynamic contours, and attachment needs. The emotional space in the medicine session can feel more immersive compared to standard psychotherapy as participants are supported through the tension between surrender and resistance. It can feel as though the emotional space is deeply shared between participant and guide, and there can be contact lows as well as contact highs.

This discussion draws from supervision sessions with therapists from a clinical research trial of psilocybin in treatment-resistant depression at Imperial College London and from the retreat teams at Synthesis in the Netherlands, where the consumption of psilocybin truffles is legal. The treatment at Imperial College involved two guides working with each depressed participant for two psychedelic sessions, each participant being randomized to high dose or low dose of psilocybin. The participants in the Netherlands were screened to exclude psychiatric disorders, and their medicine session occurred in a group setting. Both settings involved careful preparation and integration.

TRIGGERS: MESSENGERS FROM THE DEEP

A trigger is an external event that causes a reaction in the internal world, which manifests as an emotion, a behavior, or a somatic response. We are constantly triggered to some extent in everyday life, but holding the space for people having psychedelic experiences inevitably increases our own sensitivity, especially in a retreat setting with multiple interactions over an extended time frame. Triggers may have a deeply positive emotional tone; indeed, the contact high puts us in touch with feelings of love, compassion, and connection. Even such positive mood states may have side effects, but here we will focus on those triggers that affect us deeply because they illuminate a wound, which in turn provides us with a valuable opportunity for learning and healing. We manage this in the same way that we might treat a psychedelic experience, by leaning into it gently with compassion and curiosity. Rather than recoiling from the difficult emotions and feelings that arise or employ our usual defenses, we watch what is arising in ourselves and we try to make sense of it.

Triggers provide us with a window into the complexities of the deep psyche but only if properly processed. Supervision needs to facilitate a *culture of vulnerability* so that people feel safe enough to share the experiences of and learnings from triggers, while not necessarily revealing deeply personal information.

Any supervision arrangement needs to have a hierarchy of trigger management.

1. Self-management while in a professional role
2. Debriefing after the session or retreat, often brief
3. Formal supervision to allow more detail and consideration of content
4. Further attention if the material aroused is intense and problematic
5. Signposting to appropriate further work

When we are triggered in our role as guide, sitter, or therapist, the primary task is to continue in our professional role and maintain our compassionate, attentive, responsible presence for those in our care. At such times, rather than giving priority to our own process, we need to employ self-management skills, while making a mental note to unpack the learning process at a later stage.

Self-management while in role can be challenging as it may not be clear at the time that one has been triggered. Any intense emotion, perspective shift, or somatic event that arises while you are in the role of therapist should be carefully considered. Giving the feeling a name or shape is helpful. Identifying to yourself that you've been triggered (such as by saying "I've been triggered" to yourself mentally) enables you to shift from a passive role to a more active role and engage in the integrative process. In a retreat setting, it is often helpful to share with a colleague that you have been triggered and perhaps identify the nature of the trigger briefly, but given the highly sensitive and perceptive quality of the space, the primary task is always to avoid destabilizing the participants' process or undermining colleagues. Taking a brief period of time-out may be helpful to rebalance as long as this does not decrease the safety of the setting. However, sometimes a time-out can be counterproductive as it may increase feelings of alienation and inadequacy.

Triggers typically reactivate traumas of commission (things that were done to you) and traumas of omission (care deficits). A trauma in this context is something that causes a level of psychological distress that feels unbearable. We all have our areas of trauma in our psyche, and we are all vulnerable to triggers. Traumas may be events that we can remember linked to patterns of emotional response that we are familiar with, or they may be mysterious, inaccessible to conscious memory, lying within the preverbal realm. Descriptions of triggered feelings include:

- Shame: feeling useless or worthless
- Paranoia: suddenly not a safe place, feeling hated
- Anxiety: edge of panic
- Deprivation, abandonment: "everyone else is getting the good stuff"
- Anger: ugly mood, vindictive
- Cynicism: "don't want to be here"
- Somatic reaction: heavy body, clumsy, nausea,
- Visionary experience: "like an ayahuasca flashback"
- Regression: "triggered feelings from when I was three and now it's hard not to behave like a three-year-old"
- Ego inflation, grandiosity: "felt that I was so gifted in this work"

Every piece of therapeutic work is an opportunity for both therapist and client to explore, discover, and be changed. Usually the triggered material has some familiarity and settles fairly soon, but sometimes the trigger can open a reservoir of pain or a deep wound, such as the futile position (see page 77), which can cause persistent distress and require careful attention and ongoing inner work. The following story is an example of a session that triggered an expression of the futile position in the therapist.

Holding Space in the Dark

During a psilocybin ceremony, a woman in her fifties entered a place of deep anger and self-disgust. After I invited her to allow herself to more fully experience and release this anger, her experience transformed into the dark night of the soul—a place of hopelessness, nihilism, and the ultimate truth of deep suffering. My encouragement to allow these feelings to emerge and be present seemed hollow, and all my support seemed futile. As I sat with her, reassuring her that "everything will be all right," I became increasingly aware that I, too, carried a similar wound to which I had no answer.

After the ceremony and the retreat had ended, she had not emerged from this place of futility and despair. We offered additional support, but her state was deeply concerning. Afterward and during subsequent retreats, I, too, found myself in similar territory. My restlessness transformed into a disconnected, self-deprecating menace that was overwhelming. I had frequent feelings of being deeply unloved and lonely and having no place in this world.

During supervision, I realized more clearly how my own unresolved psychic wounds had been triggered. Rather than trying to bypass the experience, I needed to work on it, deepen to it. I learned to emphasize amplification in the service of resolution in such situations with participants. Personally, having reopened that wound, I consider the profundity and impact of this experience to be deeply valuable to my continuing growth as a facilitator and as a person.

RELATIONAL ASPECTS OF PSYCHEDELIC THERAPY

Everyone working with expanded states needs a basic understanding of transference, projective mechanisms, and the value of careful consideration of the countertransference. Many sessions will be uncomplicated by transference, but often such mechanisms are amplified by the psychedelic state, the duration of the session, and the intimacy of the setting. The combination of a male-female therapist dyad in some settings mimics the parental dyad, which will have profound implications for some participants. Any strong or unusual thoughts, feelings, impulses, or behaviors that we have in connection with a participant may be giving us important information about a person's internal world.

- **Transference** refers to the repetition of past patterns of relating in the present. Experiences in early life create templates that determine how we perceive and respond to current circumstances.
- **Countertransference** is the unconscious emotional response elicited in us by others through the process of projection; it informs our "gut feelings" or how we intuit something about another's emotional state.
- **Projection** is the unconscious way in which feelings are externalized into others around us, for example by attributing one's own hostility to another and denying any aggression within oneself. Projection has both an evacuative aspect and a communicative aspect. The evacuation is a means of getting rid of aspects of the self that we deem undesirable, while the communicative aspect is how we let others know about our emotional states.
- **Projective identification** refers to our identification with a projection from another. It is powerful and feels intrusive: we may feel controlled by the countertransference in a way that blindsides us.

It can be difficult as a therapist or guide to distinguish what may be our own psychological issues, what belongs to our clients, and how these two fields may mingle, causing a shared psychological space that can carry some challenge and weight. This is why doing our own psychological work is of the utmost importance if we are to become more skillful in navigating this terrain. Supervision works best when people attending feel safe enough to reflect on this. It does not (usually) involve divulging deeply personal information but does require honest examination of some issues that may feel uncomfortable. This culture of vulnerability seems to flourish in psychedelic supervision, perhaps reflected by the way in which intentional and integrated use of psychedelics seem to enhance connectivity and decrease our tendencies to narcissism in the service of the therapeutic task. Consider the following example, which shows how supervision allowed one therapist to reflect on her reactions to a particular patient.

Hostility in Countertransference

I was aware that I had a hostile reaction to Simon. I noticed that he addressed everything to my male cotherapist, and I experienced him as misogynistic and contemptuous. I was not sure that I could work with him. I took this to supervision as it is unusual for me to have such a strong reaction to a participant, although I knew my sensitivity was heightened being midway through my menstrual cycle. I spoke about how I can feel intimidated by high achievers and find it harder to be compassionate to those from a more privileged background. I struggled with Simon's tendency to see the male as in charge. Being able to flesh out my transferential issues around privilege and class helped.

In our discussion, it became clearer that Simon was reenacting some powerful dynamics from his childhood with a depressed, unempathic mother and a charismatic father whom he wanted to emulate. Different team members had different perceptions of him, and teasing this apart helped me to understand how his spikiness and apparent contempt covered his deep vulnerability in relation to early attachment.

On my next contact with him, I was able to see how difficult it was for him to tolerate his feelings, and as our rapport developed, he spoke of his feelings of disconnection, sadness, and regrets. His

spikiness seemed to dissolve, and I felt increasingly warm toward him.
He expressed gratitude for the opportunity to be on the trial and told
us that he felt safe with us both.

In a clinical research setting, we have found that the projective processes can be complex, multiple, and intrusive. There are the expectations of the participants, who have high hopes of relief but who may be
randomly allocated a low dose. The academic establishment, with its
research protocol, has its own agenda. There may be envy from some
colleagues, antagonism from others, and interest from the media. The
therapist and guides have to find their feet as a clinical team in this
complex territory, while holding the responsibility of taking vulnerable
people into deep and uncharted waters.

Group Processes

The clinical team met for supervision in the room where the psilocybin
sessions took place. This room was deep in the interior of a research
facility where the team had experienced some organizational and
cultural tensions. During the team's formative stages, concern about
their capacity to contain anxieties was softened by returning to this
room. The sense of safety created for participants' vulnerable surrender
to their experiences—in a physical and psychic space akin to a womb—
shaped the development of the reflective space. The group developed a
neologism, "wahanji," to denote "bad" energy, such as what felt like
envious attacks from the outside but also the group's own projections.
As a concept and metaphor, wahanji fortified group cohesiveness,
serving as a vessel to project out potential contaminants of the
therapeutic and creative processes and as a humorous acknowledgment
of the group's partial identification with healing approaches outside the
biomedical mainstream, symbolized by the research facility's coldness
and emotional sterility.

The capacity to think psychodynamically about transference and
countertransference phenomena was enhanced by the group's growing
understanding of each member's attachment and personal history.

This understanding was in part fostered in several group Holotropic Breathwork sessions. These sessions offered a training as both guide and breather and powerfully enhanced feelings of mutual trust through a culture of shared vulnerability. The team members' empathic understanding of their own wounds and healing journeys added depth to the group's understanding of participant sessions.

Technical and Ethical Issues in Clinical Research Trials

Clinical research trials using psychedelics raise additional issues. The participants have conditions that may be severe and longstanding. They may have high expectations of the treatment, even a feeling of desperation, but they are randomly allocated according to the study design and may receive a placebo, a low dose, or a high dose. Some such studies have a crossover design where every participant will eventually have the experimental treatment, while other studies do not.

Some issues may have no clear answers. The role of the reflective space is to carefully consider the questions, develop models of best practice, and share the emotional burden so it does not feel overly located in one team member.

- How do we manage the disappointment of the low-dose group, for whom this may be the latest on a long series of abandonments?
- When are intensification strategies helpful?
- In what circumstances and in what manner is physical support provided?
- How appropriate is it to encourage a full surrender to inner process when we think the unfolding therapeutic process may involve more sessions than the protocol allows?
- What is the duty of care after the conclusion of the program?
- How do we hold the tension between the interests of the academic program and the needs of the participant?

The following story demonstrates a therapist's reflection with her supervision group regarding the challenging dynamics of clinical trials.

What Is in the Medicine Capsule?

Her story touched me, resonating with some themes of my own childhood. I felt very aware of the depths of her suffering. She spoke tearfully of her desperation for change, and how devastated she would feel if the treatment didn't work. I really wanted her to benefit from it. The first dosing session was disappointing for her; we thought she had received the low dose. She felt damaged, and I felt guilty. The second session had the intensity of a high dose, bringing up feelings that oscillated between deep grief and barren emptiness. There was something very dark and distressing about what I was witnessing that left me feeling deeply worried and disconnected from her. Her depression felt like a heavy weight in our follow-up sessions.

In supervision, I shared with the group my feelings of ineptitude and hopelessness. I felt poisoned after her sessions and half-joked that I needed an exorcism. I realized how much my own guilt and anxiety about the darkness of her depression had pulled me into the familiar role of trying to fix things for her. I worried I had missed an important opportunity to help her work with her pain, and we discussed the pros and cons of intensification strategies for difficult feelings. We reflected on the challenges of not knowing what was in the capsules and the resonance with themes of abandonment and rejection for those participants who thought they had received the low dose.

Endings

The end of the professional relationship is a major event in psychotherapy. Endings have a powerful resonance with previous loss life-events and attachment traumas. Like all psychological wounds, once exposed there is major potential for both healing work but also retraumatization. Because endings are so difficult for some clients and may activate our own unresolved loss issues, we may feel under subtle pressure to simply not address it. The danger here is that the ending may then feel abrupt, like a cliff edge—more like an abandonment. Endings always need addressing, and this means that they have to be a part of the conversation throughout the period of engagement. In wellness retreats, this may be a simple process with the closing group followed by good-byes, hugs, and the dispersal. In a research scenario, the length of the relationship may extend over several months; the attachment may have an idealized quality and the participant may feel quite bereft. The following story describes the use of the supervision group by the therapist supporting the participants who were approaching the end of the trial.

Weighed Down by Projections

Many clients in the psilocybin and depression clinical trial found real hope of a life free from depression after their treatment. But symptoms of depression would often return after a few months. In the weekly aftercare sessions, they shared their frustration that they couldn't access further psilocybin-assisted therapy due to legality or cost issues. So, despite high motivation to work on their depression, they felt thwarted.

Eventually, I found myself stuck too. I had witnessed their transformation resulting from the psilocybin treatment, and now I was witnessing the steady decline of some, as we moved toward the ending. I felt weighed down with the impossibility of their situation and paralyzed in my thinking. I empathized deeply with them and found myself without words or ideas of how to help.

Discussion in team supervision restored clarity, creativity, and hope for me. Together, we made sense of the clients' deep concerns around the ending of their relationship with the program and its implications. Further psilocybin treatment was unlikely, but if we considered each person's recovery from depression as an ongoing journey through new perspectives toward a life rich in meaning, then the participants had just opened a doorway into a new way of being. There was so much to explore. I felt released from the weight of the projections and felt renewed possibility and hope. I found that working from this perspective with clients has been very helpful for their separation from the study with forward momentum for their recovery.

Erotic Transference

Feelings of romantic love are not uncommon in psychotherapy and may be a particular feature of psychedelic therapy. This is not surprising as work with expanded states often induces a heightened sense of connectivity, compassion, and love. This more transpersonal aspect of love can become conflated with personal and relational needs and clients suffering from depression may be particularly deprived, attachment hungry, and connection seeking. A useful strategy is to shift the focus away from the personal relationship in the outside world back to the inner journey—while acknowledging the grace and depth of the therapeutic relationship. This is potentially hazardous territory, and any supervision arrangement has to feel safe enough to address the many manifestations of the erotic transference, a situation the next story addresses.

A Confusion of Levels

In his psilocybin session, he entered a beautiful space of love that felt deeply healing for him, even divine, and this felt profound for us to witness as his guides. He told another team member that he had developed feelings for me after the session, so I had the opportunity to discuss in supervision ahead of our final integration session. In supervision, we reflected on the "confusion of levels," where a numinous experience with a love-filled quality can be projected onto an individual so that the transpersonal becomes confused with the personal. Our final integration session was thoughtful, as we bowed to his gratitude toward the treatment and his therapists but also reestablished his inner connection with the loving peaceful space from his psilocybin session. It felt important to both of us that he could carry this loving presence forward with him.

THE EXTRAORDINARY RANGE OF PSYCHEDELIC EXPERIENCE

Therapists from a traditional psychology or mental health background will find that the conventional paradigms of their training do not begin to cover the complexity and range of the psychedelic experience. The paradigm leap required has been compared to the discovery of quantum physics, the transition from a universe of discrete particles and forces to an infinitely more mysterious web of dynamic energy. Transpersonal experiences are common in expanded states and may challenge the conventional wisdom that consciousness is limited to neuronal processes or exists only during the passage from our first breath to our last. The two stories that follow offer a flavor of this complex territory.

Death of a Father

Her father died in a fire when she was little: he was a firefighter. She had no memories of him, but her mother's grief and the unfolding consequences of his death had dominated her life. In her psilocybin session, she experienced his death. It did not have an as-if or dreamlike quality. She felt that she was her father. It was a visceral and protracted reliving of his emotions, his will to live, and his fury that life was being taken from him. After the session, she felt that a part of her remained in his death. Although she quailed at the thought of another session, it seemed that the work was unfinished. I struggled to make sense of this experience, and it was helpful in supervision to hear of other accounts of ancestral memories and to think about what might arise in the next session.

Death of a Mother

He told the integration group that during his psilocybin session he met his mother again. She was deceased, and there had been tensions between them when she died. They were able to have the conversation that they had never had in life, and she told him something of her journey after her death. After the session he felt great relief—and he had lost his fear of death.

How then do we work toward a deeper understanding of such powerful and complex experiences? Some understanding of psychodynamics is fundamental, and we also need to be familiar with the psychedelic literature, the evidence base, the history of the work, and the theories of mind that have developed from the study of expanded states. But we should not be limited to this; we can usefully draw from philosophy, mythology, thanatology, anthropology, literature, comparative religion, and more. It is an important function of the reflective space to honor this complexity, to participate in the unfolding mystery of the work. We may wish to find answers, to say definitively that something is *this* or is derived from *that*. But pulls toward reductionism and seeking definitive answers generally need to be reshaped into tolerating uncertainty and framing even bigger questions.

In the same way that integration after a psychedelic experience encourages a mindset of curiosity, an emphasis on meaning, and a continuation of the inner journey, supervision should create the gentle space, the fertile soil, to encourage, suggest, and explore. This does not mean that critical faculties are lost or that previous skills are discarded; it's more that a new synthesis emerges. Working with psychedelics changes paradigms and ways of being in the world, and the supervision structure needs to support and honor this.

26

Toward an Ecology
of Ethics

Maria Papaspyrou

Working therapeutically with people in expanded states shares the same fundamental ethical principles as any other therapeutic work. The core ethics of caring for our participants while acting in support of their well-being, holding a safe space for them to explore their inner worlds, and respecting their emotional, mental, physical, and spiritual autonomy are just as relevant, if not more. And while we may not need an entirely new set of ethical codes for working with expanded states, the intensity and complexities of this work call for an even finer attunement to the ethical pitfalls along the way.

Sometimes the work takes place in legally sanctified environments, and other times it unfolds in underground therapeutic practices. The illegal status of these healing substances has led practitioners who deeply believe in the power of this work to take great personal risks to make it available. This means they are left to operate on the margins of what society deems acceptable, and in doing so, they carry extra risks and further ethical vulnerabilities. Psychedelic therapists are responsible and accountable for their own groundwork and for the participant's selection, preparation, session, and integration. We need a wide enough framework of accountability to prepare for the fullness and gravity of such a commitment.

The deeply intimate space we share with people in expanded states can amplify the transferential elements of the work.* In addition, the high degree of participant vulnerability and suggestibility in expanded states requires trustworthy, capable, reflective practitioners who continuously engage with their own inner process. In a space where the boundaries between inner and outer, self and other dissolve, it is not just our participants that come to reveal themselves deeply, we as facilitators also come to be profoundly seen and witnessed. This intimate exchange requires of practitioners well-developed ethics of care alongside the readiness, openness, and resilience to meet and show ourselves fully. It requires that we have delved deep within our own psyches, have become acquainted with our inner terrain, and have sufficiently processed our wounds and shadow.

Ethics are not just about being aware of what we shouldn't do; they are just as much about actively engaging with the things we should be doing to cultivate right relationship to self, to others, and to our work. And while ethical codes cannot always guarantee that practitioners will be prevented from engaging in unethical behavior, as a community we must actively educate one another and raise awareness on the conditions that might foster the potential for harm and malpractice in this field.

ETHICAL VULNERABILITIES

Most ethical breaches arise from the therapist's unresolved personal issues, inadequate self-care, and insufficient, or insufficiently used, professional support resources. I am not addressing here the ethical breaches that occur out of conscious and deliberate predatory behavior, devoid of

---

*I use the term *transferential elements* for brevity throughout the text; it includes transference, countertransference, projection, and projective identification. For definitions, see chapter 25.

empathy, that seek one's own gratification at the expense of others. I am addressing practitioners who deeply care about the work they do and the people they work with, highlighting ethical pitfalls we are all vulnerable to, either out of ignorance of the extraordinary complexities of this work or out of unresolved wounds and hidden blind spots.

Resolving our early childhood traumas, our attachment difficulties, our deep-seated fears and desires and being attentive to any imbalances in our current life help us develop a solid enough container so that when the material that emerges from the participant touches on our own issues, we are able to respond rather than react. Unless we have done the deeper inner work required, our capacity to be present and available as a relational object for the participant's process, or to respond effectively to the transferential elements of the work, might be severely limited.

The energy that work in expanded states requires comes from a deep well within ourselves that needs to be replenished through self-care and sufficient professional support. We need enough personal nourishment for our needs outside work so that we have sufficient resources for our participants. When our workloads exceed the right balance, our vulnerabilities and shortcomings may rise to the surface, and we may lose our presence and containing capacity, which might, indeed, reenact the participant's early relational experiences.

Ongoing supervision, peer support, and professional development will keep us plugged into a network of growth, mirroring back to us our resources as well as our blind spots and areas of potential learning and development. In addition, we need a safe community where we can meet and move together toward maintaining the integrity of this field. Being threaded into a wider network encourages accountability. A community that operates from a place of curiosity rather than judgment and encourages learning from our own and others' mistakes is able to attend to the very delicate processes of fracture and repair. None of us are perfect human beings or therapists, and in community and sharing we can dispel such idealized notions. In isolation, it is easier to bypass our shadow; in relationships and community, we are inevitably invited to go to the darker corners of Self and grapple with ways to grow from there. It is in collaborative and cocreative communities that we can built healthy, vibrant, resilient ecologies of ethics.

RIGHT RELATIONSHIP TO POWER

The power complex is central to our competitive, capitalist-driven societies, pervasive to all structures of life, and the therapeutic space is no exception. On a personal level, the lure of the power complex is fed unconsciously by the facilitator's longing to be in control as a safeguard against vulnerability and masks an underlying anxiety and fear around the process of change. Such misalignment with the movements of change, conscious or unconscious, can co-opt the whole therapeutic enterprise.

By default, the power dynamic between therapist and participant tends to be one of helper and helped, which, unless processed, can leave the therapist defensively attached to the empowered part of the archetype and the participant left to occupy the vulnerable, damaged, and needy end of the spectrum. Such dynamics also run across culture, class, race, gender identity, sexual orientation, and religion. When we bring these unseen dynamics into consciousness, we allow them to inform and support the work. In order to acknowledge and address the inherent power differentials and dynamics, facilitators must be able to work in multiculturally competent and informed ways, assess and challenge their own belief systems, reflect in an ongoing way on matters of power and privilege, and be aligned with social justice as an indispensable aspect of any healing process.

Participants can idealize facilitators and attribute the benefits that have emerged from their work to the facilitator's exceptional psychic gifts and great knowledge. The facilitator that accepts such projections becomes grandiose and omnipotent. If we accept power that is not ours, we have disempowered its true source—the participant's psyche. Facilitators need to be open and available for the wide range of projections they might be required to receive and hold, critically aware of their tendencies to readily accept the idealized projections and to distance themselves from the negative ones. It is important to remember that any archetypal energy we attach to has a positive and a negative pole. The counterbalance of the magician, the healer, or the hero is, according to Adolf Guggenbühl-Craig (2015), the charlatan, who is not to be trusted and cannot be counted upon. Lest we forget, we are not there to do magic tricks; we are there to be a containing and compassionate human presence, witnessing the participant's precious journey into the deep Self. Our power as facilitators is to be used to reassure, support, and empower our participants as they venture forth to what is unknown, to them and us.

Kylea Taylor (2017) has a wonderful suggestion for working with idealized projections that the participant refuses to withdraw from us: to pass on the devotion that has been transferred to us to a higher source that aligns with our spiritual belief system and can accommodate such powerful projections, thereby clearing our own energies for being present and available to the work.

WORKING WITH EROS

Sexual enactment is the highest reported ethical violation and the area of greatest concern for boundary breaches and professional malpractice in therapy. Beyond the inviolable principle that prohibits sexual relationships between therapists and participants, it is important that facilitators understand the nature of erotic dynamics in the work. In the intensity of expanded states, the energies surrounding Eros are ever more powerful and potentially destructive.

"Love is the emotional attention by which we take each other seriously and bring soul to presence between us" (Haule 1996, 106). While love has a very significant place in the therapeutic process, it is not to be confused with the sexual manifestations of Eros. The archetypal Greek god Eros was a dynamic force, "oldest and yet youngest of all the gods, at the beginning of all things and ever-renewing, ever-emergent" (Hollis 1994, 28). Interpreting the energies of Eros in a sexualized way truncates and misdirects his true purpose and power into the physical dimension.

Eros's presence brings vitality to the therapeutic field and sustains the potential for change. The true nature of such feelings can be of a spiritual dimension, where the divine is projected onto the facilitator. Or they can represent an inner drive and pull from the participant's and/or the facilitator's psyche toward union and integration, which becomes concretized as a longing for a sexual act between them. Or they can be a reenactment of early attachment dynamics or sometimes early sexual violations. Or they can spring from a part of the participant's psyche that tries to distract from the difficulties of inner work or tries to frustrate and attack the therapeutic process alongside the facilitator, becoming a vessel for unintegrated destructive and aggressive energies. Unless erotic, romantic, and sexual tansferential dynamics are held and understood through a therapeutic frame, they can be extremely compelling and perilous. To reduce these processes to an embodied act is to literalize the psychological unfolding, lose our foothold on the internal process, and disrupt the soul making that is underway.

Facilitators who have not attended to their own attachment, self-esteem, confidence, or narcissistic issues might actually believe that a participant is attracted to them and commit the hubris of appropriating archetypal energies that belong to the divine and the soul. Sexual acting out emerges out of the woundedness of both participant and facilitator, under a power dynamic where the facilitator can exert a powerful influence over the participant and within a context where the facilitator is the one responsible for the participant's well-being and for holding the therapeutic frame in place and the therapeutic process in progress. There is no question that sexual acting out can be immensely wounding to our participants, besides ourselves.

Such energies can be extremely difficult to navigate and contain in therapy and even more so in expanded states work. Working in groups or cofacilitating can support the diffusion of such energies and render such dynamics safer. Ongoing supervision will support the therapist to process such material. Attending to the discomfort, remaining conscious of our true place and size, and holding the tension rather than collapsing it by literalizing and physicalizing can support us in utilizing the inherent messages and growth-oriented potential of Eros in expanded work.

ETHICS FOR WORKING IN
EXPANDED STATES

To guide psychedelic-assisted sessions, often additional training is required to inform practitioners on how to work specifically with the power and intensity of psychedelic experiences. Work in expanded states can only be supported by what Taylor (2017) calls "theoretical elasticity," which requires being informed and able to operate from therapeutic model with enough breadth and depth to encompass the varied range of experiences that can emerge.

The most fundamental ethical requirement for facilitating such work safely and effectively is for the practitioner to have had his or her own extensive experiences in expanded states within a therapeutically informed set and setting and to have put in the time and effort required for processing and integrating these. Familiarity with these inner and far-out landscapes is where we cultivate our conceptual and experiential understanding of these spaces, how we slowly carve and shape a compatible belief system that supports such experiences, how we cultivate our relationship with the inner healing intelligence, how we open up to the level and degree of inner work required for being safe and competent facilitators, and how we learn to trust the healing potency of experiences in expanded states. Only then can we freely follow our participants to often frightening and challenging spaces where they come to face their deep grief, rage, and pain, loss of control and even sanity, and symbolic death and rebirth. Such material can be powerfully triggering if we have left behind us difficult experiences that are unintegrated and unresolved. Doing our inner work means processing our wounds and shadow and becoming conscious of our vulnerabilities, inner resources, and deeper unconscious motivations for doing this work. The degree of our theoretical and inner groundwork will determine our capacity to surrender to the creative and regenerative chaos that expanded work inevitably invites and relies upon.

Preparation ethics require that we select, prepare, and inform the participant for the work that lays ahead in ways that will prime the individual to stay open and surrender to the experience as it unfolds. The facilitator's capacity to discuss the potential difficulties and challenges he or she and the participant might be called to navigate in the work ahead will introduce the participant to the facilitator's openness and trust in the process.

Determining the suitability of the participant and identifying those that might be at risk is a significant responsibility. People who might be not ready for such an opening are those who exhibit a limited capacity for self-reflection, present immaturely, have a history of impulsive or violent behaviors, are suicidal, have a history of losing their connection with reality and their sense of self, or those who we feel in our gut, perhaps for reasons we cannot put into words, that we shouldn't work with.

If the session is part of an ongoing therapeutic relationship, negotiating the shifting boundaries of the transition to expanded states work and the subsequent return to ordinary states work will be essential for preserving the therapeutic container. If facilitator and participant are not already working together, this is the time to develop a sense of connection and rapport between them; we must not underestimate the layers of trust required for the level of surrendering necessary from both participant and facilitator in this work; such trust requires relationship.

Informed consent while in liminal expanded states will be a difficult negotiation to navigate. It is therefore imperative that we agree and contract explicitly in ordinary states of consciousness any boundaries regarding the setting, the use of touch and physical support, erotic feelings and expressions, aggressive and violent urges, or the impulse to abort the session prematurely. Touch is an area with a significant impact on the transferential elements of the work that requires careful and appropriate measuring and handling, as errors of both omission and commission are grave. To offer inappropriate touch at times when the participant is working through experiences where personal boundaries may have been invaded or to refuse physical support at times when the participant may be recalling early experiences of abandonment or loss would be inappropriate and unethical. The therapeutic relationship, contract, and intentions will be the anchors that steady the ship in turbulent waters, there for both facilitator and participant to return to at times of challenge for restoring their direction or resolve in engaging with the process.

During the session, the facilitator is required to be highly attentive to everything that emerges in the field alongside the safety needs of the participant. It is essential that the facilitator is able to tolerate uncertainty and to operate from the awareness that he or she is not there to "do the healing," as this is guided by the plant or substance medicines and the inner healing intelligence. Nature and soul are leading the way. Change can only emerge from these deeper sources—indeed in such complex, original, creative, and unique ways that our linear thinking modes are often unable to fully capture and comprehend. Ego must be set aside and disentangled from its pull toward control and power, to allow what is ripe to emerge forth from the unknown.

The diffusion of boundaries between self and other during expanded states opens the space to amplified transferential dynamics. In such intense states, the potential to collude with or abuse the transference is a real danger. "Professional abuses of client transference can include coercion, sexual seduction, or influencing the client to perform some behavior or act, which she would not have done otherwise" (Spence 1982, 175). Working one-on-one in expanded states work is not an ideal or recommended setting as the facilitator has to work unsupported under lengthy, intense, and demanding circumstances.

The highly perceptive quality of such experiences makes the participant greatly attuned to the unseen and that includes the unseen aspects of the facilitator. If we operate from an inauthentic inner place or from a compensating place where we need to be needed or to be heroic, masterful, or magical, we can contaminate the level of trust and safety required. Our capacity to be present stems from our capacity to be seen, which stems from our capacity to be intimate, which stems from our capacity to be vulnerable. Being available on all these levels throughout the session places enormous demands on the facilitator to withdraw the barriers that keep one's own experience as separate from the participant's. Facilitator and participant can then cojourney in deeper, more intimate, and more meaningful ways.

Closure ethics are about attending to the participant's transition from expanded states back into ordinary consciousness, as well as supporting the integration process, either as therapists ourselves or by appropriate signposting. At a most fundamental level, the facilitator must ensure the participant is sufficiently able to engage with ordinary reality; until then, the facilitator is responsible for the participant's care, well-being, and safety. If the participant's sense of self remains overwhelmed or disoriented, the facilitator must ensure the appropriate holding spaces to support this process from a nonpathologizing framework; occasionally, it can take longer than anticipated for a participant to land back into her or his sense of self. These situations require careful tending, sufficient understanding from the practitioner, and a reliable referral network that can adequately support the participant's needs. When the session has taken place in the context of an already established therapeutic relationship, the facilitator-therapist is responsible for attending to the integration and the return of the relationship to a therapeutic framework, with its own set of boundaries and safety nets.

MAINSTREAMING ETHICS

Psychedelic work in expanded states rests within the wider political, social, cultural, legal, economic, and medical systems of a time and a place, all with their own sets of values, biases, and influences. In our work as facilitators and therapists, we need to engage with the complex wider realities that shape our work. We are currently in a transitional period as psychedelic medicines may be nearing decriminalization, legalization, medical approval, and mainstreaming. These developments were a faraway dream for the first generation of psychedelic explorers and activists, yet as they are drawing nearer, we come to recognize just how difficult and fragile these transitions are, fraught with ethical concerns and requirements. As the tide turns, the diverse psychedelic community is coming into close contact with the very capitalist structures it has traditionally opposed. As psychedelics collide with Big Pharma, venture capital, and data and compound exclusivity, the inherent tensions increase and the stakes escalate. As we stand at these crossroads, which values will serve us best as we move forward?

The greatest ethical concern arising is money and the power attached to financial structures. As major investors move in, the values they bring are not always aligned with the values of the wider psychedelic and plant medicine communities. There will inevitably be compromises ahead. Being able to discern the compromises that will retain the essence of the work and psychedelic values at large versus those that will absorb the potential for healing into systems and frameworks that inherently promote illness and disease will be essential.

Some in the psychedelic field are trying to redefine capitalism through more ethical avenues, hoping to withstand the inherent tensions between capitalism and ethics. Can *conscious capitalism* find a balance between ethical integrity versus greed and opportunism, or are we dealing with a Trojan horse? Whether the psychedelic movement can be adapted to capitalist structures and still maintain psychedelic values, prioritizing benefit and accessibility over profit, remains to be seen.

INDIGENOUS RIGHTS AND RECIPROCITY

Indigenous communities are the original guardians and stewards of these ancestral medicines, uniquely knowledgeable and connected to their sacred qualities. The protection of biocultural indigenous community resources from appropriation is of essence for the psychedelic field, if we are to extricate from the legacy of generations of systematic indigenous colonization, oppression, and genocide. Western interest in plant medicines and their traditional contexts has already impacted negatively upon indigenous communities and their practices through psychedelic tourism. The current research wave aiming toward medicalization, decriminalization, or legalization of psychedelic compounds could have even more serious consequences on indigenous lands, plants, practices, and social order through a larger scale commodification of their sacred plants and practices. Respect for indigenous sovereignty and indigenous communities' inalienable right to self-determination requires including their active consultation and consent on decisions surrounding any part of the mainstreaming process that involves the harvesting of sacred plants and/or the appropriation of their sacred practices.

Reciprocity and inclusivity are deeply aligned with plant medicine wisdom and values. To decolonize the psychedelic movement, we must reflect on our collective shadow—our deeply entrenched attitudes of extraction, appropriation, and commodification—and strive to develop respectful collaborative models instead of bypassing indigenous involvement through scientific protocols and ethnocentric bias. If we aim to monetize and profit from indigenous sacred technologies, active reciprocity in forms that directly benefit, support, and empower their communities is an essential part of this process, in deep recognition and respect to the sacredness of the exchange and to where the knowledge we are trying to commercialize truly comes from. These people are the ancient roots of the psychedelic world; unless we tend to and nourish the roots, no tree can ever flourish and thrive.

SUSTAINABILITY ETHICS

Matters of sustainability are of crucial importance and consequence. The term *sustainable use* is defined by the 1992 *Convention on Biological Diversity* as "the use of components of biological diversity in a way and at a rate that does not lead to the long-term decline of biological diversity, thereby maintaining its potential to meet the needs and aspirations of present and future generations" (United Nations 1992, 4).

There are significant concerns regarding overharvesting and the sustainability of peyote (Davis 2017), iboga (Faura, Langlois, and Bouso

2020), *Bufo alvarius* (Kronenfeld 2019), and *Banisteriopsis caapi* in some areas (Stanley 2019). The slow growth cycles of these resources are met with high extraction demands, which could potentially get higher if pharmaceutical interests evolve. The National Council of Native American Churches and the Indigenous Peyote Conservation Initiative have issued a statement requesting that decriminalization efforts do not mention peyote explicitly in any list of plants and fungi (NCNAC and IPCI 2020). We need to properly acknowledge the scarcity alongside indigenous voices and rights to self-determination. These plants are an intrinsic part of wider natural and social ecosystems, and any threats to them carry broad ramifications. While we might be ready to proclaim that nature belongs to us all, it might well be that these sacred plants require protection from deeply ingrained unsustainable, exploitative, and unethical Western attitudes.

ETHICS OF EQUITY, INCLUSIVITY, AND ACCESSIBILITY

As the movement toward mainstreaming gains momentum, matters of inclusivity are taking center stage. Who holds the power? Who controls the narrative? Who influences and makes decisions? Whose voices are included and who benefits? Whose voices are missing and excluded? While the wider psychedelic community is comprised of extremely diverse populations, the current Western psychedelic representation is primarily white, male, and middle class, lacking diversity in terms of sexual orientation, gender identity, social status, and race. The underrepresentation of women's voices in the field has been a long-standing issue that has given rise to initiatives like the Women's Visionary Congress and the Femtheogen Collaborative.

This book was edited during the time of COVID-19, which has brought the impact of generations of discrimination and racial inequalities to stark view, as communities of color are disproportionately affected by the virus. The psychedelic community is no different; the evident underrepresentation of BIPOC (black, indigenous, and people of color) in research settings as either researchers or participants and at academic conferences excludes their particular experiences and ways of engaging with these medicines from the wider narratives (Michaels at al. 2018; Neitzke-Spruill 2019; Williams and Leins 2016). We need to address the realities of privilege and power that are embedded in the Western psychedelic field if we are to move toward racial and social justice and true collective healing.

Given that the War on Drugs has primarily stigmatized, targeted, and marginalized racial minority communities, it is no surprise that there are significant barriers and taboos in BIPOC communities for engaging with these substances either as advocates or as potential treatment participants. Effective outreach work needs to support and include their voices as the field develops and to strive to make these treatments available as safe and viable options for marginalized communities. Matters of social justice and accessibility should be at the forefront of the psychedelic field's concerns and aligned efforts as the truest aims and values of any inner work. We can only leverage privilege through diversity, equity, and inclusion. We are in urgent need of structures and frameworks that bring all the disparate voices together, in ways that can hold complexity and richness. When we remove the invisible but all too real obstacles for marginalized voices and communities to come to the table and participate, coinform, and cocreate, we can facilitate deep change.

FRACTAL ETHICS

A fractal is a geometric figure where small-scale and large-scale structures resemble and reflect one another, while holding infinite complexity. Chaos theory reveals the deep interconnection between parts of the whole, exposing the inherent order in chaos, in line with the alchemical dictum of *as above so below, as within so without.* This theory, when applied to work in expanded states, dissolves the illusion of separateness between facilitator and participant, revealing a deep underlying connection between the two in terms of process. It places their respective psyches in dialogue and cocreation, within the field of transformation.

As facilitators we can only facilitate surrendering insofar as we are resourced enough to surrender ourselves. We can only support our participants to face their deepest, darkest aspects inasmuch as we engage ourselves with the bravery and courage required to doing so in our own lives. We can only support the participant's deep inner work to the extent we are intimately involved with our own. Our intentions in doing this work can be as potent in the process as the participant's intentions. How we show up in any part of the process will reflect how we show up in the rest of the process.

On a metalevel this also applies to this chapter's distinct parts, the ethics surrounding the actual work and the ethics surrounding the psychedelic field at this point in time. These two are also fragments of a fractal, and when we step in one—whether we attend to it or not—we have stepped in the other. Any separation or fragmentation between the two is arbitrary and limiting.

There is a deep synchronicity between our own growing edges and those wounds our participants bring forth to the work. When we prepare participants for the work ahead, we are inherently also cultivating our own preparation. We are tasked with integrating the impact of the participants' journey on ourselves, just as we ask participants to engage with their integration. In doing so, we acknowledge the complex interrelational field that we and the participants have entered as part of the work. To step into service of the therapeutic work of others is for many of us an intrinsic and inextricable part of our own ongoing inner work and process.

The Closing Circle

Maria Papaspyrou and Tim Read

Each journey to the deep needs a proper ending, not just a turning of the last page but an ending that honors and anchors. In ceremonies, retreats, and workshops, we celebrate our emergence from the chrysalis of the expanded state in a closing circle. The circle has a poignancy too, holding its own death and rebirth: we know that this will be the ending of our time together. As we speak in the circle, we distill the essence and wisdom of our journey. As we listen, we honor the speaker with our undivided attention; we bring our full presence as we witness their pain, their ecstasy, and their flowering. Above all, the circle is a place of connection and love. As we close this book, we extend an invitation to join us in this tender, germinative place.

It is a complex journey that we walk through in this work. We accompany our clients to deep places, and we go to deep places ourselves. We enjoy those beautiful moments of connection, compassion, and spirit, and we enter those darker places of disconnection, unlove, grief, and despair that have such profound healing potential when allowed to flow toward resolution, becoming fertile soil for new layers of growth and life. Above all, therapeutic work in expanded states departs from the model of *treatment* by moving toward *healing*. This is a fundamental paradigm change; while treatment rests on the principles of exclusion, healing relies on the powers of inclusion. In treatment, what is seen as painful and undesirable is fragmented from the whole and treated in isolation. In healing work, we follow the movements of inclusion, honoring our symptoms as messengers of the soul, in service of our own unconscious depths. In the treatment paradigm, the agency is located primarily outside us, placed upon doctors or pills; while in the healing paradigm, we ourselves are the primary agent of change as the healing journey takes place firmly within.

The psychedelic experience, with intention and the right containers, can facilitate such growth, and yet, as with any movement toward greater awareness and consciousness, our experiences in expanded states require our full participation. The extraordinary depth of the psychedelic experience requires skill and presence by the facilitators if we are to meet and support its healing potential. The journey ahead to bring expanded states to validation and recognition will require all of us that have witnessed the potency of such work to bring our voices to the emergent wider narratives—to break the barriers and to recognize that healing is an indispensable birthright for us all.

On a collective level, as we journey into the gloaming of our moment in history, we remember that in these dark places, we may be guided by our own inner healing intelligence—the truest, deepest part of us. The more open we are, the more available our inner healing intelligence becomes in the service of healing our collective wounds. As we accelerate our journey ahead, our capacity to be anchored to our inner wisdom will be indispensable to us. A world that is aching requires more of us to be available as a resource for its healing processes. We can only do so by growing from a narrow to a broader sense of self, by opening up to greater inner and outer wholeness. From this space, we can come to witness our inherent interconnectedness and interdependence and recognize that to be in service of life we need to cultivate reciprocal collaborative partnerships with the world around us.

In closing this book, we would like to offer our deep gratitude to all that has brought us to this path, whether adversity or resource, for it has opened us up to truly meaningful encounters with ourselves and others. We wish to honor our ancestors, whose stories have laid the deeper foundations for our own life paths, as well as our past, present, and future guides and teachers who cultivate the soil of curiosity and knowing within us; our colleagues along the way with whom we have shared the journey; and, of course, our clients and students who have trusted us with their life stories and allowed us to walk alongside them in their search for healing and purpose. We deeply thank our partners, Stuart Griggs and Jo O'Reilly, for all their patience, love, and support as we have midwifed this book into the world. We are grateful to Inner Traditions for believing in this project and resourcing it to come into reality. In particular, we thank Jon Graham for supporting our initial vision; Jeanie Levitan, Patricia Rydle, Kate Mueller, and Kayla Toher for their patient and astute editing guidance; the production team for designing and typesetting our book to perfection; and John Hays, Manzanita Carpenter Sanz, Kelly Bowen, and Erica Robinson, who held space for the wider support of this project. We express our deep gratitude to the authors for their contribution to this book, the rigor of their work and the quality of their company. And finally, we honor you, the reader: we bow to you as you take this work forward and sow onward these seeds of love.

Contributor Biographies

John Ablett is a registered social worker and certified Holotropic Breathwork practitioner. For the last ten years, he has worked in very ordinary states of consciousness with homeless people, where he is able to make use of transpersonal perspectives to relate to experiences of alienation and drug-induced psychosis. His 2020 account of integrating his own psychospiritual crisis as a young man is published in the collection *Breaking Open: Finding a Way Through Spiritual Emergency.*

Deanne Adamson, M.A., with a master's in mental health counseling, is the founder and president of Being True To You, an online transformational coaching organization. Since 2010, Being True To You has provided holistic addiction recovery coaching and preparation and integration services surrounding psychedelic experiences to people around the world. Deanne's transformational recovery model extends support across one's greater journey of healing and growth, helping clients integrate psychedelic experiences to ensure lasting results. Through her intensive coach training program at Being True To You, Deanne certifies top coaches in addiction recovery and psychedelic integration and has built a worldwide network of coaches to support this movement with integrity, neutrality, and compassion.

Christopher M. Bache, Ph.D., is professor emeritus in philosophy and religious studies at Youngstown State University in Ohio where he taught for thirty-three years. He is also adjunct faculty at the California Institute of Integral Studies, Emeritus Fellow at the Institute of Noetic Sciences, and on the advisory board of Grof Legacy Training. An award-winning teacher and international speaker, Chris has written four books: *Lifecycles,* a study of reincarnation in light of contemporary consciousness research; *Dark Night, Early Dawn,* a pioneering work in psychedelic philosophy and collective consciousness; *The Living Classroom,* an exploration of teaching and collective fields of consciousness; and *LSD and the Mind of the Universe,* the story of his twenty-year journey with LSD.

Michelle Baker-Jones is an integrative psychotherapeutic counselor in private practice, based in London. She is also a member of the psychedelic research team at Imperial College. Michelle was a lead guide on the most recent Imperial College RCT trial, which compared psilocybin to antidepressants as a form of treatment for depression (PSILODEP II). She also offers individual psychedelic integration for people who are struggling to process psychedelic experiences and cofacilitates a monthly psychedelic integration group. Michelle is presently writing on the subject of embodiment as an adjunct to the ACE therapy model and is also exploring its wider implications for psychedelic therapy as a whole. www.mbjcounselling.co.uk

Jerome Braun, M.A., LMFT, IAAP, is a bilingual Spanish- and English-speaking Jungian psychoanalyst practicing in San Francisco, California, offering pre- and postpsychedelic integration psychotherapy oriented in depth psychology. He trained and taught at the C. G. Jung Institute Kusnacht, Zurich, Switzerland, and he completed his training in the Psychedelic-Assisted Therapies and Research Certificate Program at the California Institute of Integral Studies in San Francisco, California. Jerome is intricately involved in the Shipibo ancestral lineage of healing through medicinal, psychedelic, and sacred plants in the Peruvian Amazon.

Shannon Clare Carlin, M.A., LMFT, is a psychotherapist and the director and head of training and supervision at MAPS Public Benefit Corporation where she oversees the MDMA Therapy Training Program. Shannon received her master's in integral counseling psychology from the California Institute of Integral Studies. She began working at MAPS in 2011 and has served as a cotherapist on two MAPS-sponsored clinical trials with MDMA-assisted therapy. She also provides ketamine-assisted psychotherapy through the California Center for Psychedelic Therapy. Shannon is committed to supporting experiences of safety, acceptance, and love, through expanding access to care, clinical training in ethics, efficacy, and quality, promoting cultural awareness and community engagement, and cultivating relationship with psychedelic medicines and inner healing intelligence. She lives in sunny San Diego, California.

Andrew Feldmar is a psychotherapist based in Vancouver, Canada, with over fifty years of experience. His interest in psychedelics, entheogens, empathogens, and plant medicines started in 1967. With MAPS, he and Dr. Ingrid Pacey started the first government-sanctioned MDMA research with people suffering from intractable PTSD. The Feldmar Institute in Budapest has facilitated the publication of over thirty books and countless videos. For details, see his biography on Wikipedia as well as andrewfeldmar.com.

Holly Harman has a first degree in psychology and is a registered mental health nurse. She has worked in acute mental health settings within the National Health Service for over twenty years and is currently working independently. Holly is a certified Holotropic Breathwork facilitator and director of HolotropicUK (www.holotropicuk.co.uk). Over the last ten years, she has offered Holotropic Breathwork events in the UK and has traveled extensively with Grof Transpersonal Training, leading and facilitating Holotropic Breathwork trainings and events around the world. Holly was an associate director for Grof Transpersonal Training, and she also worked for and alongside Stan and Christina Grof for a number of years.

Rachel Harris, Ph.D., is a psychologist with both a research and a clinical background. She was in the 1968 residential program at Esalen Institute, Big Sur, California, and remained on the staff for a number of years. During the decade she worked in academic research, Rachel received a New Investigator's Award from the National Institutes of Health and published over forty scientific studies in peer-reviewed journals. She also worked as a psychological consultant to Fortune 500 companies including the UN. Rachel was in private psychotherapy practice for thirty-five years, specializing in people interested in psychospiritual development. Rachel is the author of *Listening to Ayahuasca: New Hope for Depression, Addiction, PTSD, and Anxiety.* Visit Rachel at her website, www.listeningtoayahausca.com.

Renee Harvey is a clinical psychologist who has recently relocated to Australia after a long career in the UK as a consultant in the National Health Service and more recently as an Honorary Research Fellow at Imperial College London in the study of psilocybin for treatment-resistant depression. She was responsible for leading service development for people with complex emotional needs in the UK and specialized in training clinicians for this work. Renee was a key member of developing psychedelic interest groups and in establishing and running a psychedelic Integration Circle in Brighton prior to leaving the UK. She is currently based in Melbourne, Australia, and is supporting the development of training programs in psychedelic-assisted therapies.

Scott J. Hill, Ph.D., returned to graduate studies in 2002 to inquire into the nature of his own traumatic yet ultimately life-enhancing psychedelic experiences in 1967. After exploring a wide range of theoretical perspectives, he constructed a Jungian framework for understanding difficult psychedelic experiences. Scott currently lives in Sweden, where he conducts scholarly research on the intersection between psychedelic studies and Jungian psychology. He holds degrees from the University of Minnesota (B.A., psychology; M.A., educational psychology) and the California Institute of Integral Studies (Ph.D., philosophy and religion). He is the author of *Confrontation with the Unconscious: Jungian Depth Psychology and Psychedelic Experience.*

Lisa Marie Jones, M.D., is a physician working in hospital and clinic settings. She has completed a training in underground psychedelic psychotherapy.

Sven Kimenai is a highly curious adventurist who has spent years traversing the world, experimenting and challenging himself. After his psychobiology studies and working as a supplement developer, he went on a path of self-healing and exploration, venturing through his inner landscapes using science-based methods. He became a Wim Hof method instructor and a breathwork facilitator and started studying and working with psychedelics for transformational healing. He emphatically empowers others to step out of their comfort zones and supports them on their inner journeys. Working with these tremendous tools, he aims to catalyze personal growth, insight, and human connection.

Jonny Martell, M.D., grew up on the edge of the Pennines in Northumberland, UK. He is a National Health Service psychiatrist currently training in general adult psychiatry and medical psychotherapy with a special interest in psychedelic research. He is a member of the Centre for Psychedelic Research at Imperial College London. He worked as a study doctor and guide in PSILODEP II, the psilocybin versus escitalopram for depression trial at Imperial College London. He lives in Devon with his family.

Gabor Maté, M.D., is a retired Canadian physician, public speaker, and bestselling author published internationally in over twenty-five languages. His most recent book is the award-winning *In the Realm of Hungry Ghosts: Close Encounters with Addiction.* For twelve years Gabor worked in Vancouver's Downtown Eastside with patients challenged by hard-core drug addiction, mental illness, and HIV, including at the Vancouver Supervised Injection Site. His other interests encompass childhood developmental issues, mind/body health, trauma, psyche-delic healing, and parenting. He has received an Outstanding Alumnus Award from Simon Fraser University and an honorary degree in law from the University of Northern British Columbia. For his ground-breaking medical work and writings, he has been given the Order of Canada and the Civic Merit award from his home city of Vancouver.

Daniel McQueen, M.A., is the executive director of the Center for Medicinal Mindfulness and is a professional psychedelic therapist and guide. He has a master's degree in transpersonal counseling psychology from Naropa University and over twenty years' experience exploring psy-chedelic medicines, including ten years working as a professional facili-tator. In 2012, he cofounded the Center for Medicinal Mindfulness with his wife, Alison McQueen, MA, LPC, ATR, as a psychedelic harm-reduction program in Boulder, Colorado, and the program has since evolved into a psychedelic therapy center and international psy-chedelic therapy training program focusing on Cannabis-Assisted Psychedelic Therapy, Cannabis-Assisted Psychotherapy, and Ketamine-Assisted Psychotherapy. Daniel lives with his family in Boulder and is a proud father, a writer, and a psychedelic community organizer. www.medicinalmindfulness.org

Friederike Meckel Fischer, M.D., trained as a medical doctor in Germany and retrained as a medical psychotherapist. She trained as a Holotropic Breathwork facilitator with Stanislav Grof from 1989 to 1991 and completed a psychedelic psychotherapy training in Switzerland in the early 1990s. She also trained as a couple's therapist, a family ther-apist, and a family constellation worker. In the mid-1990s, she intro-duced the use of psychedelics into her psychotherapy practice, working underground with specifically chosen clients in groups. In 2009, she and her husband were arrested, and in 2010, she was sentenced to a con-ditional prison term of sixteen months with a probationary period of two years for "dealing" LSD. She was explicitly acquitted for her thera-peutic work. Her book *Therapy with Substance* was published in 2015.

Roberta Murphy, M.D., is a psychiatrist based in London. She is currently training as a medical psychotherapist in South West London and St. George's National Health Service Trust. She is a member of the Centre for Psychedelic Research at Imperial College London. Roberta worked as a study doctor and guide on PSILODEP II, a research trial investigating the use of psilocybin for moderate to severe depression and on INSIGHT, a healthy volunteer psilocybin study. She is interested in alternative approaches to severe and enduring mental health issues. Roberta has trained and works in open dialogue therapy, which offers a systemic-based approach to mental health crisis and psychosis in particular.

Ashleigh Murphy-Beiner was an assistant psychologist on PSILODEP II, the Psilocybin for Depression Study in the Psychedelic Research Group at Imperial College London. She is now training as a clinical psychologist at the Royal Holloway University of London. Ashleigh is trained as a mindfulness meditation teacher and has developed and led mindfulness sessions to support preparation and integration in ceremonies in Peru. She has also published research examining the therapeutic potential and mechanism of action of ayahuasca for treating depression and anxiety.

Marianne Murray, Ph.D., has a doctorate in transformative learning and change in human systems from California Institute of Integral Studies (CIIS) and master's degrees in transpersonal psychology and mindfulness-based psychotherapy. She is a certified Holotropic Breathwork facilitator, having trained with Stanislav Grof in the 1990s. She works with Holotropic Breathwork trainings and workshops internationally as well as in the United States. Marianne is based in the Southwestern US where for the past twenty years she has worked with groups and individuals in the field of transformative learning.

Svea Nielsen is a psychologist who has studied ethnopsychiatry. Following her experience in harm reduction services in trance festivals, she coedited *The Manual of Psychedelic Support,* published by MAPS (2017). Then, feeling the call to work in a sacred therapeutic setting, the sacred wood came to find her. An elder "sister" offered her all her knowledge and expertise to support people in search of personal development, and drug addicts seeking an off-switch. In Switzerland, Svea cofounded the psychedelic association Eleusis (www.eleusis-society.ch). There she leads integration groups to provide a sharing space for people who have their psychedelic experiences on their own. This reflects her commitment to link the psychedelic renaissance with a communal tribal experience, healing the isolation that our Western existence has confined us to.

Jo O'Reilly, M.D., is a medical doctor, psychiatrist, and psychoanalyst. She is a consultant medical psychotherapist in a National Health Service post in London and is on the executive committee of the medical psychotherapy faculty at the Royal College of Psychiatrists. She is coeditor of *Seminars in Psychotherapy* (2021).

Ingrid Pacey, MBBS, FRCPC, is a psychiatrist based in Canada. She specialized in the treatment of trauma disorders, initially using traditional psychotherapy. She began training in Holotropic Breathwork with Dr. Stanislav Grof and Christina Grof in 1987 after a pivotal experience. This deepened her interest in the therapeutic power of expanded states of consciousness, and from 1990 to 2004, Ingrid and her partner offered Holotropic Breathwork groups to trauma survivors. She was principal investigator of the Phase 2 MDMA-assisted psychotherapy research study with trauma survivors in Vancouver from 2012 to 2016. Ingrid is now retired from clinical practice but mentors therapists working with Holotropic Breathwork and psychedelic substances.

Maria Papaspyrou is an integrative psychotherapist, clinical supervisor, and systemic family constellations facilitator based in Brighton, UK. She coedited the book *Psychedelic Mysteries of the Feminine* and is cofounder and codirector of the Institute of Psychedelic Therapy (https://instituteofpsychedelictherapy.org). You can find out more about her work at towardswholeness.co.uk

Natasja Pelgrom is a sacred medicine woman, mystic, devotional creative, and visionary who leads spiritual alchemy journeys, providing a compassionate space for healing and remembering. She is the creatrix of the Phoenix Rising Course, the six month in-person Awaken Self-Love course, and the tailor-made Psychedelic Integration Journey as well as the founder of Awaken the Medicine Within Retreats. Natasja is also a founding member of the Synthesis Institute; she leads the psilocybin-assisted Wellness retreats, is a key influencer in the development of the online Wellness program, the Psychedelic Practitioner Training, and is the cocreatrix of the Women's Leadership Retreat. www.natasjapelgrom.com.

Tim Read, M.D., is a medical doctor, psychiatrist, and psychotherapist based in London. He led psychiatric services at the Royal London Hospital for twenty years and held academic positions at London University. He has trained in psychoanalytic therapy (IGA) and in transpersonal therapy (GTT) with Stanislav Grof. He is a certified facilitator of Holotropic Breathwork and has an active clinical and supervisory role in the therapeutic use of psychedelics. His books include *Walking Shadows: Archetype and Psyche in Crisis and Growth* and *Breaking Open: Finding a Way through Spiritual Emergency,* coedited with Jules Evans. With Maria Papaspyrou, he is a director of the Institute of Psychedelic Therapy.

Leor Roseman, Ph.D., is a postdoc at the Centre for Psychedelic Research, Imperial College London, where he also received his doctorate and MRes, under the supervision of Robin Carhart-Harris and Professor David Nutt. His research interests are diverse and cover neuroscientific, phenomenological, anthropological, therapeutic, and psychosocial aspects of psychedelic use. Currently, Leor is investigating relational processes and group dynamics in psychedelic rituals. His main line of research is examining the potential of psychedelics for peace building. While his research is currently focused on the Palestinian-Israeli conflict, he and his collaborators are hoping to develop an approach that is applicable in other contexts as well.

Nir Tadmor, M.Sc., is a transpersonal psychotherapist and a cofounder of a psychedelic education, harm-reduction, and peer-support project called Safe Shore. He holds a master's in transpersonal psychology from Middlesex University (through the Alef Trust) and trained in Hakomi mindfulness-based psychotherapy. During the last six years, Nir worked as a mental health guide in various alternatives to psychiatric hospitalization, supported and supervised hundreds of psychedelic crises in parties and festivals, trained more than seven hundred psychedelic harm reduction sitters in Israel, the UK, and The Netherlands through Safe Shore's Holding Space workshop, and gave talks in international conferences about psychedelic integration, psychedelic crisis intervention, and transpersonal psychiatry. Visit www.nirtadmor.com and www.psychedelicare.com.

Becca Tarnas, Ph.D., is a scholar, artist, and editor of *Archai: The Journal of Archetypal Cosmology.* She received her doctorate in philosophy and religion from the California Institute of Integral Studies (CIIS), with her dissertation titled *The Back of Beyond: The Red Books of C. G. Jung and J. R. R. Tolkien.* Her research interests include depth psychology, literature, philosophy, and the ecological imagination. Becca teaches at both Pacifica Graduate Institute and CIIS, and is the author of *Journey to the Imaginal Realm: A Reader's Guide to J. R. R. Tolkien's The Lord of* *the Rings*. She lives in northern California, where she has an astrological counseling practice. Her website is www.BeccaTarnas.com.

Bruce Tobin, Ph.D., is a Canadian clinical psychologist and registered art therapist in private practice in Victoria, British Columbia, Canada. He is a founder and honorary lifetime member of the BC Art Therapy Association and taught expressive therapies for twenty-five years at the University of Victoria. He is founder and chair of the board of TheraPsil, a patient rights group advocating for access to psilocybin-assisted psychotherapy for palliative patients suffering from end-of-life distress. On August 4, 2020, Health Canada granted approvals for TheraPsil's first four patient applicants. On August 12, 2020, Bruce conducted Canada's first legal psilocybin psychotherapy session.

Rosalind Watts trained as a clinical psychologist at University College London and practiced psychotherapy for six years before joining the Centre for Psychedelic Research at Imperial College London as clinical lead of Imperial's clinical depression psilocybin trial, PSILODEP II. Rosalind developed the psychedelic therapy model ACE (accept, connect, embody), based on acceptance and commitment therapy. She is currently clinical director for Synthesis Retreats. She is committed to building structures to safeguard the ethical expansion of psychedelic therapy and sits on Usona Institute's Clinical Advisory Board.

Bibliography

Ablett, John. 2020. "The Accidental Guru." Chap. 2 in *Breaking Open: Finding a Way through Spiritual Emergencies,* edited by Jules Evans and Tim Read, 11–24. London: Aeon Books.

Alderson, Phil. 2004. "Absence of Evidence Is Not Evidence of Absence." *British Medical Journal* 328 (476): 476–77.

Bache, Christopher M. 2008. *The Living Classroom: Teaching and Collective Consciousness.* Albany: SUNY Press.

———. 2019. *LSD and the Mind of the Universe.* Rochester, Vt.: Inner Traditions.

Bakan, David. 1967. *On Method: Toward a Reconstruction of Psychological Investigation.* San Francisco, Calif.: Jossey-Bass.

Bernstein, Amit, Yuval Hadash, Yael Lichtash, Galia Tanay, Katherine Shepherd, and David M. Fresco. 2015. "Decentering and Related Constructs: A Critical Review and Metacognitive Process Model." *Perspectives on Psychological Science* 10 (5): 599–617.

Bick, Esther. 1968. "The Experience of the Skin in Early Object Relations." *International Journal of Psychoanalysis* 49 (2): 484–86.

Bowlby, John. 1969. *Attachment and Loss: Volume 1, Attachment.* New York: Basic Books.

Buber, M. (1923) 1970. *I and Thou.* New York: Charles Scribner's Sons.

Carhart-Harris, Robin L., and Karl J. Friston. 2010. "The Default-Mode, Ego Functions and Free Energy: A Neurobiological Account of Freudian Ideas." *Brain* 133: 1265–83.

Carhart-Harris, Robin L., Robert Leech, Peter J. Hellyer, Murray Shanahan, Amanda Feilding, Enzo Tagliazucchi, Dante R. Chialvo, and David Nutt. 2014. "The Entropic Brain: A Theory of Conscious States Informed by

Neuroimaging Research with Psychedelic Drugs." *Frontiers in Human Neuroscience* 8: 1–22.

Castaneda, Carlos. 1990. *The Teachings of Don Juan: A Yaqui Way of Knowledge.* London: Penguin Books.

Cutner, Margot. 1959. "Analytic Work with LSD-25." *Psychiatric Quarterly* 33 (4): 715–57.

Dahl, Cortland J., Antoine Lutz, and Richard J. Davidson. 2015. "Reconstructing and Deconstructing the Self: Cognitive Mechanisms in Meditation Practice." *Trends in Cognitive Science* 19: 515–23.

Davis, Dawn D. 2017. "How My Elder's Sacred Peyote Is Disappearing." Chacruna: Institute for Psychedelic Plant Medicines (website).

Dickins, Robert, and Tim Read. 2015. *Out of the Shadows: A Cornucopia from the Psychedelic Press.* London: Muswell Hill Press.

Edinger, Edward. 1992. *Ego and Archetype: Individuation and the Religious Function of the Psyche.* Boston: Shambhala. First published 1972.

Emerson, Amy, Linnae Ponté, Lisa Jerome, and Rick Doblin. 2014. "History and Future of the Multidisciplinary Association for Psychedelic Studies (MAPS)." *Journal of Psychoactive Drugs* 46 (1): 27–36.

Estés, Clarissa P. 2003. *The Beginner's Guide to Dream Interpretation.* Read by the author. Audiobook, 1 hr., 19 min. Louisville, Colo.: Sounds True.

Evans, Jules, and Tim Read. 2020. *Breaking Open: Finding a Way through Spiritual Emergency.* London: Aeon Books.

Fadiman, James. 2005. "Transpersonal Transitions: The Higher Reaches of Psyche and Psychology." In *Higher Wisdom,* edited by Roger Walsh and Charles S. Grob, 21–46. Albany, N.Y.: SUNY Press.

Fadiman, James, and Sophia Korb. 2017. "Creative Problem-Solving: High Doses Then, Microdoses Now." Breaking Convention Conference. YouTube video, 26 mins.

Faura, Ricard, Andrea Langlois, and José C. Bouso. 2020. "Expanding Ancestral Knowledge Beyond the Sale of Molecules: Iboga and Ibogaine in the Context of Psychedelic Commercialization." *MAPS Bulletin Spring 2020* 30 (1): 42–44.

Feduccia, Allison A., and Michael C. Mithoefer. 2018. "MDMA-Assisted Psychotherapy for PTSD: Are Memory Reconsolidation and Fear Extinction Underlying Mechanisms?" *Progress in Neuro-Psychopharmacology & Biological Psychiatry* 84: 221–28.

Feldmar, Andrew. 2001. "Entheogens and Psychotherapy." Academia (website).

Felitti, Vincent J., Robert F. Anda, Dale Nordenberg, David F. Williamson, Alison M. Spitz, Valerie Edwards, Mary P. Koss, and James S. Marks. 1998. "Relationship of Childhood Abuse and Household Dysfunction to Many of the Leading Causes of Death in Adults. The Adverse Childhood Experiences (ACE) Study." *American Journal of Preventive Medicine* 14 (4): 245–58.

Ferrer, Jorge. 2002. *Revisioning Transpersonal Theory: A Participatory Vision of Human Spirituality*. Albany, N.Y.: SUNY Press.

———. 2011. "Participatory Spirituality and Transpersonal Theory: A Ten Year Retrospective." *Journal of Transpersonal Psychology* 43 (1): 1–34.

Ferrer, Jorge, and Justin Sherman, eds. 2008. *The Participatory Turn*. Albany, N.Y.: SUNY Press.

Foucault, Michel. 1983. "The Meaning and Evolution of the Word 'Parrhesia.'" In "Discourse and Truth: The Problematization of Parrhesia," six lectures given by Michel Foucault. University of California at Berkeley. Foucault. info (website).

Freud, Sigmund. 1917. "Mourning and Melancholia." *International Journal for Medical Psychoanalysis* 4 (6): 288–301.

———. 1938. "An Outline of Psycho-Analysis." In *Moses and Monotheism: An Outline of Psycho-Analysis and Other Works,* 139–208. Vol. 23 of *The Standard Edition of the Complete Psychological Works of Sigmund Freud*. London: Hogarth Press.

Fussell, Paul. 2013. *The Great War and Modern Memory*. New York: Oxford University Press.

Gearin, A. 2015. "'Whatever You Want to Believe': Kaleidoscopic Individualism and Ayahuasca Healing in Australia." *The Australian Journal of Anthropology* 26 (3): 442–55.

Gendlin, Eugene T. 1981 *Focusing*. New York: Bantam. First published 1978.

Ginot, Efrat. 2012. "Self-Narratives and Dysregulated Affective States." *Psychoanalytic Psychology* 29: 59–80.

Gorman, Peter. 2010. *Ayahuasca in My Blood*. Iquitos, Peru: Gorman Bench Press.

Granqvist, Pehr, Mario Mikulincer, and Phillip R. Shaver. 2010. "Religion as Attachment: Normative Processes and Individual Differences." *Personality and Social Psychology Review* 14: 49–59.

Griffiths, Roland R., Matthew W. Johnson, William A. Richards, Brian D. Richards, Robert Jesse, Katherine A. MacLean, Frederick S. Barrett,

Mary P. Cosimano, and Maggie A. Klinedinst. 2018. "Psilocybin-Occasioned Mystical-Type Experience in Combination with Meditation and Other Spiritual Practices Produces Enduring Positive Changes in Psychological Functioning and in Trait Measures of Prosocial Attitudes and Behaviors." *Journal of Psychopharmacology* 32 (1): 49–69.

Grof, Stanislav. 1975. *Realms of the Human Unconscious: Observations From LSD Research*. New York: Viking.

———. 1978. (1980). *LSD Psychotherapy*. Pomona, Calif.: Hunter House.

———. 1988. *The Adventure of Self-Discovery: Dimensions of Consciousness and New Perspectives in Psychotherapy and Inner Exploration*. Albany, N.Y.: SUNY Press.

———. 1996. *Transpersonal Psychotherapy: Second Edition*. Albany, N.Y.: SUNY Press.

———. 2001. *LSD Psychotherapy: Exploring the Frontiers of the Hidden Mind*. Sarasota, Fla.: Multidisciplinary Association for Psychedelic Studies.

———. 2005. "The Great Awakening: Psychology, Philosophy and Spirituality in LSD Psychotherapy." In *Higher Wisdom,* edited by Roger Walsh and Charles S. Grob, 119–50. Albany, N.Y.: SUNY Press.

———. 2009. "Holotropic Research and Archetypal Astrology." *Archai: The Journal of Archetypal Cosmology* 1: 65–85.

———. 2010. *Holotropic Breathwork: A New Approach to Self-Exploration and Therapy*. Albany, N.Y.: SUNY Press.

———, ed. 2019. *The Way of the Psychonaut: Encyclopedia for Inner Journeys*. 2 vols. Santa Cruz, Calif.: MAPS.

Guggenbühl-Craig, Adolf. 2015. *Power in the Helping Professions*. Thompson, Conn: Spring Publications.

Hari, Johann. 2015. "Everything You Think You Know about Addiction Is Wrong." TED Talk. TEDGlobalLondon, 14 mins.

———. 2018. *Lost Connections: Why You're Depressed and How to Find Hope*. London: Bloomsbury.

Harris, Rachel. 2017. *Listening to Ayahuasca: New Hope for Depression, Addiction, PTSD, and Anxiety*. Novato, Calif.: New World Library.

Harris, Rachel, and Lee Gurel. 2012. "A Study of Ayahuasca Use in North America." *Journal of Psychoactive Drugs* 44: 209–15.

Haule, John R. 1996. *The Love Cure: Therapy Erotic and Sexual*. Woodstock, Conn.: Spring.

Herman, Judith Lewis. 1992. *Trauma and Recovery: The Aftermath of Violence—From Domestic Abuse to Political Terror.* New York: Basic Books.

Hill, Scott. 2019. *Confrontation with the Unconscious: Jungian Depth Psychology and Psychedelic Experience.* London: Aeon Books. First published 2013.

Hoffer, Abram, and Andrew Saul. 2008. *Orthomolecular Medicine for Everyone: Megavitamin Therapeutics for Families and Physicians.* Laguna Beach, Calif.: Basic Health Publications

Hofmann, Albert. 1979. *LSD: My Problem Child.* Sarasota, Fla.: MAPS.

Holland, Julie. 2010. "Cannabinoids and Psychiatry." In *The Pot Book: A Complete Guide to Cannabis,* edited by Julie Holland, 282–94. Rochester, Vt.: Park Street Press.

Hollis, James. 1994. *Under Saturn's Shadow: The Wounding and Healing of Men.* Scarborough, Ontario, Canada: Inner City Books.

Johnson, Richard E. 1971. *Existential Man: The Challenge of Psychotherapy.* Oxford: Pergamon Press.

Jung, Carl Gustav. 1966. "The Therapeutic Value of Abreaction." In *Practice of Psychotherapy,* 129–38. Vol. 16 of *The Collected Works of C. G. Jung.* Princeton, N.J.: Princeton University Press.

———. 1966a. "The Practical Use of Dream Analysis." In *Practice of Psychotherapy,* 139–61. Vol. 16 of *The Collected Works of C. G. Jung.* Princeton, N.J.: Princeton University Press.

———. 1968. "Individual Dream Symbolism in Relation to Alchemy." In *Psychology and Alchemy,* 39–472. Vol. 12 of *The Collected Works of C. G. Jung.* Princeton, N.J.: Princeton University Press.

———. 1969. "Psychoanalysis and the Cure of Souls." In *Psychology and Religion: East and West.* Vol. 11 of The *Collected Works of C. G. Jung.* 2nd ed. Princeton, N.J.: Princeton University Press.

———. 1969a. "The Transcendent Function." In *Structure and Dynamics of the Psyche,* 67–91. Vol. 8 of *The Collected Works of C. G. Jung.* Princeton, N.J.: Princeton University Press.

———. 1969b. "The Psychological Foundation of Belief in Spirits." In *Structure and Dynamics of the Psyche,* 301–18. Vol. 8 of *The Collected Works of C. G. Jung.* Princeton, N.J.: Princeton University Press.

———. 1969c. "Spirit and Life." In *Structure and Dynamics of the Psyche,* 319–37. Vol. 8 of *The Collected Works of C. G. Jung.* Princeton, N.J.: Princeton University Press.

———. 1969d. "A Review of the Complex Theory." In *Structure and Dynamics of the Psyche*, 92–104. Vol. 8 of *The Collected Works of C. G. Jung*. Princeton, N.J.: Princeton University Press.

———. 1969e. "Psychological Factors Determining Human Behavior." In *Structure and Dynamics of the Psyche*, 114–25. Vol. 8 of *The Collected Works of C. G. Jung*. Princeton, N.J.: Princeton University Press.

———. 1971. *Psychological Types*. Vol. 6 of *The Collected Works of C. G. Jung*. Princeton, N.J.: Princeton University Press.

———. 1972a. "The Psychology of Dementia Praecox." In *Psychogenesis of Mental Disease*, 1–151. Vol. 3 of *The Collected Works of C. G. Jung*. Princeton, N.J.: Princeton University Press.

———. 1972b. "Schizophrenia." In *Psychogenesis of Mental Disease*, 256–72. Vol. 3 of *The Collected Works of C. G. Jung*. Princeton, N.J.: Princeton University Press.

———. 1973a. "Association, Dream, and Hysterical Symptom." In *Experimental Researches*, 353–407. Vol. 2 of *The Collected Works of C. G. Jung*. Princeton, N.J.: Princeton University Press.

———. 1973b. "Appendix Four: On the Doctrine of Complexes." In *Experimental Researches*, 598–604. Vol. 2 of *The Collected Works of C. G. Jung*. Princeton, N.J.: Princeton University Press.

———. 1976. *C. G. Jung Letters, Volume 2: 1951–1961*. Edited by Gerhard Adler. Translated by Jeffrey Hulen. Bollingen Series XCV:2. Princeton, N.J.: Princeton University Press.

Kalsched, Donald. 1996. *The Inner World of Trauma: Archetypal Defenses of the Personal Spirit*. New York: Routledge.

———. 2003. "Response to James Astor." *Journal of Analytical Psychology* 48: 201–5.

———. 2013. *Trauma and the Soul: A Psycho-Spiritual Approach to Human Development and Its Interruption*. New York: Routledge.

Kaptchuk, Ted J. 2011. "Placebo Studies and Ritual Theory: A Comparative Analysis of Navajo, Acupuncture and Biomedical Healing." *Philosophical Transactions of the Royal Society of London Series B: Biological Sciences* 366: 1849–58.

Kettner, H., F. Rosas, C. Timmermann, L. Kärtner, R. Carhart-Harris, and L. Roseman. 2021. "Psychedelic Communitas: Intersubjective Experience during Psychedelic Group Sessions Predicts Enduring Changes in Psychological Wellbeing and Social Connectedness." *Frontiers in Pharmacology*. Further publication detail not available at publication.

Kirkpatrick, Lee A. 2005. *Evolution and the Psychology of Religion*. New York: Guilford Press.

Klein, Melanie. 1959. "Our Adult World and Its Roots in Infancy." *Human Relations* 12 (4): 291–303.

Kronenfeld, Jeff. 2019. "Is the Juice Worth the Squeeze: The Impact of Climate Change, Development, and Psychonauts on the Sonoran Desert Toad." *Psychedelics Today,* December 17, 2019.

Laing, R. D. 1965. "Practice and Theory—The Present Situation." *Psychotherapy and Psychosomatics* 13 (1/3): 58–67.

———. 1987. "Hatred of Health." *Journal of Contemplative Psychotherapy* IV: 77–86.

Laval-Jeantet, Marion. 2006. *Iboga Invisible et Guérison: Une Approche Ethnopsychiatrique*. Paris: Paris-Musees Association.

Le Grice, Keiron. 2009. "The Birth of a New Discipline: Holotropic Research and Archetypal Astrology." *Archai: The Journal of Archetypal Cosmology* 1 (1): 65–85.

Leuner, Hanscarl. 1983. "Psycholytic Therapy: Hallucinogens as an Aid in Psychoanalytically Oriented Psychotherapy." In *Psychedelic Reflections*, edited by L. Grinspoon and J. Bakalar, 177–92. New York: Human Sciences Press.

Levine, Peter A. 2008. *Healing Trauma: A Pioneering Program for Restoring the Wisdom of Your Body*. Boulder, British Columbia, Canada: Sounds True.

Levine, Peter A., and Anne Frederick. 1997. *Waking the Tiger: Healing Trauma*. Berkeley, Calif.: North Atlantic Books.

Lingis, Alphonso. 2018. *Irrevocable: A Philosophy of Mortality*. Chicago: University of Chicago Press.

Lommel, Pim van. 2010. *Consciousness Beyond Life*. New York: Harper Collins.

Lotsof, Howard S., and Norma E. Alexander. 2001. "Case Studies of Ibogaine Treatment: Implications for Patient Management Strategies." Chap. 16 in *The Alkaloids: Chemistry and Biology,* vol. 60, edited by Geoffrey A. Cordell, 293–313. San Diego, Calif.: Academic Press

McQueen, Daniel. 2021. *Psychedelic Cannabis: Therapeutic Methods and Unique Blends to Treat Trauma and Transform Consciousness*. Rochester, Vt.: Park Street Press.

Meckel Fischer, Friederike. 2015. *Therapy with Substance.* London: Muswell Hill Press.

Merton, Thomas. 1958. *Thoughts in Solitude.* New York: Farrar, Straus & Cudahy.

Michaels, Timothy I., Jennifer Purdon, Alexis Collins, and Monnica T. Williams. 2018. "Inclusion of People of Color in Psychedelic-Assisted Psycho-Therapy: A Review of the Literature." *BMC Psychiatry* 18 (245): 1–15.

Milner, Marion. 1950. *On Not Being Able to Paint.* London: Heinemann Educational Books.

Mithoefer, Michael C. 2019. *MDMA-Assisted Psychotherapy Treatment Manual.* With contributions by Annie Mithoefer, Lisa Jerome, June Ruse, Rick Doblin, Elizabeth Gibson, Marcela Ot'alora G., and Evan Sola. MAPS.

Mogenson, Greg. 2005. *A Most Accursed Religion: When Trauma Becomes God.* Putnam, Conn.: Spring.

Naranjo, Claudio. 1969. "Psychotherapeutic Possibilities of New Fantasy-Enhancing Drugs." *Clinical Toxicology* 2: 209–24.

NCNAC and IPCI. 2020. "Official Statement of National Council of Native American Churches & Indigenous Peyote Conservation Initiative on the 'Decriminalization' Efforts of Peyote and Other Sacred Plants." *Journal of Native Sciences.*

Neitzke-Spruill, Logan. 2019. "Race as a Component of Set and Setting: How Experiences of Race can Influence Psychedelic Experiences." *Journal of Psychedelic Studies* 4 (2): 1–10.

Nielson, E. M. 2018. "The Influence of Therapists' First-Hand Experience with Psychedelics on Psychedelic-Assisted Psychotherapy Research and Therapist Training." *Journal of Psychedelic Studies* (2): 64–73.

O'Brien, Melissa, and Jason McDougall. 2018. "Cannabis and Joints: Scientific Evidence for the Alleviation of Osteoarthritis Pain by Cannabinoids." *Current Opinion in Pharmacology* 40: 1049.

O'Carroll, Sean. 2015. "Ayahuasca Is My Therapist (Or Is It?)." Psychotherapy. net (website).

Papaspyrou, Maria. 2015. "Femtheogens: The Synergy of Sacred Spheres." In *Out of the Shadows: A Cornucopia from the Psychedelic Press,* edited by Robert Dickins and Tim Read, 125–36. London: Muswell Hill Press.

———. 2019. "Femtheogenic Consciousness: Archetypal Energies of Regeneration."

In *Psychedelic Mysteries of the Feminine,* edited by Maria Papaspyrou, Chiara Baldini, and David Luke, 10–25. Rochester, Vt.: Park Street Press.

Perry, John Weir. 1999. *Trials of the Visionary Mind: Spiritual Emergency and the Renewal Process.* Albany, N.Y.: SUNY Press.

Phelps, Janis. 2017. "Developing Guidelines and Competencies for the Training of Psychedelic Therapists." *Journal of Humanistic Psychology* 57 (5): 450–87.

Pietromonaco, Paula R., and Lisa Feldman Barrett. 2000. "The Internal Working Models Concept: What Do We Really Know about the Self in Relation to Others?" *Review of General Psychology* 4: 155–75.

Rancière, Jacques. 1991. *The Ignorant Schoolmaster: Five Lessons in Intellectual Emancipation.* Stanford, Calif.: Stanford University Press.

Read, Tim. 2014. *Walking Shadows: Archetype and Psyche in Crisis and Growth.* London. Muswell Hill Press.

Roseman, L., D. J. Nutt, and R. L. Carhart-Harris. 2017. "Quality of Acute Psychedelic Experience Predicts Therapeutic Efficacy of Psilocybin for Treatment-Resistant Depression." *Frontiers in Pharmacology* 8 (January 17): 974.

Roseman, L., Y. Ron, A. Saca, N. Ginsberg, L. Luan, N. Karkabi, R. Doblin, and R. Carhart-Harris. 2021. "Relational Processes in Ayahuasca Groups of Palestinians and Israelis." *Frontiers in Pharmacology.* Further publication detail not available at publication.

Sandison, Ronald A. 1954. "Psychological Aspects of the LSD Treatment of the Neuroses." *Journal of Mental Science* 100: 508–15.

Schore, Allan N. 2011. "The Right Brain Implicit Self Lies at the Core of Psychoanalysis." *Psychoanalytic Dialogues* 21: 75–100.

Shulgin, Alexander T. S., and Anne Shulgin. 2005. "Frontiers of Pharmacology: Chemistry and Consciousness." In *Higher Wisdom,* edited by Roger Walsh and Charles S. Grob, 69–90. Albany, N.Y.: SUNY Press.

Siegel, Daniel J. 2010. *The Mindful Therapist: A Clinician's Guide to Mindsight and Neural Integration.* New York: W. W. Norton.

Smith, Huston. 2005. "Do Drugs Have Religious Import? A Forty Year Follow-Up." In *Higher Wisdom,* edited by Roger Walsh and Charles S. Grob, 223–40. Albany, N.Y.: SUNY Press.

Solomon, Linda. 2007. "LSD as Therapy? Write about It, Get Barred from US: BC Psychotherapist Denied Entry after Border Guard Googled His Work." *The Tyee.*

Spence, D. P. 1982. *Narrative Ttruth and Historical Truth: Meaning and Interpretation in Psychoanalysis.* New York: Norton.

Spezanno, Charles. 2005. "Intersubjectivity." In *Textbook of Psychoanalysis,* edited by Glenn Gabbard, Bonnie E. Litowitz, and Paul Williams, 77–92. Washington, D.C.: American Psychiatric Publishing.

Spiller, Jan. 1997. *Astrology for the Soul.* New York: Bantam Books.

Stanley, Bob Otis. 2019. "Ethical and Sustainable Access to Entheogenic Plants." Chacruna: Institute for Psychedelic Plant Medicines (website).

Swann, W. B., J. Jetten, A. Gómez, H. Whitehouse, and B. Bastian. 2012. "When Group Membership Gets Personal: A Theory of Identity Fusion." *Psychological Review* 119 (3): 441.

Tafur, Joseph. 2017. *Fellowship of the River: A Medical Doctor's Exploration into Traditional Amazonian Plant Medicine.* Phoenix, Ariz.: Espiritu Books.

Tarnas, Richard. 2006. *Cosmos and Psyche: Intimations of a New World View.* New York: Viking.

———. 2019. "Epilogue: Psyche and Cosmos." In *The Way of the Psychonaut,* vol. 2, edited by Stanislav Grof, 290–91. Santa Cruz, Calif.: MAPS.

Taylor, Kylea. 2017. *The Ethics of Caring: Finding the Right Relationships with Clients.* Santa Cruz, Calif.: Hanford Mead.

Thorner, Isidor. 1965. "Prophetic and Mystic Experience: Comparison and Consequences." *Journal for the Scientific Study of Religion* 5 (1): 82–96.

Turner, E. 2012. *Communitas: The Anthropology of Collective Joy.* New York: Palgrave Macmillan.

Turner, V. (1969) 2017. *The Ritual Process: Structure and Anti-Structure.* Abingdon: Routledge.

United Nations. 1992. *Convention on Biological Diversity.* Legal document.

Van der Kolk, Bessel A. 2014. *The Body Keeps the Score.* New York: Penguin.

Walsh, Roger, and Charles S. Grob. 2005. *Higher Wisdom.* Albany, N.Y.: SUNY Press.

Wampold, Bruce E. 2015. "How Important Are the Common Factors in Psychotherapy? An Update." *World Psychiatry* 14: 270–77.

Waters, Frank. 1970. *Masked Gods.* New York: Ballantine Books.

Williams, Monnica T., and Chris Leins. 2016. "Race-Based Trauma: The Challenge and Promise of MDMA-Assisted Psychotherapy." *Multidisciplinary Association for Psychedelic Studies Bulletin* 26 (1): 32–37.

Wolff, Jeremy. 2010. "Thots on Pot." Chap. 35 in *The Pot Book: A Complete*

Guide to Cannabis, edited by Julie Holland, 387–94. Rochester, Vt.: Park Street Press.

Young, Jeffrey E., and Janet S. Klosko. 1993. *Reinventing Your Life: The Breakthrough Program to End Negative Behavior and Feel Great Again.* New York: Plume.

Zendo Project. 2017. *Zendo Psychedelic Harm Reduction Training Manual.* MAPS.

Index

BOOKS OF RELATED INTEREST

Psychedelic Medicine
The Healing Powers of LSD, MDMA, Psilocybin, and Ayahuasca
by Dr. Richard Louis Miller

Plants of the Gods
Their Sacred, Healing, and Hallucinogenic Powers
by Richard Evans Schultes, Albert Hofmann, and Christian Rätsch

The Psychedelic Explorer's Guide
Safe, Therapeutic, and Sacred Journeys
by James Fadiman, Ph.D.

DMT: The Spirit Molecule
A Doctor's Revolutionary Research into the Biology of
Near-Death and Mystical Experiences
by Rick Strassman, M.D.

Grandmother Ayahuasca
Plant Medicine and the Psychedelic Brain
by Christian Funder

LSD and the Mind of the Universe
Diamonds from Heaven
by Christopher M. Bache, Ph.D.
Foreword by Ervin Laszlo

Psychedelics and Spirituality
The Sacred Use of LSD, Psilocybin, and MDMA
for Human Transformation
Edited by Thomas B. Roberts, Ph.D.

Cannabis and Spirituality
An Explorer's Guide to an Ancient Plant Spirit Ally
Edited by Stephen Gray

INNER TRADITIONS • BEAR & COMPANY
P.O. Box 388 • Rochester, VT 05767
1-800-246-8648 • www.InnerTraditions.com

Or contact your local bookseller